Asterion
The Practical Handbook of
ANATOMY

AF070322

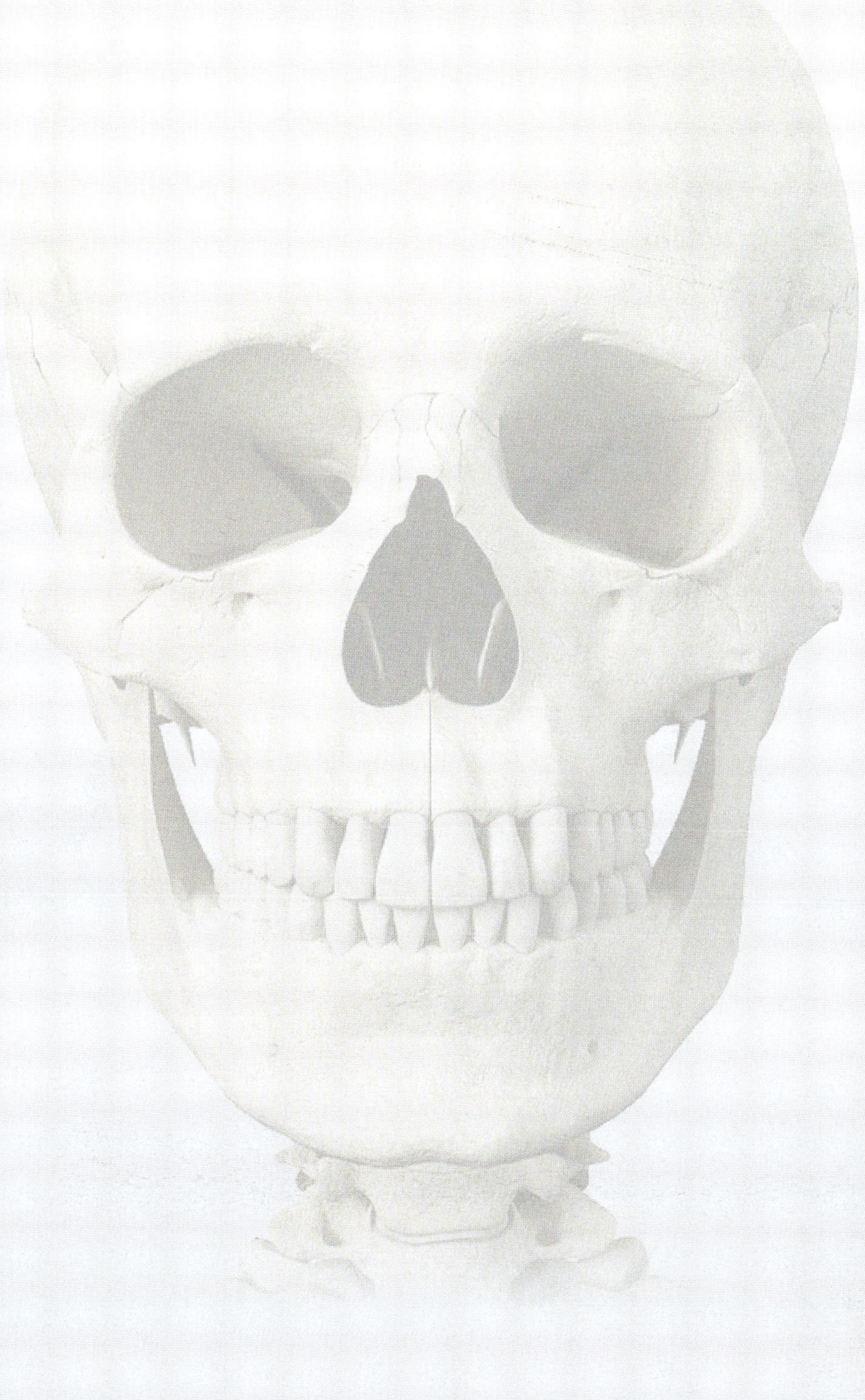

Asterion
The Practical Handbook of
ANATOMY

As per the Competency-Based Medical Education Curriculum (NMC)

Third Edition

Editors

Harishanker JS MBBS
Postgraduate student MBA
Kozhikode, Kerala, India

Ajai Sasi MBBS
Postgraduate Student MD (Pediatrics)
KMCT Medical College
Kozhikode, Kerala, India

Aswathy BI MBBS
Postgraduate Student MPH
Sree Chitra Tirunal Institute for Medical Sciences and Technology (SCTIMST)
Thiruvananthapuram, Kerala, India

Forewords

Kanchan Kapoor
VS Akbar Sherif

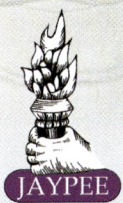

JAYPEE BROTHERS MEDICAL PUBLISHERS
The Health Sciences Publisher
New Delhi | London

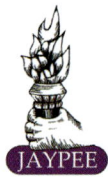
Jaypee Brothers Medical Publishers (P) Ltd

Headquarters
Jaypee Brothers Medical Publishers (P) Ltd
EMCA House, 23/23-B
Ansari Road, Daryaganj
New Delhi 110 002, India
Landline: +91-11-23272143, +91-11-23272703
+91-11-23282021, +91-11-23245672
Email: jaypee@jaypeebrothers.com

Corporate Office
Jaypee Brothers Medical Publishers (P) Ltd
4838/24, Ansari Road, Daryaganj
New Delhi 110 002, India
Phone: +91-11-43574357
Fax: +91-11-43574314
Email: jaypee@jaypeebrothers.com

Overseas Office
J.P. Medical Ltd
83 Victoria Street, London
SW1H 0HW (UK)
Phone: +44 20 3170 8910
Fax: +44 (0)20 3008 6180
Email: info@jpmedpub.com

Website: www.jaypeebrothers.com
Website: www.jaypeedigital.com

© 2023, Jaypee Brothers Medical Publishers

The views and opinions expressed in this book are solely those of the original contributor(s)/author(s) and do not necessarily represent those of editor(s) and publisher of the book.

All rights reserved. No part of this publication may be reproduced, stored or transmitted in any form or by any means, electronic, mechanical, photocopying, recording or otherwise, without the prior permission in writing of the publishers.

All brand names and product names used in this book are trade names, service marks, trademarks or registered trademarks of their respective owners. The publisher is not associated with any product or vendor mentioned in this book.

Medical knowledge and practice change constantly. This book is designed to provide accurate, authoritative information about the subject matter in question. However, readers are advised to check the most current information available on procedures included and check information from the manufacturer of each product to be administered, to verify the recommended dose, formula, method and duration of administration, adverse effects and contraindications. It is the responsibility of the practitioner to take all appropriate safety precautions. Neither the publisher nor the author(s)/editor(s) assume any liability for any injury and/or damage to persons or property arising from or related to use of material in this book.

This book is sold on the understanding that the publisher is not engaged in providing professional medical services. If such advice or services are required, the services of a competent medical professional should be sought.

Every effort has been made where necessary to contact holders of copyright to obtain permission to reproduce copyright material. If any have been inadvertently overlooked, the publisher will be pleased to make the necessary arrangements at the first opportunity.

Inquiries for bulk sales may be solicited at: jaypee@jaypeebrothers.com

Asterion—The Practical Handbook of Anatomy

First Edition: 2013
Second Edition: 2015
Third Edition: **2023**
ISBN: 978-93-5465-920-1

Printed at: Samrat Offset Pvt. Ltd.

Dedicated to

All COVID warriors for their selfless service during the pandemic
Our Family and Friends for continuous support at all times.

"Learn to see, learn to hear, learn to feel, learn to smell, and know that by practice alone can u become expert"

—Sir William Osler

Foreword

It is my privilege to write the foreword for the *Asterion—The Practical Handbook of Anatomy* (3rd edition) for the undergraduate students, written by Dr Harishanker JS, Dr Ajai Sasi and Dr Aswathy BI who are dedicated professionals.

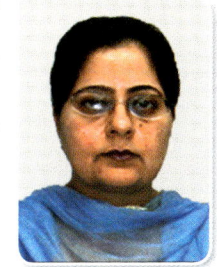

The book is meant for ready reference to the histology especially in practical where they have to replicate the histology images which aims at fulfilling the academic needs of the MBBS 1st professional students. The highlight of the book is its rich illustrations which are very clear and precisely labeled. The diagrams are set against the black background which enhances the aesthetic value of the book. Another aspect worth mentioning is a separate heading of briefly written applied anatomy. At the end of each chapter the questions and answers for viva voce are added which would serve as ready reference at the time of practical examination.

Chapters on embryology, osteology, radiology and surface markings with images are helpful for students and serves as ready reckoner during various theory and practical examinations.

I congratulate Dr Harishanker JS and his team for his efforts and attention to all details. I wish the book a great success.

Kanchan Kapoor PhD MNAMS
Professor and Head
Department of Anatomy
Government Medical College and Hospital
Chandigarh, India

Foreword

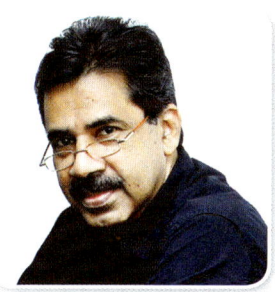

I am very much delighted to know that Dr Harishanker JS, Dr Ajai Sasi, and Dr Aswathy BI are coming up with the third edition of their book: *Asterion—The Practical Handbook of Anatomy*. During their college days when they approached me with the idea of Asterion, I readily welcomed that idea. The editors have seen that the book is concise and student friendly. Various sections of the book covering histology, embryology, osteology, radiology and surface marking will make a quick reference for the exam-going students and gives them an upper edge over the topics and also help them dedicate more time for the gross and applied anatomy topics. In this latest update of the book, the editors have made sure that the book is compliant with the latest curriculum and crisper and more concise.

I am using this opportunity to congratulate Dr Harishanker JS, Dr Ajai Sasi and Dr Aswathy BI for their dedicated efforts in bringing the thoroughly revised and updated version of this book. I wish them all the success for this venture.

VS Akbar Sherif MBBS MS MCh
Pediatric Surgeon
Former Principal, Malabar Medical College
Calicut, Kerala, India

Preface to the Third Edition

It seems like only a short time has passed since the second edition of this book was published. We are very much delighted to announce the new revised and updated third edition of *Asterion—The Practical Handbook of Anatomy*. The overwhelming response of first and second editions were the greatest encouragement in bringing out the latest edition of the *Asterion*. Due to the immense responses and outstanding feedback from all around, we have made sure that the necessary revisions and updates were made along with making it compliant with various curriculum. We have again left the basic plan of the book unchanged. We have also corrected any mistakes and elucidated any obscurities which may have creeped up in the earlier editions. Each and every chapter has been updated carefully with finer images and utmost details.

We hope the latest edition of *Asterion* prepares each and every student to face the exam confidently and give them an upper hand in their examination.

Harishanker JS
Ajai Sasi
Aswathy BI

Preface to the First Edition

Every tributary of anatomy confluent to form "Asterion". It is the right solution for all the last minute queries of every student just before the examination. It is an exclusive handout focusing mainly on practical anatomy.

A need of such a book will be felt maximum as we approach our university examination, a point of time when we get lost completely but keep staring at Histology, Radiology, Osteology, etc., with a heavy heart full of fear and anxiety. Such a fear was there indeed in our heart too, which gave us the spark of compiling all these together, and this gave birth to our Asterion.

Asterion covers all practical aspects of anatomy comprising Histology, Embryology, Osteology, Radiology and Surface Marking. It is only a preparatory manual for undergraduates (UG), not a complete textbook. It is a very student-friendly concise book which will make you so confident that you can spot the toughest of spotters with no time. It gives you the exact idea for facing every exam—be it viva or theory at most precision, thus helping you to leave the exam hall with a smile.

One of the marking features of Asterion is that it presents you "The Red Alert" section which gives you the most probable theory questions from the gross anatomy section, thereby clearing away your vague minds and promising you a sure shot at the exam.

Now everything is set. Here we present you so gladly and proudly the magical wand of anatomy "Asterion". So take away the wand and cast your spell on the examiner, so that everyone of you have a magical result.

Harishanker JS
Ajai Sasi
Avinash N

Acknowledgments

We are very grateful to the whole team of M/s Jaypee Brothers Medical Publishers (P) Ltd, New Delhi, India, who helped and guided us, Shri Jitendar P Vij (Group Chairman), Mr Ankit Vij (Managing Director), Mr MS Mani (Group President), Dr Madhu Choudhary (Director–Educational Publishing), Ms Pooja Bhandari (Production Head), Ms Sunita Katla (Executive Assistant to Group Chairman and Publishing Manager), Ms Samina Khan (Executive Assistant to Director–Educational Publishing), Dr Aditya Tayal (Team Lead–UG Publishing), Mr Rajesh Sharma (Production Coordinator), Ms Seema Dogra (Cover Visualizer), Ms Geeta Barik (Proofreader), Mr Deep Dogra (Typesetter), Mr Rakesh Kumar (Graphic Designer) and their team members, for all their support to work in this project and make it a success. Without their cooperation, we could not have completed this project.

We also extend our sincere thanks to Dr VS Akbar Sherif for being our inspiration, lighting our path in dark times.

We are heartily thankful to Dr Kavya P Valsaraj for taking care of the diagrams with utmost sincerity and dedication.

We would also like to thank Dr Shabeeb PK for helping us update our radiology section by providing new images.

We sincerely thank to all the anatomy students and teachers who gave their valuable feedback and suggestions from time to time which helped us immensely in updating this new edition.

We would also like to express our deep gratitude to our family who has helped and supported us throughout the entire making process. And above all without the blessing of God Almighty this book would not have been a complete one.

Contents

1. **Histology** 1

   Microscope 2
   - Parts of microscope 2
   - Slide preparation and staining 2

   Epithelium 3
   - General functions of epithelial cells 3
   - Simple squamous epithelium 4
   - Simple cuboidal epithelium 4
   - Simple columnar epithelium 7
   - Surface specializations of the epithelial cells 7
   - Pseudostratified columnar epithelium 8
   - Stratified epithelium 8
   - Transitional epithelium 8

   Cartilage 11
   - General aspects 11
   - Hyaline cartilage 12
   - Elastic cartilage 15
   - Fibrocartilage 16

   Bone 19
   - General aspects 19
   - Bone transverse section 19
   - Bone longitudinal section 20

   Muscle 23
   - General aspects 23
   - Skeletal muscle 23
   - Smooth muscle 24
   - Cardiac muscle 27

   Blood Vessels 28
   - General aspects 28
   - Arteries 28
   - Large artery or elastic artery 28
   - Medium-sized artery 31
   - Veins 32
   - Large vein 32
   - Medium-sized vein 35

   Lymphoreticular System 36
   - Lymph node 36
   - Palatine tonsil 39
   - Spleen 40
   - Thymus 43

   Nervous Tissue 44
   - Nerve fiber 44
   - Spinal ganglion 47
   - Sympathetic ganglion 48

   Oral Cavity 51
   - Serous salivary gland 51
   - Mucous salivary gland 52
   - Mixed salivary gland 55
   - Tongue 56

   Alimentary System 59
   - General aspects 59
   - Esophagus 59
   - Stomach fundus 60
   - Stomach pylorus 63
   - Small intestine 64
   - Duodenum 64
   - Jejunum 67
   - Ileum 68
   - Colon 71
   - Appendix 72

   Liver and Pancreas 75
   - Liver 75
   - Gallbladder 76
   - Pancreas 79

   Respiratory System 80
   - Trachea 80
   - Lung 83

   Renal System 84
   - Kidney 84
   - Ureter 87
   - Urinary bladder 88

   Skin 91
   - General aspect 91
   - Thick skin 91
   - Thin skin 92

   Special Senses 95
   - Cornea 95
   - Retina 96
   - Optic nerve 99

   Female Reproductive System 100
   - Mammary gland 100
   - Ovary 103
   - Fallopian tube 104
   - Uterus 107
   - Placenta 108
   - Umbilical cord 111

   Male Reproductive System 112
   - Testis 112
   - Epididymis 115
   - Vas deferens 116
   - Prostate gland 119

   Endocrine System 120
   - Adrenal gland 120
   - Thyroid gland 123

- Parathyroid gland 123
- Pituitary gland 124

Central Nervous System 127
- Spinal cord 127
- Cerebellum 128
- Cerebrum 131

2. Embryology 133

General Embryology 134
- Embryogenesis 134
- Implantation 134
- Decidua 135
- Embryonic disc and germ layers 135
- Intraembryonic mesoderm 135
- Somites 136
- Notochord 136
- Neurulation 136
- Neural crest 137
- Lamina terminalis 137
- Placenta 137

Systemic Embryology 138
- Pharyngeal arches 138
- Palate 138
- Face 140
- Upper lip 140
- Tongue 141
- Thyroid gland 141
- Lungs 141
- Heart tube 142
- Right atrium 142
- Interatrial septum 142
- Fallot's tetralogy 143
- Diaphragm 143
- Gut 143
- Esophagus 143
- Stomach 143
- Meckel's diverticulum 144
- Pancreas 144
- Liver and gallbladder 144
- Kidney 144
- Urinary bladder 145
- Uterus 145
- Uterine tube 145
- Development of gonads (testis and ovaries) 146
- Rectum and anal canal 147
- Prostate 147
- Amniocentesis 147

Genetics 149
- Barr body (sex chromatin) 149
- Chromosome banding 149
- Karyotyping 149
- Nondisjunction 150
- Klinefelter syndrome 150
- Turner's syndrome 150
- Down syndrome 151

3. Radiology 153

Basics 154
- Imaging modalities 154

Imaging Modalities with Ionizing Radiations 154
- Concept of radio-opacity 154
- Plane radiography 154
- How to read a chest radiograph (PA view)? 155
- Contrast radiography 156
- Barium studies 156
- Barium swallow 156
- Barium meal 157
- Barium enema 157
- Iodine studies 157
- Intravenous pyelography 158
- Water-soluble contrast study 158
- Hysterosalpingography 158
- Computed tomography 158
- Positron emission tomography scan 159

Imaging Modalities with Nonionizing Radiations 159
- Ultrasonography 159
- Doppler studies 159
- Magnetic resonance imaging 159

4. Osteology 177
- Introduction to bones 178
- Markings on the bones 178
- Age and sex determination with bones 179
- Clinical aspects of osteology 179

5. Surface Marking 203

Upper Limb 204
- Axillary artery 204
- Brachial artery 204
- Radial artery 204
- Ulnar artery 204
- Axillary nerve 204
- Median nerve 204
- Musculocutaneous nerve 205
- Radial nerve 205
- Ulnar nerve 205
- Flexor retinaculum 205
- Extensor retinaculum 205
- Superficial palmar arch 206
- Deep palmar arch 206

Lower Limb 206
- Femoral artery 206
- Popliteal artery 206
- Posterior tibial artery 206
- Dorsalis pedis artery 206
- Saphenous opening 206
- Great saphenous vein 206
- Sciatic nerve 207
- Superior extensor retinaculum 207
- Inferior extensor retinaculum 207
- Flexor retinaculum 207

Thorax   208
- Heart   208
- Arch of aorta   208
- Lungs   208
- Pleural reflection   209
- Esophagus   209
- Thoracic duct   210

Abdomen and Pelvis   210
- Abdomen planes and quadrants   210
- Inguinal canal   210
- Stomach   211
- Liver   211
- Fundus of gallbladder   211
- Abdominal aorta   212
- Spleen   212
- Root of mesentery   212
- McBurney's point   212
- Kidney   212
- Ureter   212

Head and Neck   213
- Common carotid artery   213
- External carotid artery   213
- Facial artery   213
- Facial vein   213
- Internal jugular vein   213
- External jugular vein   213
- Facial nerve   214
- Parotid gland   214
- Parotid duct   214

6. Spotters and Discussion Topics............215

Spotters   216
- Upper limb   216
- Lower limb   216

- Thorax   217
- Abdomen and pelvis   218
- Head and neck   218
- Brain   220

Discussion Topics   220
- Discussion topics   220

7. Red Alert..221

Anatomy Examination Paper 1—
Important Topics   222
- Upper limb   222
- Lower limb   222
- Thorax   223
- General histology   223
- General embryology   223
- General anatomy   223

Anatomy Examination Paper 2—
Important Topics   224
- Head and neck   224
- Neuroanatomy   224
- Abdomen and pelvis   225
- Histology   225
- Systemic embryology   226

Important Diagrams   227
- Upper limb   227
- Thorax   227
- Lower limb   227
- Abdomen and pelvis   227
- Head and neck   228

Index 229

Competency Table

Number	COMPETENCY The student should be able to	Chapter Number	Page Number
AN9.2	Describe microanatomy of breast	1	100
AN 25.1	Identify, draw and label a slide of trachea and lung	1	80
AN43.2	Identify, describe and draw the microanatomy of pituitary gland, thyroid, parathyroid gland	1	123
	Identify, describe and draw the microanatomy of tongue, salivary glands, tonsil		51
	Identify, describe and draw the microanatomy of epiglottis, cornea, retina		95
AN43.3	Identify, describe and draw microanatomy of optic nerve	1	99
AN52.1	Describe and identify the microanatomical features of gastrointestinal system: esophagus, fundus of stomach, pylorus of stomach, duodenum, jejunum, ileum, large intestine, appendix, liver, gallbladder, pancreas	1	53
	Describe and identify the microanatomical features of suprarenal gland		120
AN52.2	Describe and identify the microanatomical features of: Urinary system: Kidney, ureter and urinary bladder	1	84
	Male reproductive system: Testis, epididymis, vas deferens, prostate and penis		112
	Female reproductive system: Ovary, uterus, uterine tube, cervix, placenta and umbilical cord		103
AN64.1	Describe and identify the microanatomical features of spinal cord, cerebellum and cerebrum	1	127
AN65.1	Identify epithelium under the microscope and describe the various types that correlate to its function	1	3
AN67.1	Describe and identify various types of muscle under the microscope	1	23
AN68.1	Describe and identify ganglia, peripheral nerve	1	44
AN69.1	Identify elastic and muscular blood vessels, capillaries under the microscope	1	28
AN70.2	Identify the lymphoid tissue under the microscope and describe microanatomy of lymph node, spleen, thymus, tonsil and correlate the structure with function	1	36
AN71.1	Identify bone under the microscope; classify various types and describe the structure—function correlation of the same	1	19
AN71.2	Identify cartilage under the microscope and describe various types and structure-function correlation of the same	1	11
AN72.1	Identify the skin and its appendages under the microscope and correlate the structure with function	1	91
AN73.1	Describe the structure of chromosomes with classification	2	149
AN73.2	Describe technique of karyotyping with its applications		
AN75.1	Describe the structural and numerical chromosomal aberrations		
AN76.1	Describe the stages of human life	2	134
AN77.4	Describe the stages and consequences of fertilization	2	134
AN78.1	Describe cleavage and formation of blastocyst	2	134
AN78.2	Describe the development of trophoblast	2	134
AN78.3	Describe the process of implantation and common abnormal sites of implantation	2	134

Competency Table

Number	COMPETENCY The student should be able to	Chapter Number	Page Number
AN78.4	Describe the formation of extra-embryonic mesoderm and coelom, bilaminar disc and prochordal plate	2	134
AN79.1	Describe the formation and fate of the primitive streak	2	134
AN79.2	Describe formation and fate of notochord	2	134
AN79.3	Describe the process of neurulation	2	134
AN79.4	Describe the development of somites and intra-embryonic coelom	2	134
AN80.1	Describe formation, functions and fate of-chorion: amnion; yolk sac; allantois and decidua	2	134
AN80.3	Describe formation of placenta, its physiological functions, foetomaternal circulation and placental barrier	2	134
AN25.2	Describe development of pleura, lung and heart	2	141
AN43.4	Describe the development and developmental basis of congenital anomalies of face, palate, tongue, branchial apparatus, pituitary gland, thyroid gland and eye	2	138
AN52.4	Describe the development of anterior abdominal wall	2	143
AN52.6	Describe the development and congenital anomalies of: Foregut, midgut and hindgut		
AN52.7	Describe the development of urinary system	2	144
AN52.8	Describe the development of male and female reproductive system	2	145
AN13.5	Identify the bones and joints of upper limb seen in anteroposterior and lateral view radiographs of shoulder region, arm, elbow, forearm and hand	3	138
AN20.6	Identify the bones and joints of lower limb seen in anteroposterior and lateral view radiographs of various regions of lower limb	3	160
AN25.7	Identify structures seen on a plain X-ray chest (PA view)	3	163
AN25.8	Identify and describe in brief a barium swallow	3	171
AN43.7	Identify the anatomical structures in: (1) Plain X-ray skull, (2) AP view and lateral view, (3) Plain X-ray cervical spine—AP and lateral view, (4) Plain x-ray of paranasal sinuses	3	169
AN54.1	Describe and identify features of plain X-ray abdomen	3	163
AN54.2	Describe and identify the special radiographs of abdominopelvic region (contrast X-ray barium swallow, barium meal, barium enema, cholecystography, intravenous pyelography and hysterosalpingography)	3	171
AN8.1	Identify the given bone, its side, important features and keep it in anatomical position of upper limb	4	185
AN14.1	Identify the given bone, its side, important features and keep it in anatomical position of lower limb	4	189
AN26.1	Demonstrate anatomical position of skull, Identify and locate individual skull bones in skull	4	180
AN 21.1	Identify and describe the salient features of sternum, typical rib, Ist rib and typical thoracic vertebra	4	195
AN 21.2	Identify and describe the features of atypical rib	4	196
AN 26.5	Describe features of typical and atypical cervical vertebrae (atlas and axis)	4	197
AN 26.7	Describe the features of the 7th cervical vertebra		
AN 30.1	Describe the cranial fossae and identify related structures	4	182
AN 30.2	Describe and identify major foramina with structures passing through them		
AN13.7	Identify and demonstrate surface projection of cephalic and basilic vein, palpation of brachial artery, radial artery	5	204

Competency Table

Number	COMPETENCY The student should be able to	Chapter Number	Page Number
AN20.9	Identify and demonstrate palpation of vessels (femoral, popliteal, dorsalis pedis, post tibial), mid inguinal point, surface projection of: femoral nerve, saphenous opening, sciatic, tibial, common peroneal and deep peroneal nerve, great and small saphenous veins	5	206
AN25.9	Demonstrate surface marking of lines of pleural reflection, lung borders and fissures, trachea, heart borders, apex beat and surface projection of valves of heart	5	208
AN43.6	Demonstrate surface projection of: Parotid gland and duct, pterion, common carotid artery, internal jugular vein, subclavian vein, external jugular vein, facial artery in the face and accessory nerve	5	213
AN55.1	Demonstrate the surface marking of: Regions and planes of abdomen, superficial inguinal ring, deep inguinal ring, McBurney's point	5	210
AN55.2	Demonstrate the surface projections of: Stomach, liver, fundus of gall bladder, spleen, duodenum, pancreas, ileocaecal junction, kidneys and root of mesentery		

Histology

OUTLINE

- Microscope
- Epithelium
- Cartilage
- Bone
- Muscle
- Blood Vessels
- Lymphoreticular System
- Nervous Tissue
- Oral Cavity
- Alimentary System
- Liver and Pancreas
- Respiratory System
- Renal System
- Skin
- Special Senses
- Female Reproductive System
- Male Reproductive System
- Endocrine System
- Central Nervous System

MICROSCOPE

A microscope is basically used to magnify and see small objects which otherwise cannot be seen properly with naked eyes. In histology, a light microscope is routinely used. Light microscope uses visible light to illuminate the object.

PARTS OF MICROSCOPE

- **Eye piece lense**: It is the lense on which we place our eye to see through the microscope. It can magnify objects from 10X to 15X times.
- **Objective lense:** Objects are being illuminated and magnified by objective lense and being projected onto eye piece lense. It has lenses that can magnify objects up to 10X, 40X and even 100X times.
- **Condenser**: It has a lense that focuses light onto the specimen.
- **Light source**: For this purpose, a built-in light source is used. Alternatively, natural light can also be used with the help of a concave mirror.
- **Focusing knobs**: They are used for both fine and coarse adjustment by adjusting the distance between the objective lense and the object.
- **Arm:** The curved portion of a microscope that holds all the optical parts.
- **Stage:** It is the platform on which a slide is placed.
- **Base**: Part that bears the weight of a microscope.

SLIDE PREPARATION AND STAINING

- Slide preparation is a tedious process. A tissue has to go through various processes like fixation, dehydration, clearing, embedding, section cutting, staining and mounting in order.
- For staining, we use the concept that components in a cell have either acidic or basic properties. A basic dye can stain the acidic component of a cell and vice versa.
- Commonly used acidic stains are eosin, acid fuchsin, orange G, etc.
- Commonly used basic stains are hematoxylin, toluidine blue, methylene blue, etc.

Eosin (E) is an acidic dye. It stains eosinophilic/acidophilic cell components like cytoplasm, mitochondria and collagen. These parts appear as pink on staining.

Hematoxylin (H) is a basic dye. It stains basophilic nuclei of a cell due to the presence of nucleic acid. The dye gives nuclei a purple color.

EPITHELIUM

Epithelial tissue covers the body and lines the inner and outer surfaces of the organs and the body cavities. They are very tightly packed cells and lie on a thin basement membrane. Epithelial cells have capacity for faster regeneration and replace damaged cells with new cells.

GENERAL FUNCTIONS OF EPITHELIAL CELLS

Depending on the location in the body, they play different roles:
1. Protection and barrier function
2. Absorption
3. Secretion
4. Selective permeability to molecules
5. Sensory perception
6. Excretion

Epithelia broadly classified into:
1. **Simple epithelium:** Having only one layer of cells.
2. **Pseudostratified epithelium:** Entire epithelial cells are resting on the basement membrane, but not all the cells extend to the surface.
3. **Stratified epithelium:** They have two or more layers of cells.

SIMPLE SQUAMOUS EPITHELIUM

- It is composed of a single layer of flattened cells forming a continuous surface and the nuclei of the cells are flattened.
- **Functions:** The peculiar shape and arrangement of the cells helps in diffusion and filtration of molecules easily.
- **Examples:** They line the blood vessels (endothelium), body cavities such as pleural, pericardial and peritoneal cavity (mesothelium), parietal layer of Bowman's capsule (renal corpuscle in kidney).

SIMPLE CUBOIDAL EPITHELIUM

- They appear in square shape in the section drawn perpendicular to the surface of the epithelium. But on the surface, they have a polygonal shape.
- The nucleus of a cell is round and centrally placed.
- **Functions:** Normally they have a role in secretion, absorption and excretion of substances.
- **Examples:** It is present in small ducts of glands, thyroid follicles, tubules of the kidney and surface of the ovary.

SIMPLE SQUAMOUS EPITHELIUM

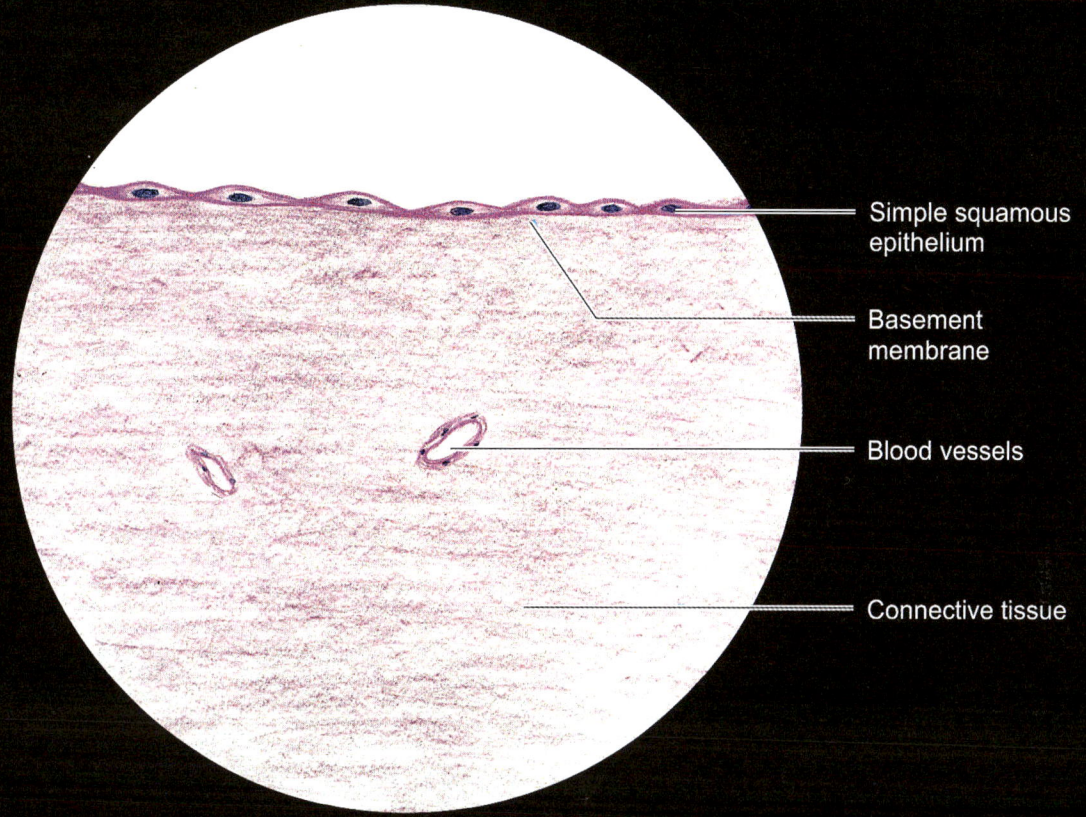

SIMPLE CUBOIDAL EPITHELIUM

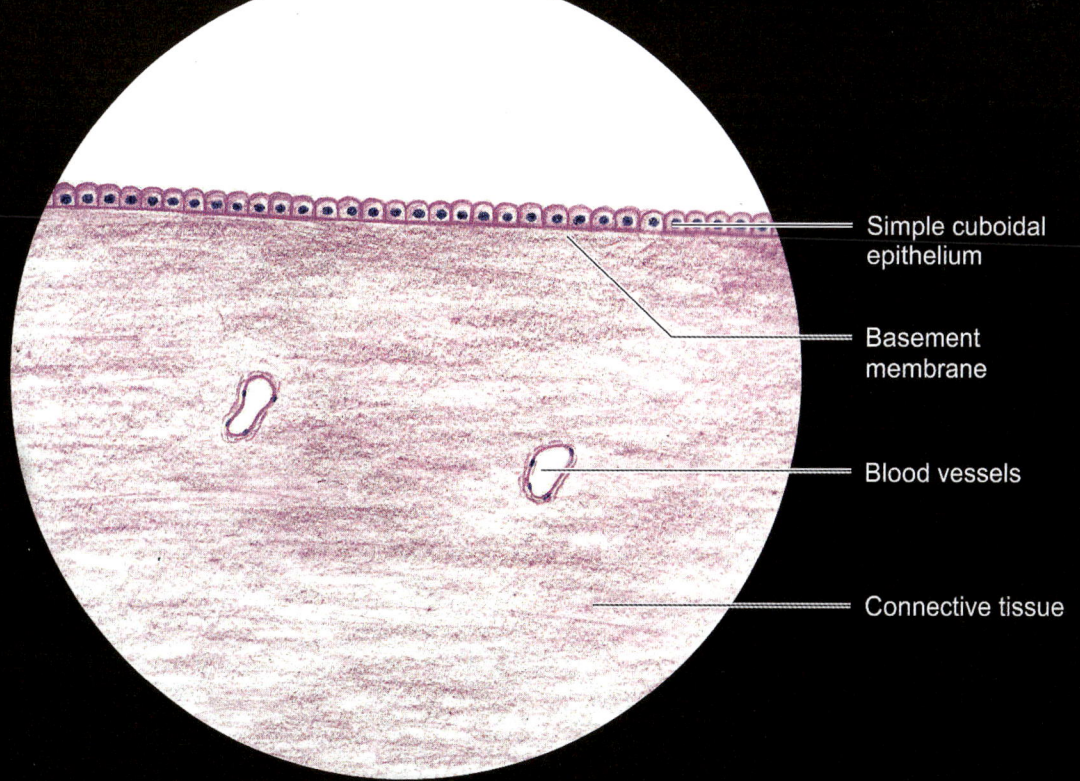

SIMPLE COLUMNAR EPITHELIUM

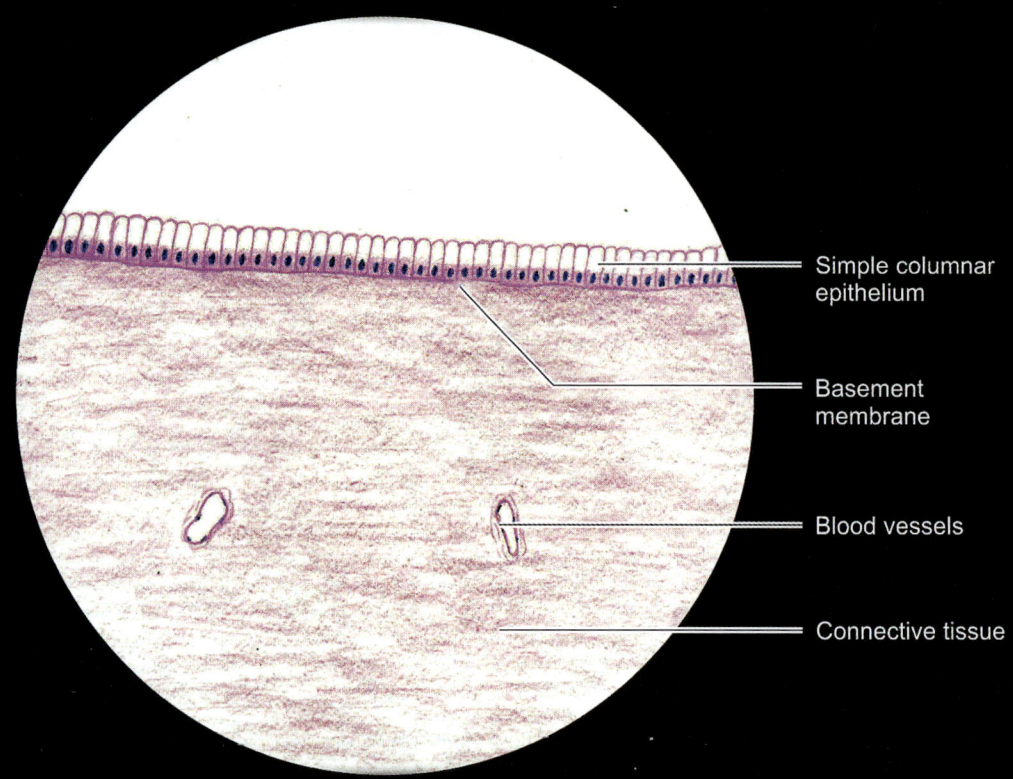

CILIATED COLUMNAR EPITHELIUM WITH GOBLET CELLS

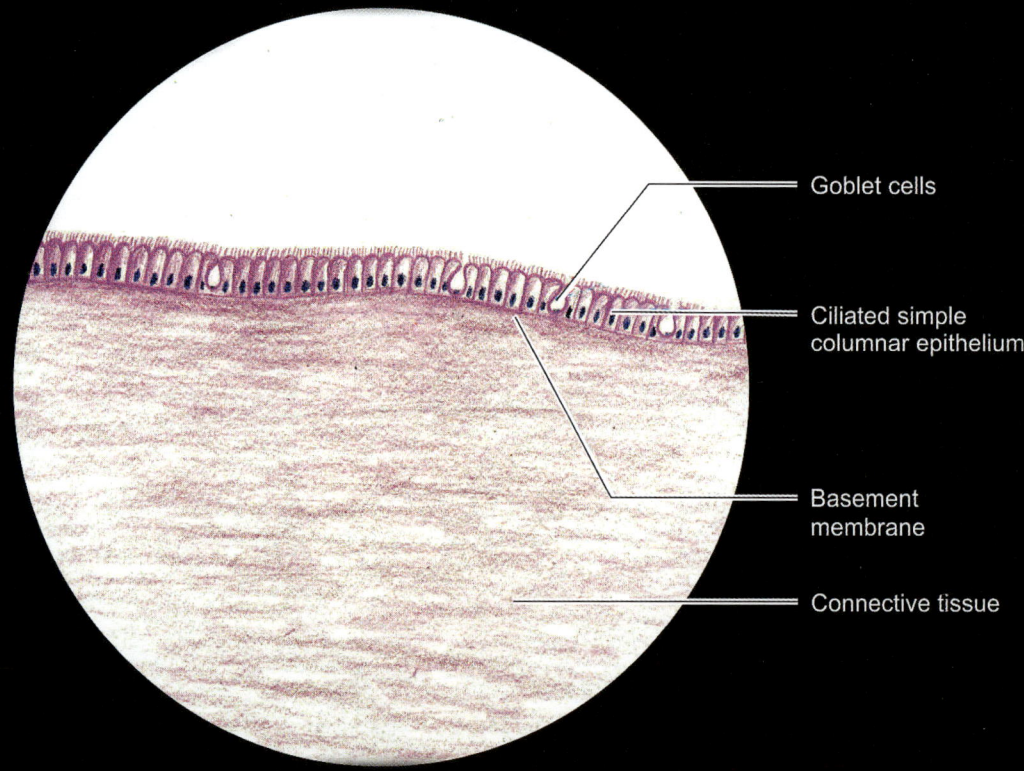

SIMPLE COLUMNAR EPITHELIUM

Height of the cell is greater than its width. Nuclei are elongated and close to the base of the cells.
- **Functions:** The main function of the simple columnar epithelium is secretion and absorption.
- **Examples:** They line the internal surface of the stomach, intestines, uterus and gallbladder.

SURFACE SPECIALIZATIONS OF THE EPITHELIAL CELLS

1. **Microvilli**: They increase the surface area of the epithelial cells they are found in epithelia specialized for absorption as in the small intestine.
2. **Stereocilia:** They are extremely long microvilli and appear like thread-shaped extensions from the epithelial cells. They are nonmotile. But helps in increasing the surface area. Found on the epithelial cells of the epididymis and hair cells in the inner ear.
3. **Cilia**: They are elongated, motile structures from the cell surface. They are present on the epithelial cells of larger airways of the respiratory tract, fallopian tube, etc., and help to propel the fluid present on the epithelial surface in a particular direction.
4. **Flagella**: They are longer than cilia spermatozoa have flagella.

PSEUDOSTRATIFIED COLUMNAR EPITHELIUM

- Here, all cells rest on the basement membrane. But only some of the cells reach the surface.
- So, the cells are of different heights and their nuclei stay at different levels. This gives a false impression that the epithelium consists of two or more layers.
- **Examples:** In the larger airways of the respiratory tract and some parts of the male reproductive system.

STRATIFIED EPITHELIUM

It contains two or more layers of cells. From the surface layer to the deep layer, cells show gradual transition from one type to another. Stratified epithelium is further classified on the basis of the shape of the cells in the topmost layer.

Stratified Squamous Epithelium

- The surface layer is of squamous type. Cells in the deepest layer are columnar or cuboidal.
- In some locations of the body, near the surface of the epithelium, cells are keratinized and make the surface dry. These cells are dead and flat in shape, without a nucleus.
- **Functions:** They provide protection against mechanical injury, act as a barrier against infection and prevent excessive water loss from the body.
- **Examples:**
    - **Keratinized sites**: It is present in skin
    - **Nonkeratinized sites**: It usually lines the wet surfaces such as oral cavity, esophagus, anal canal, vocal folds, vagina, etc.

Stratified Cuboidal Epithelium

Present in the ducts of some glands such as sweat and salivary glands.

Stratified Columnar Epithelium

Present in larger ducts of some glands and conjunctiva.

TRANSITIONAL EPITHELIUM

- It is a stratified epithelium.
- It lines most of the urinary passage, hence, it is also called urothelium. It has the capacity to stretch.
- Surface cells are large and dome shaped. Some of the surface cells may have two nuclei also.
- Going from the surface to deep, cells show gradual transition to polygonal shape.
- Basal cells are cuboidal to columnar.

PSEUDOSTRATIFIED COLUMNAR EPITHELIUM

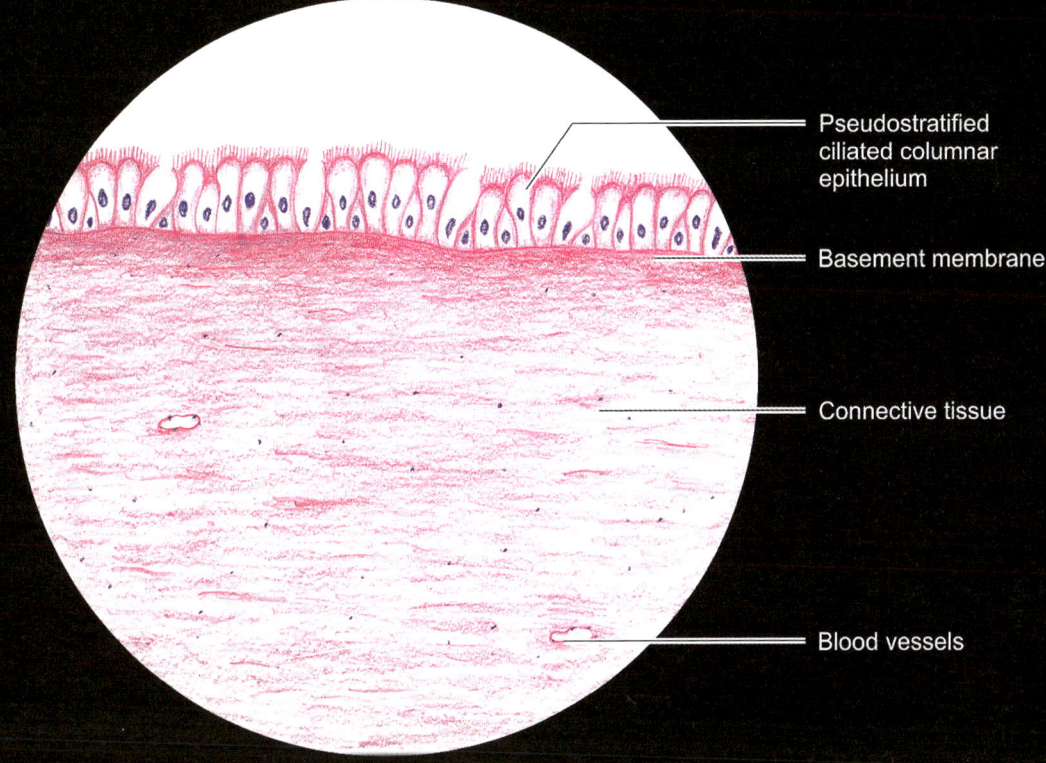

- Pseudostratified ciliated columnar epithelium
- Basement membrane
- Connective tissue
- Blood vessels

TRANSITIONAL EPITHELIUM

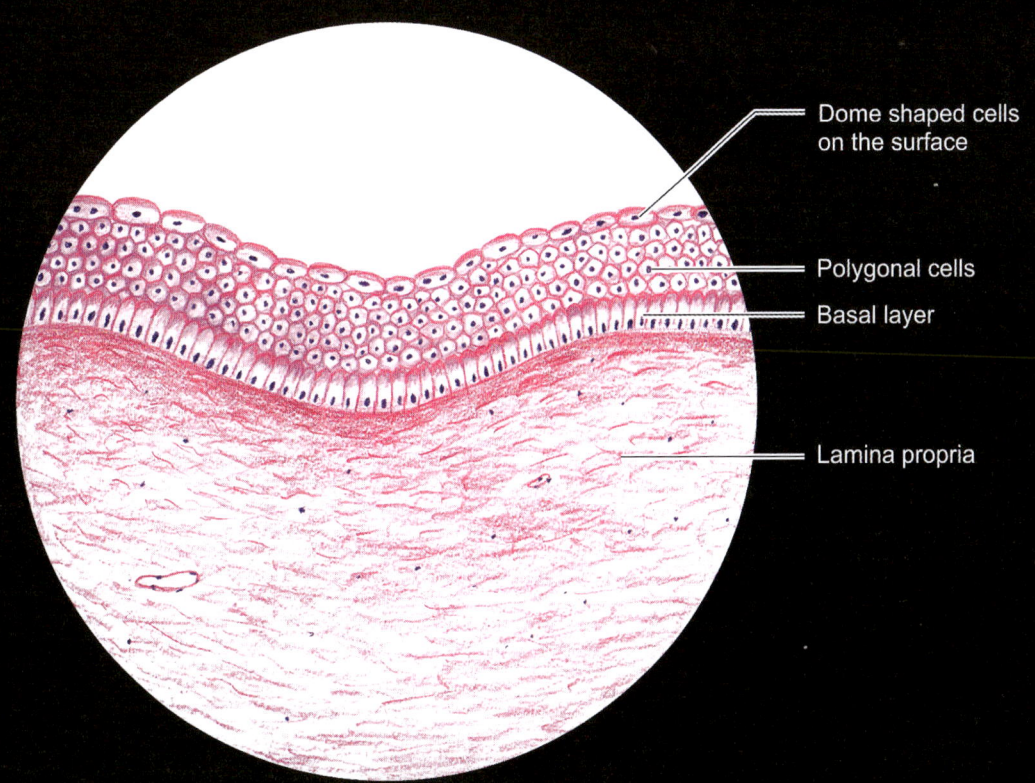

- Dome shaped cells on the surface
- Polygonal cells
- Basal layer
- Lamina propria

NONKERATINIZED STRATIFIED SQUAMOUS EPITHELIUM

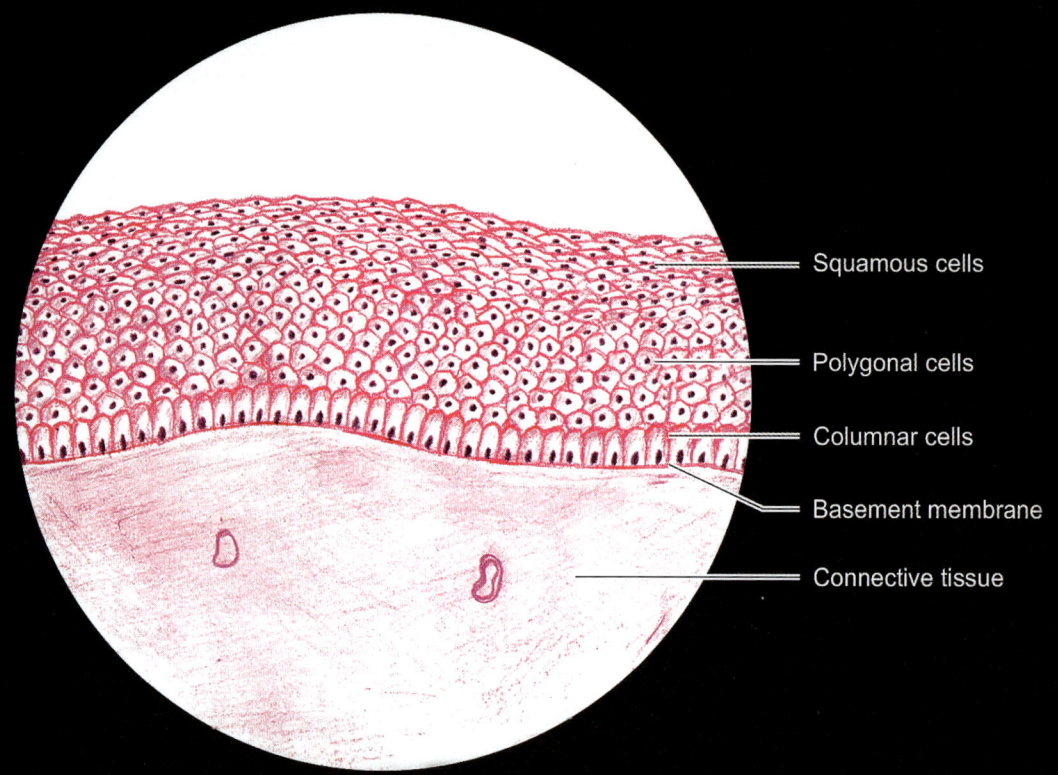

- Squamous cells
- Polygonal cells
- Columnar cells
- Basement membrane
- Connective tissue

KERATINIZED STRATIFIED SQUAMOUS EPITHELIUM

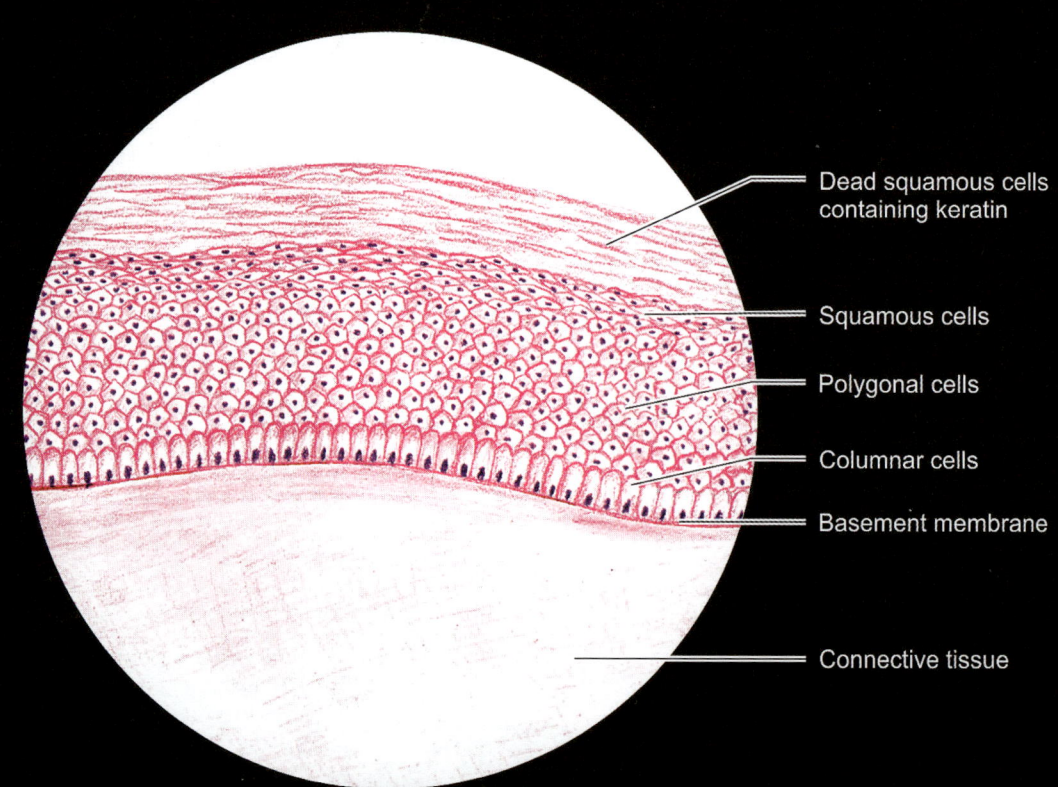

- Dead squamous cells containing keratin
- Squamous cells
- Polygonal cells
- Columnar cells
- Basement membrane
- Connective tissue

CARTILAGE

GENERAL ASPECTS

- Cartilage is a special form of dense connective tissue showing great elasticity and flexibility. It develops from primitive mesenchyme. It is of three types:
  1. *Hyaline cartilage*
  2. *Elastic cartilage*
  3. *Fibrocartilage*
- Basically, cartilage consists of **cells** and an **extracellular matrix**.
- The cells of cartilage are **chondroblasts, chondrocytes and fibrocytes**.
- The nucleus of cartilage cells are initially euchromatic, as cells start to mature the nuclei become heterochromatic.
- The extracellular matrix consists of fibers (collagen and elastic) and ground substance.
- The ground substance of cartilage is made of proteins and carbohydrates, they form a meshwork which is filled by water and dissolved salts.
- Usually, cartilage is covered by **perichondrium** (except in fibrocartilage, and hyaline cartilage at articular surfaces).
- Perichondrium consists of two layers:
  i. **Outer fibrous layer** made of **type 1 collagen fibers**.
  ii. **Inner cellular/chondrogenic layer** contains **chondroblast** cells.
- Cartilage has no blood supply, lymphatics and nerves; whereas perichondrium have all these. Hence, oxygen and metabolites diffuse from the perichondrium into the cartilage. The highly hydrated nature of ground substances helps in this diffusion.
- In articular cartilage, where there is no perichondrium, nourishment is from the synovial fluid that bathes the cartilage.
- Cartilage has poor healing capacity since it is an avascular tissue and depends on the surrounding tissue for its nourishment.
- Growing pattern are by two different ways:
  i. **Interstitial growth**: Newly formed cartilage grows by proliferation of cells throughout its substance.
  ii. **Appositional growth**: It occurs in mature cartilage. Growth of cartilage takes place by addition of new cartilage over the surface of existing cartilage.

HYALINE CARTILAGE

- **Perichondrium** is present.
- **Chondrocytes** are present as cell nests inside the lacunae and are arranged homogeneously in the matrix (because collagen fibers in the matrix have the same refractive index as that of ground substance).
- In the inner part of the cartilage chondrocytes are arranged in clusters called cell nests (isogenous groups)
- In hematoxylin and eosin staining, the matrix is basophilic (i.e., stained blue in color).
- **Chondrocytes** in the center are larger than those at the periphery.
- **Matrix** can be differentiated into two types:
  1. **Territorial matrix:** Darker matrix adjacent to chondrocytes and are newly formed without fibers.
  2. **Interterritorial matrix:** Lightly stained matrix between chondrocytes and are old with fibers.
- Ground substance consists of **type 2 collagen** fibers.
- **Examples**: Nasal septum, tracheal rings, articular surfaces of the moveable joints, costal cartilages, epiphyseal plate and costal skeleton.

Applied Anatomy

- Hyaline cartilage forms the skeleton of the fetus. The cartilage forms a framework of the bones and later endochondral ossification occurs and is replaced by bone.
- Hyaline cartilage calcifies on aging whereas elastic cartilage does not.
- Chondromas are benign tumors of cartilage, in which the chondrocytes are arranged in clusters with abundant intercellular stroma.

Viva voce

Q. Costal cartilage is composed of what type of cartilage?
Ans. Hyaline cartilage.
Q. Which is the most abundant type of cartilage in the body?
Ans. Hyaline cartilage.
Q. Which type of cartilage forms the articular surface on bones?
Ans. Hyaline cartilage.

HYALINE CARTILAGE

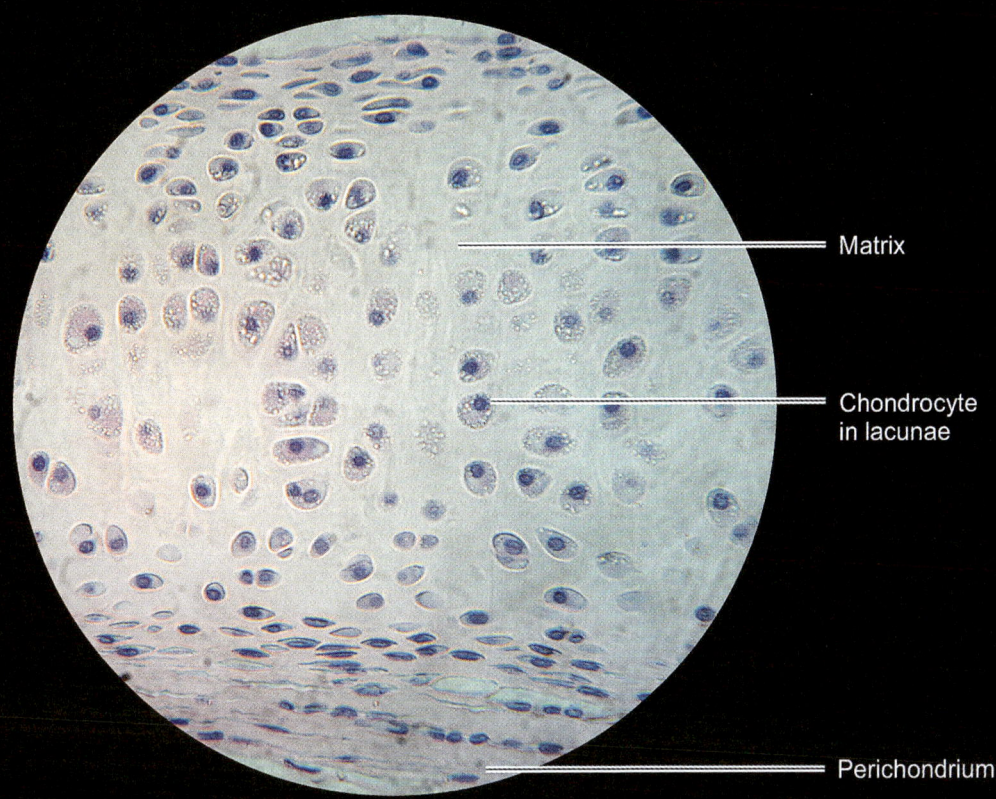

Matrix

Chondrocyte in lacunae

Perichondrium

SP:
- Cell nests of chondrocytes present.
- Territorial and interterritorial matrix present, perichondrium present.

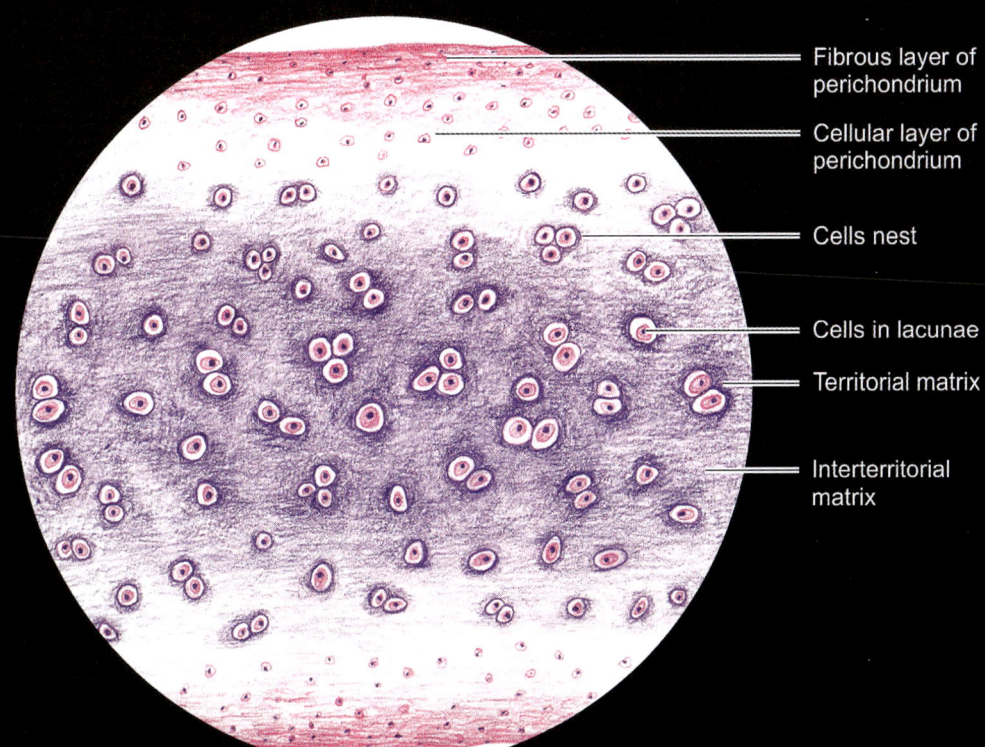

Fibrous layer of perichondrium

Cellular layer of perichondrium

Cells nest

Cells in lacunae

Territorial matrix

Interterritorial matrix

ELASTIC CARTILAGE

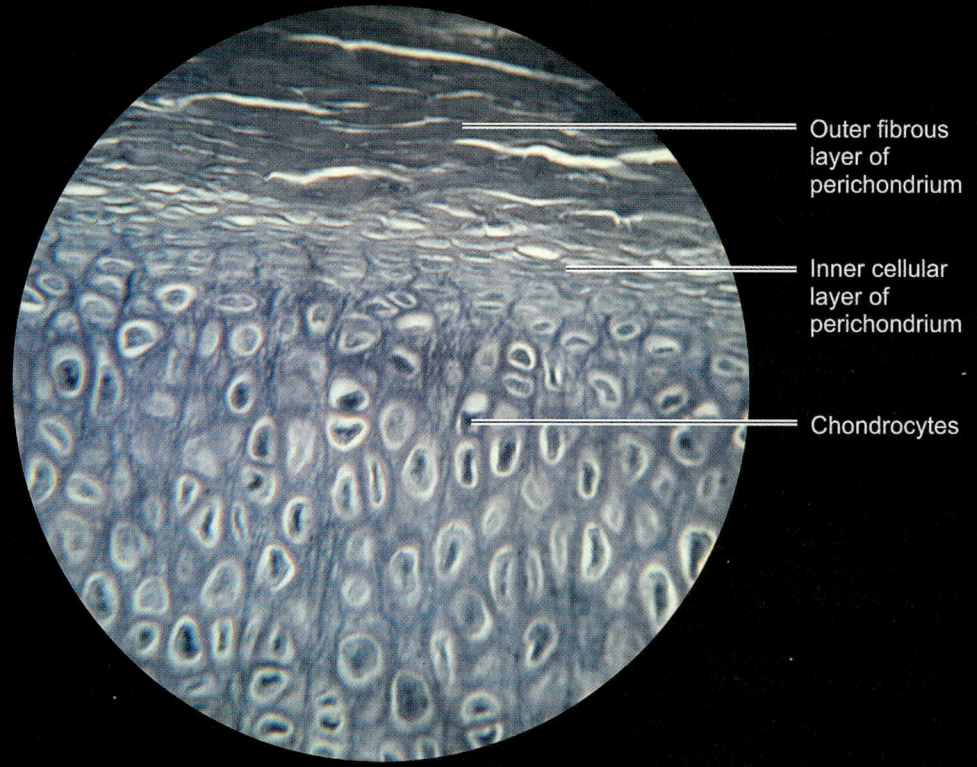

- Outer fibrous layer of perichondrium
- Inner cellular layer of perichondrium
- Chondrocytes

SP:
- Large singly arranged chondrocytes in lacunae.
- Perichondrium present.

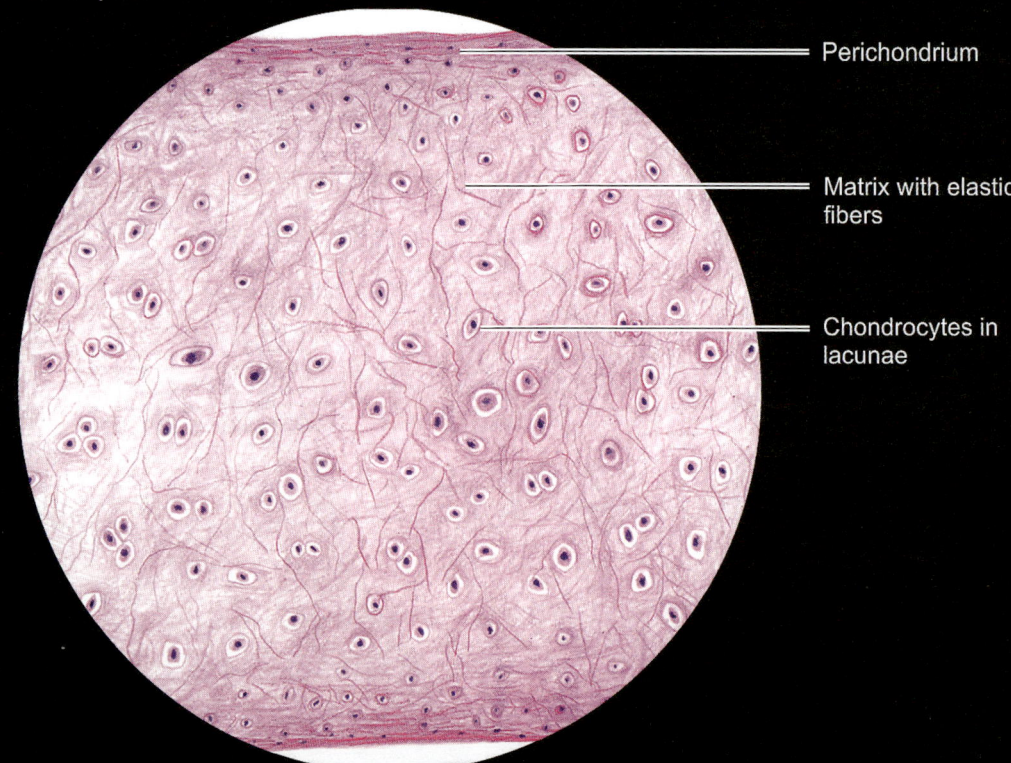

- Perichondrium
- Matrix with elastic fibers
- Chondrocytes in lacunae

ELASTIC CARTILAGE

- It is also known as **yellow fibrocartilage**.
- **Perichondrium** is present.
- Highly flexible.
- **Matrix** contains numerous **elastic fibers** instead of collagen fibers.
- **Chondrocytes** are larger, **singly arranged** and are present in lacunae.
- In H and E staining the fibers are not clearly visualized, it is better seen in special staining methods like Verhoeff's method.
- Fibers are thicker and branching in the center and thinner at the periphery.
- **Examples:** Auricle of the ear, walls of the external auditory canal, Eustachian tube and epiglottis.

Applied Anatomy

- Elastic cartilage does not calcify on aging.
- Due to its high flexibility it regains its shape quickly after being deformed.

Viva voce

Q. What stain would be best to demonstrate the elastic fibers in elastic cartilage?
Ans. Resorcin-fuchsin and orcein would best show the elastic fibers in elastic cartilage.
Q. If you bend your ear forward, it bounces back into its proper position. Why is it so?
Ans. If you bend your ear forward, it bounces back into its proper position. This is due to the elastic cartilage present in the external ear. Due to its high flexibility it regains its shape quickly after being deformed.

FIBROCARTILAGE

- It is also known as **white fibrocartilage**.
- It consists of alternating layers of cartilage matrix and thick dense layers of **type 1 collagen fibers**.
- Collagen fibers are arranged as **wavy bundles** and are oriented in the direction of stress.
- **Chondrocytes** in lacunae distributed **in rows**.
- Chondrocytes are of similar size.
- **Perichondrium is absent**, since fibrocartilage forms a transitional area between hyaline cartilage and tendon/ligament.
- Fibrocartilage provides tensile strength to the region where it is located.
- **For example,** intervertebral discs, glenoid labrum, symphysis pubis.

Applied Anatomy

It possesses great tensile strength and a considerable amount of elasticity.

Viva voce

Q. Which type of cartilage forms the intervertebral disc?
Ans. Fibrocartilage forms the intervertebral disc.
Q. How are collagen fibers arranged?
Ans. Collagen fibers are arranged as wavy bundles.
Q. Which type of collagen fibers make up the fibrocartilage?
Ans. Type 1 collagen fibers.

FIBROCARTILAGE

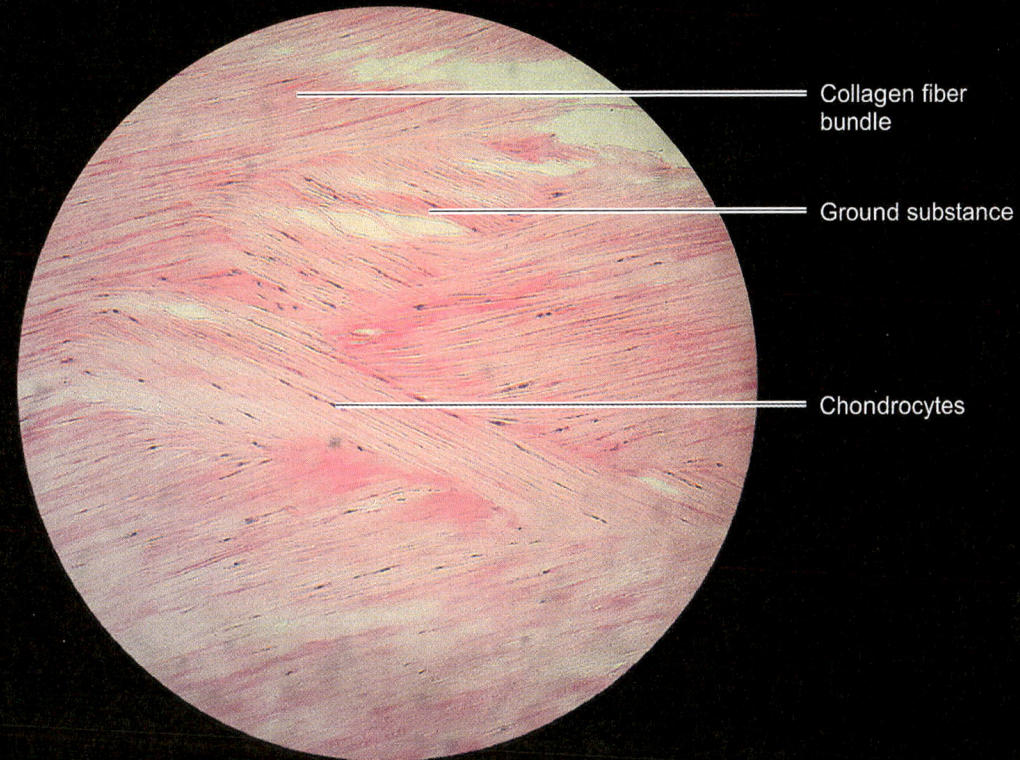

- Collagen fiber bundle
- Ground substance
- Chondrocytes

SP:
- Chondrocytes of similar size present between collagen bundles.
- Perichondrium absent.

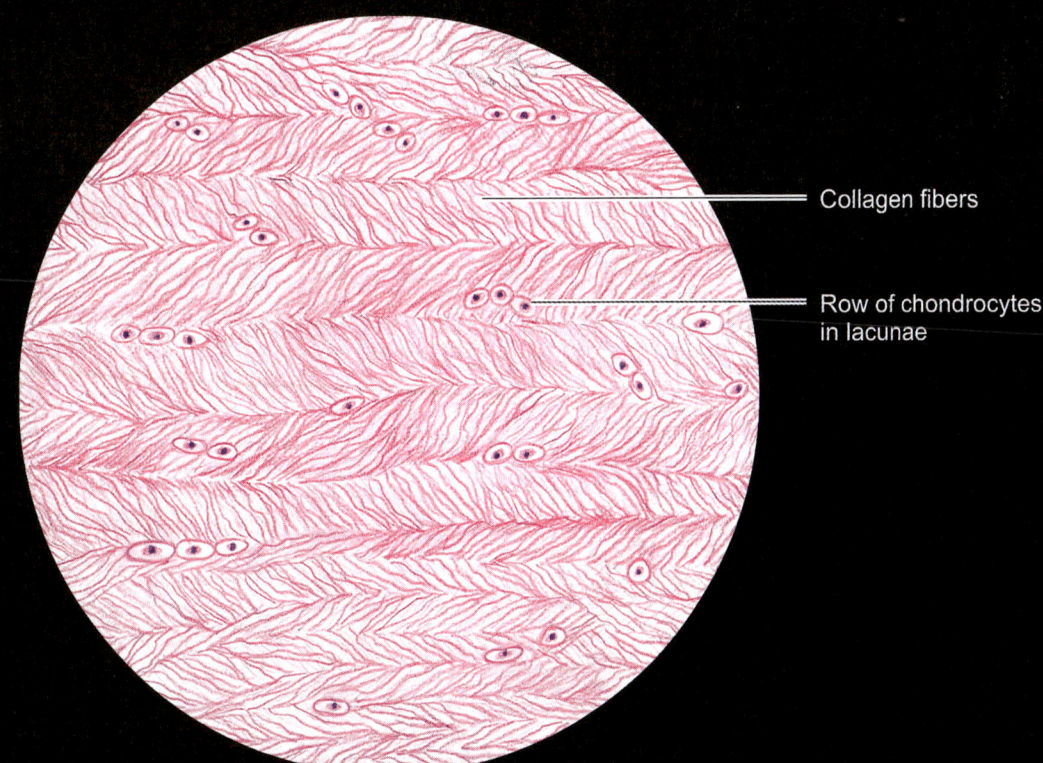

- Collagen fibers
- Row of chondrocytes in lacunae

COMPACT BONE : TRANSVERSE SECTION

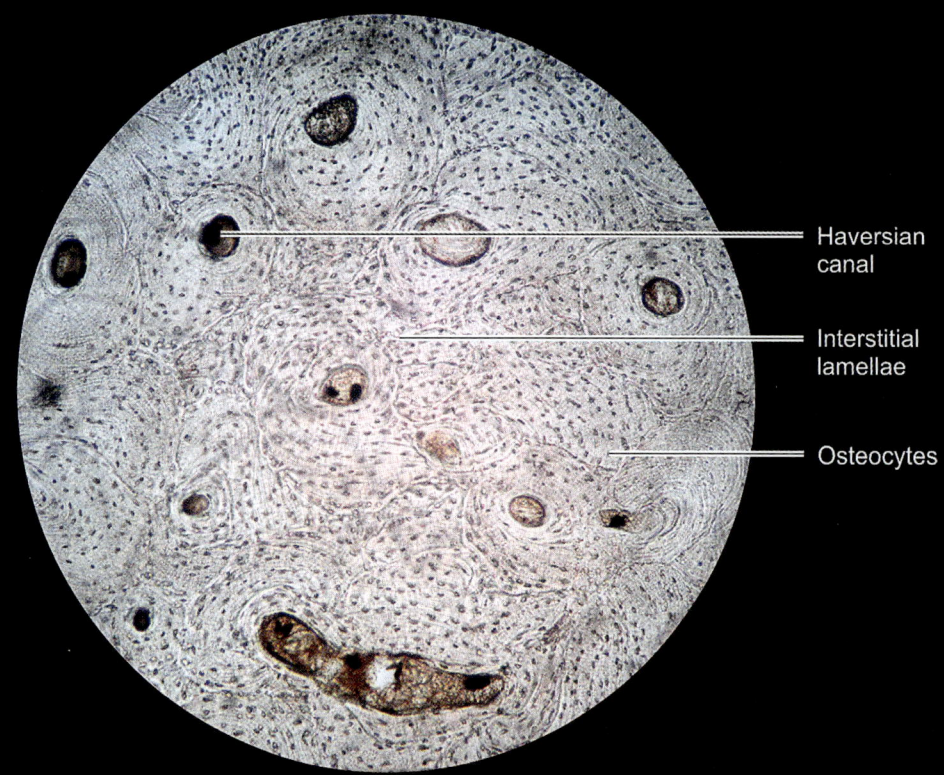

- Haversian canal
- Interstitial lamellae
- Osteocytes

SP:
- Presence of osteocytes in lacunae.
- Haversian system present with concentric lamellae.

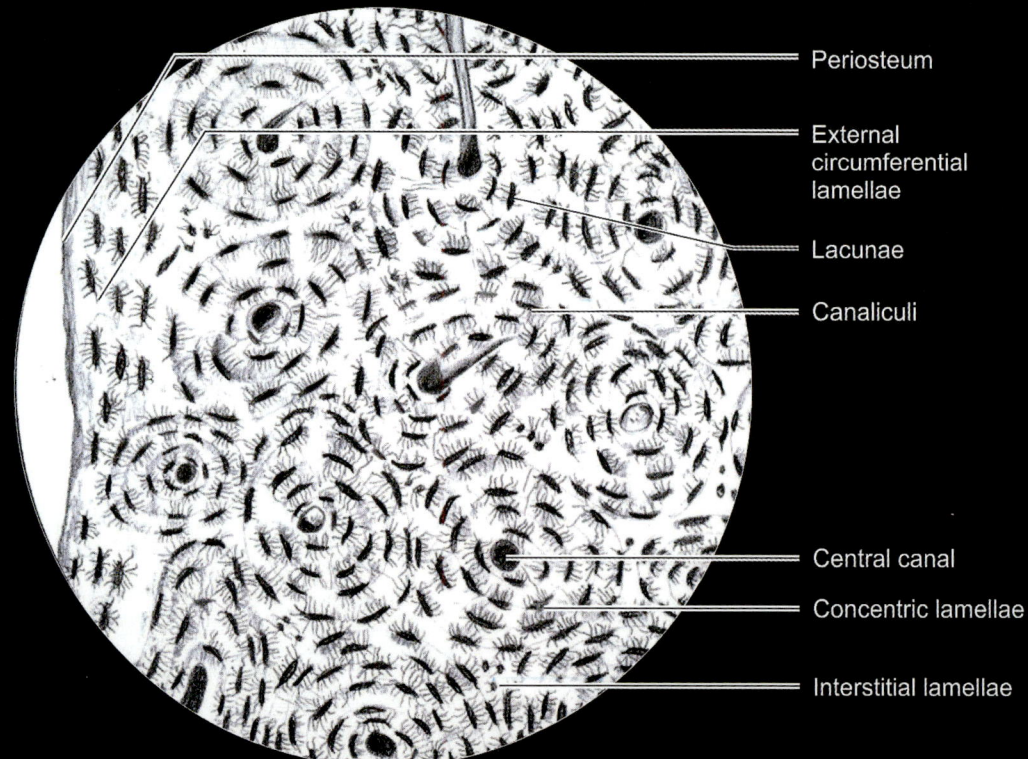

- Periosteum
- External circumferential lamellae
- Lacunae
- Canaliculi
- Central canal
- Concentric lamellae
- Interstitial lamellae

BONE

GENERAL ASPECTS

- Bone is a **dense connective tissue**.
- Bone consists of **cells** and **extracellular matrix**
- Three types of cells are there in bone: **osteoblasts, osteocytes and osteoclasts**.
- The outer and inner surfaces of the bone have coverings of connective tissue known as **periosteum** and **endosteum** respectively.

Cells in the Bone

- **Osteoblasts** synthesize organic components of the bone matrix. They later differentiate into osteocytes.
- **Osteocytes** are located in the matrix in cavities called lacunae. Normally, each lacuna contains a single osteocyte. Adjacent lacunae are connected with each other by canaliculi.
- **Osteoclasts** are involved in bone resorption.

Bone Matrix

- Matrix consists of inorganic compounds, collagen fibers and ground substance.
- Inorganic components are mainly calcium and phosphate and form hydroxyapatite crystals.
- These inorganic salts in the extracellular matrix of bone makes it hard and rigid.
- Organic components are type I collagen fibers and ground substance.
- Ground substance is composed of glycosaminoglycans, proteoglycans and some amount of water.

Coverings of Bone

- **Periosteum**: It is a layer of connective tissue that covers the external surface of the bone, except at the attachment of a muscle. It consists of two layers. The outer **fibrous layer** and the inner **osteogenic layer**. Collagen fibers binding the periosteum to the bone are called **Sharpey's fibers**.
- **Endosteum**: It lines the inner surface of the bone.

BONE TRANSVERSE SECTION

- **Haversian systems** or **osteons** are the structural units of the bone matrix.
- Each osteon is outlined by a **cement line**.
- **Osteons** are located between internal and external **circumferential lamellae**.
- It consists of layers of **concentric lamellae** arranged around a central canal.
- **Central canal** consists of blood vessels, nerves and reticular connective tissue.
- **Lamellae** contains osteocytes in spaces called **lacunae** and tiny canals radiate from lacunae known as **canaliculi**.
- Small irregular areas of bone are present between osteons, known as **interstitial lamellae** and represents remnants of eroded osteons.
- External wall is formed by **external circumferential lamellae** and the internal wall by **internal circumferential lamellae**.

BONE LONGITUDINAL SECTION

- **Osteocytes** are present.
- **Central canal** is surrounded by lamellae with **lacunae** and **canaliculi**.
- **Volkmann's canal (perforating canal)** is visible in the longitudinal section (LS).
- Volkmann's canal is formed by anastomoses between central canals.
- Volkmann's canal joins the central canal with a marrow cavity.
- **Concentric lamellae is absent** in Volkmann's canal since they directly penetrate via lamellae.
- Throughout life there is continuous destruction and rebuilding of the haversian system.

Applied Anatomy

- Inflammation of bone marrow is known as osteomyelitis.
- Ischemia results in avascular necrosis of bones which is mainly caused by fracture or dislocation.
- Osteoporosis is a condition resulting from the quantitative reduction of the normal bone.
- Osteomalacia and rickets are conditions occurring in adults and children respectively characterized by qualitative abnormality as impaired bone mineralization due to deficiency of vitamin D.
- Aneurysmal bone cyst is an expanding osteolytic lesion filled with blood.
- Osteoarthritis is a chronic disorder of synovial joints characterized by progressive degenerative changes in articular cartilage over years.
- Following an injury to bone, osteoprogenitor cells in the endosteum and periosteum differentiate into osteoblasts and they repair the damaged bone.
- Osteoclasts upon the action of parathyroid hormone, increases the bone resorption and leads to increase in the blood calcium level. But, calcitonin decreases the activity of the osteoclasts, decreases the bone resorption, hence decreases in the blood calcium level.
- Growth hormone stimulates growth of epiphyseal plates.

Viva voce

Q. What structures are found within haversian canals?
Ans. Capillaries and nerves.
Q. Is the osseous lamella adjacent to the haversian canal the youngest or the oldest lamella of a particular osteon?
Ans. The youngest.
Q. What structure in mature bone is created by the zone of resorption?
Ans. The marrow canal.
Q. What are the differences between intramembranous ossification and endochondral ossification?
Ans. **Intramembranous ossification:** Does not use a cartilage framework, bone develops directly on or within mesenchyme. Bone growth is appositional. Found in irregular bones such as the bones of the skull.
Endochondral ossification: Replaces a pre-existing cartilage framework. The bone lengthens through interstitial growth and changes diameter through appositional growth. Found in long bones.

COMPACT BONE : LONGITUDINAL SECTION

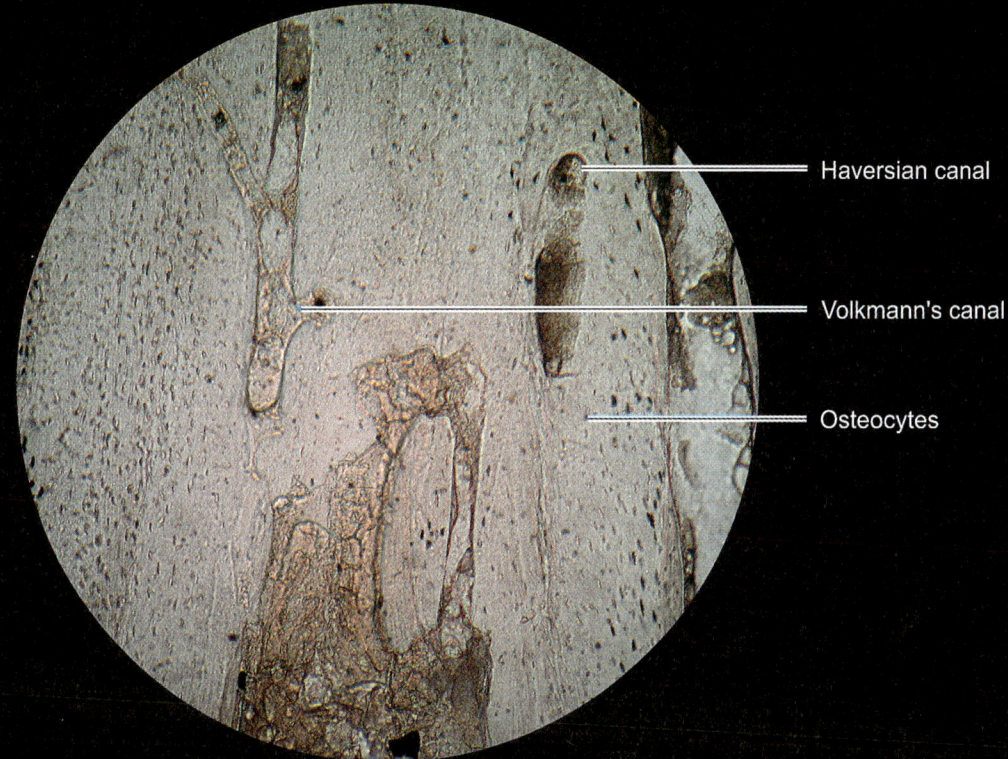

SP:
- Osteocytes present.
- Longitudinal section of haversian system and Volkmann's canal seen.

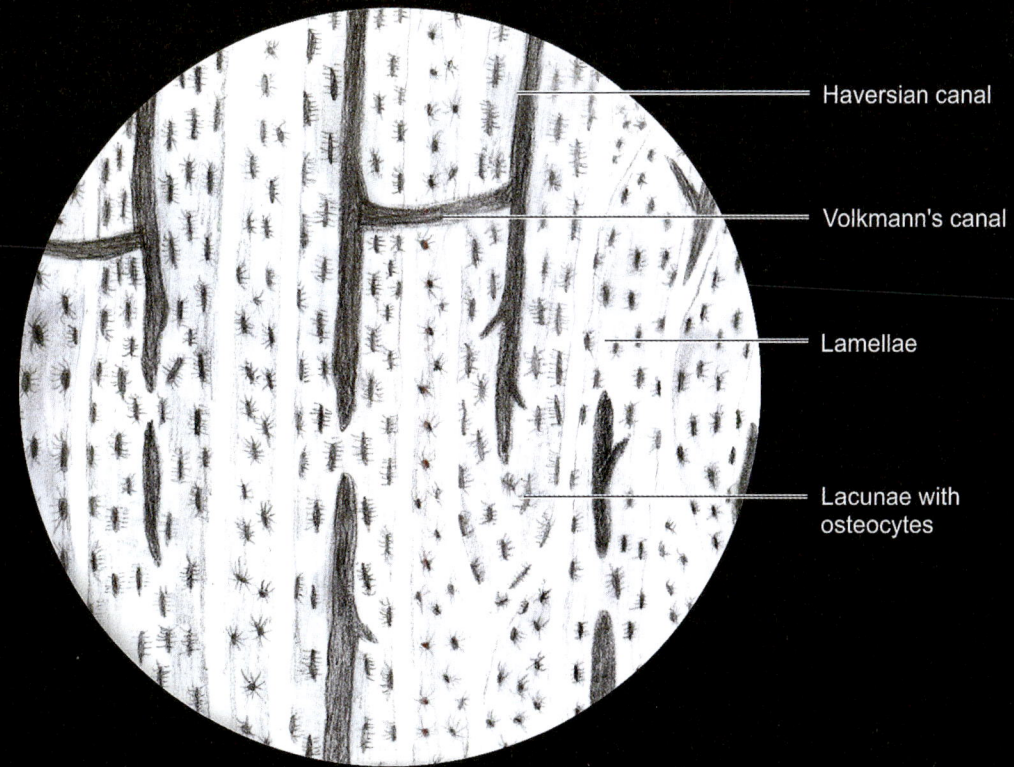

SKELETAL MUSCLE

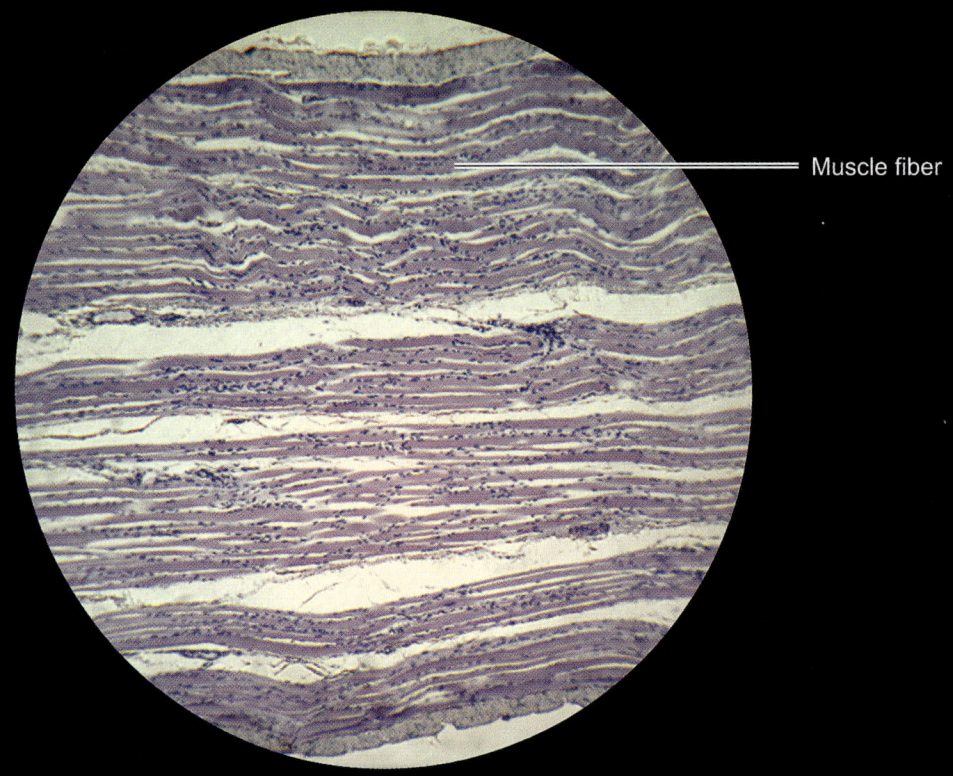

SP:
- Cylindrical muscle fibers with prominent striations.
- Presence of peripherally arranged flattened multinuclei.

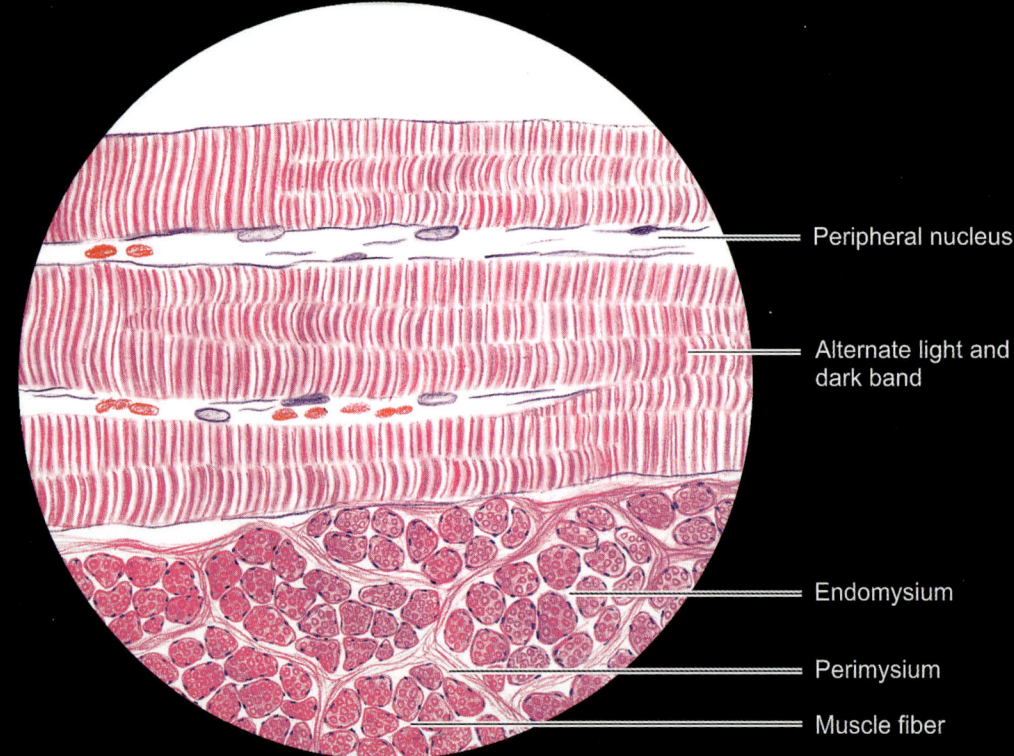

MUSCLE

GENERAL ASPECTS

- The muscle cells develop from mesoderm.
- Muscle cell cytoplasm is called sarcoplasm, cell membrane is called sarcolemma and the endoplasmic reticulum is called sarcoplasmic reticulum.
- Muscle fibers contain myofibrils.
- Myofibrils are made of contractile proteins called actin and myosin.
- Skeletal and cardiac muscles have striations.
- Smooth muscles lack striations.

SKELETAL MUSCLE

- Also known as **voluntary muscle.**
- During the development of skeletal muscle, **myoblasts** fuse together to form **multinucleated muscle cells.**
- Muscle fibers are **long, cylindrical** and **multinucleated**.
- Nuclei are arranged at the **periphery** and are **elongated**.
- In the longitudinal section, skeletal muscle fibers show alternate light and dark bands, known as **I band** and **A band** respectively, giving **striated** appearance to these muscle fibers.
- Individual muscle fibers are surrounded by connective tissue called **endomysium**.
- Muscle fibers form groups and form **fasciculus**. Each fasciculus is surrounded by connective tissue called **perimysium**.
- A muscle is formed with bundles of fasciculi and the entire muscle is covered by connective tissue called **epimysium**.

Applied Anatomy

- Heat rigor occurs above 43°C where the muscle protein gets denatured, as a result muscle remains in a contracted state.
- Skeletal muscle is capable of limited regeneration.
- When there is damage to skeletal muscles, muscle cells are stimulated. They divide, fuse with the existing muscle fibers and repair it.
- But, if large regions are damaged, regeneration does not occur and the missing muscle is replaced by connective tissue.
- Polymyositis is a disease of muscle characterized by inflammation of the muscle fibers.

SMOOTH MUSCLE

- **Involuntary** muscle.
- Present in walls of hollow viscera and blood vessels.
- **Uninucleated, spindle shaped myocytes.**
- **Centrally placed single nucleus**.
- **Nonstriated**, since actin and myosin filaments are arranged randomly and are without cross striation patterns.
- Present in arteries, veins and walls of hollow organs like gastrointestinal tract, respiratory tract and urinary tract.

Applied Anatomy

- These muscle cells divide actively and have capacity to regenerate.
- Leiomyosarcomas are malignant tumors of smooth muscle. The tumor consists of spindle cells with large hyperchromatic nuclei.
- The contraction of smooth muscle cells is slow, but they can remain contracted for long periods.
- Smooth muscle cells form the extracellular fibrous tissue components in the tunica media of blood vessels.
- Smooth muscle cells in the walls of elastic arteries regulate the blood supply to their target tissues.

Viva voce

Q. When the muscle cells are cut in the cross section, there are interruptions in the basal laminae. What is responsible for these discontinuities?
Ans. Gap junctions.
Q. Why do smooth muscle fibers in the cross section have different diameters and why do some of these fail to show nuclei?
Ans. Smooth muscle cells have tapered ends. Since the cells interdigitate different diameters would be revealed in a particular plane of section and the plane of section does not always go through the nucleus.
Q. Are myofibrils or sarcomeres present in smooth muscle fibers?
Ans. No.

SMOOTH MUSCLE

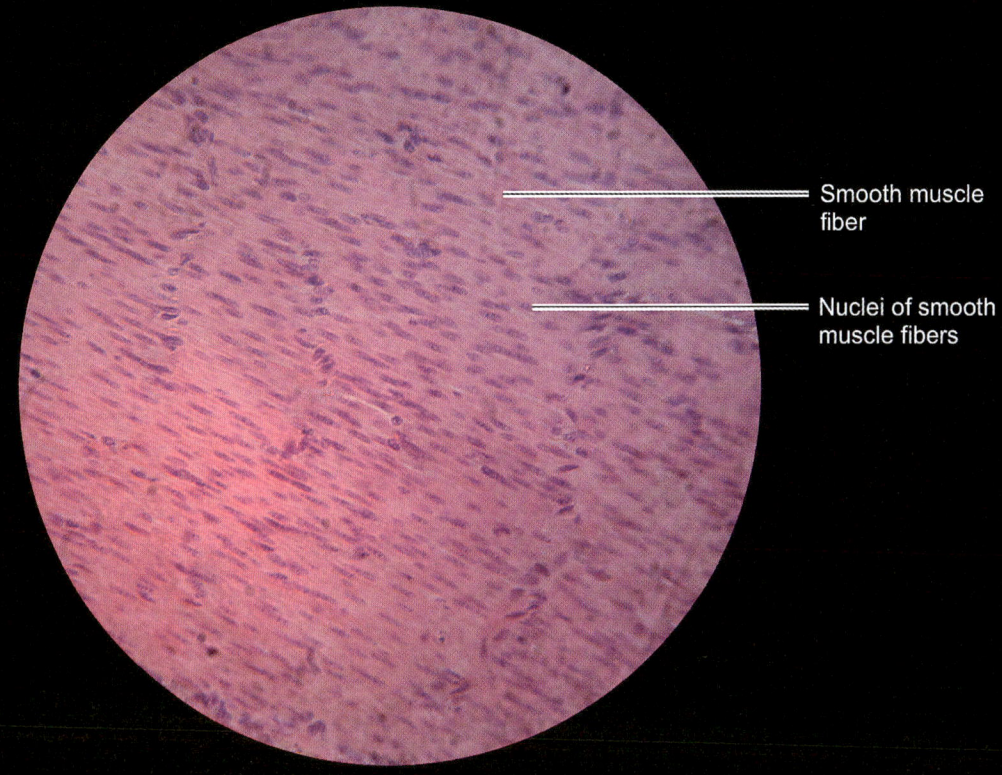

SP:
- Presence of single, uninucleated, spindle shaped fibers.
- Presence of centrally placed nucleus.

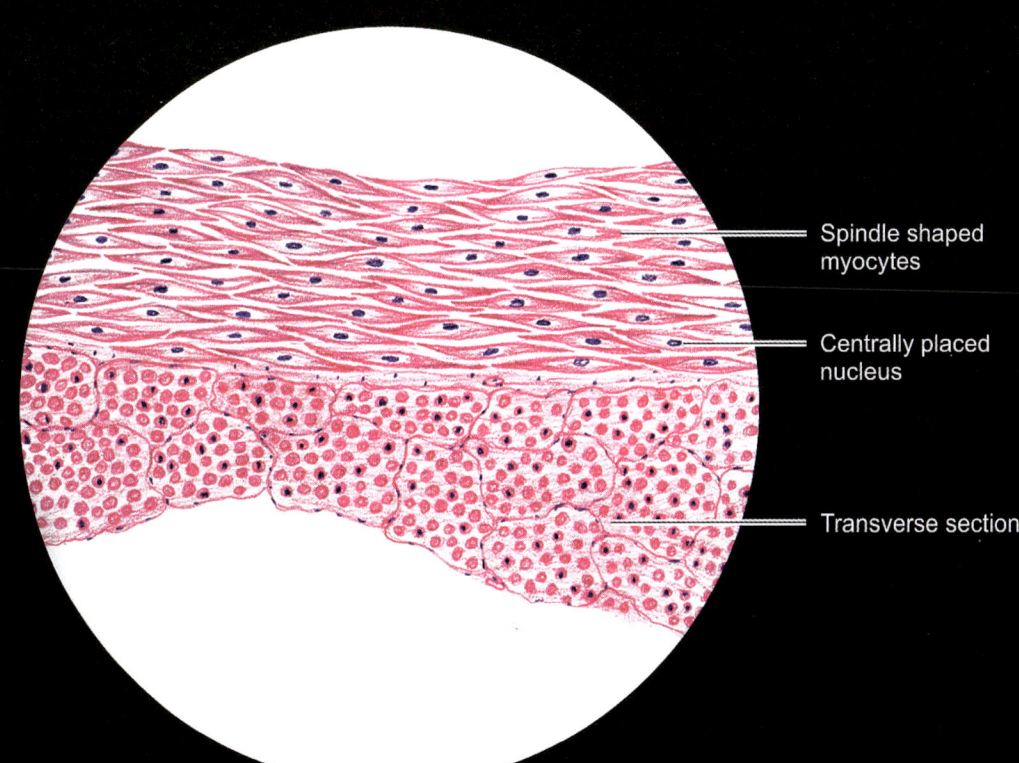

CARDIAC MUSCLE

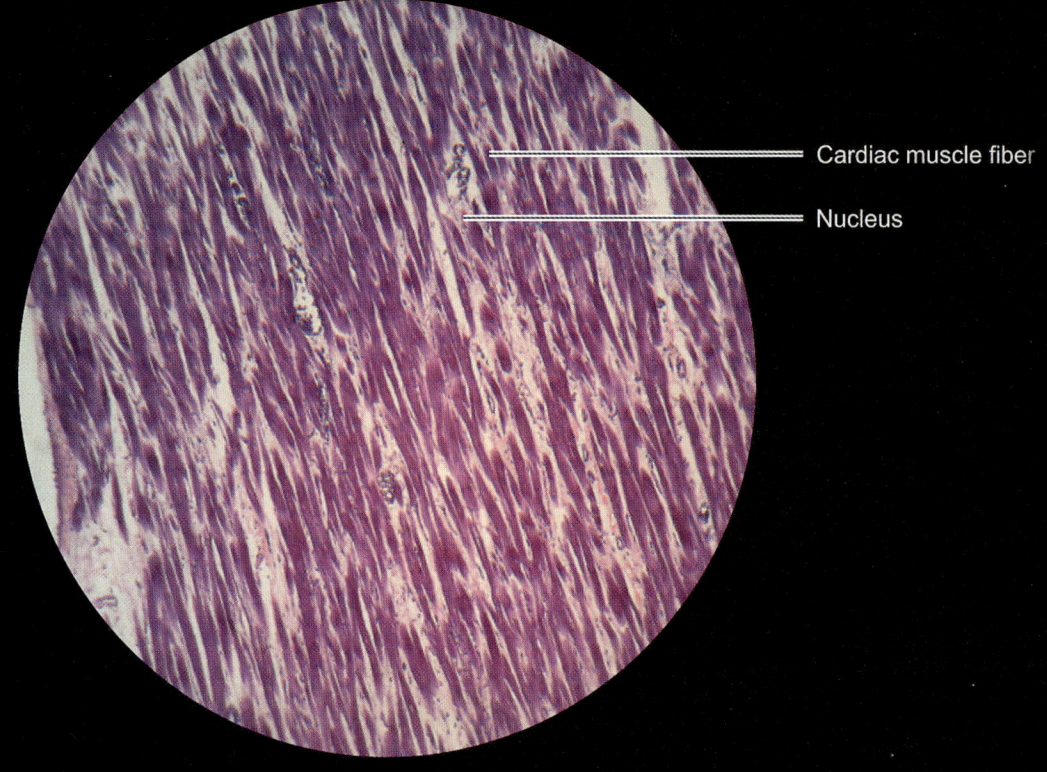

SP:
- Branching fibers with striations present.
- Intercalated discs and centrally placed nucleus present.

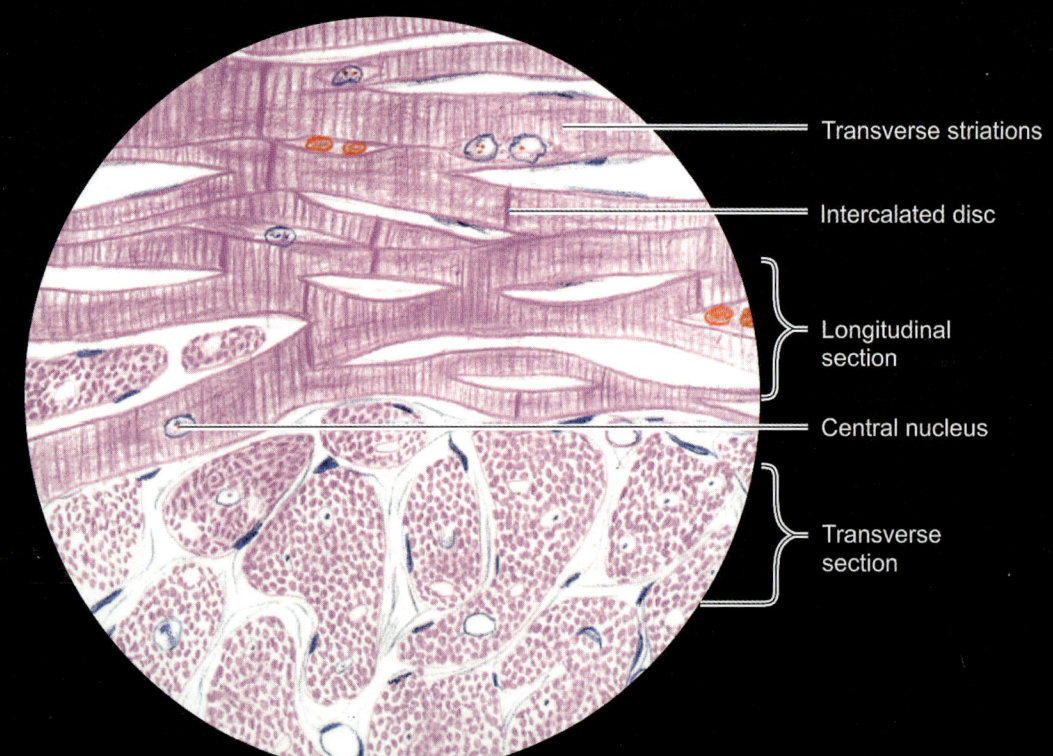

CARDIAC MUSCLE

- It is an **involuntary** muscle.
- Made up of cylindrical fibers with **striations**.
- Cardiac muscle fibers are shorter than skeletal muscle fibers.
- Contains a **single central nucleus**.
- **Binucleate muscle fibers** are occasionally seen.
- It is present in **branching anastomosis**.
- **Intercalated discs** (gap junction complex) are present at regular intervals.
- These gap junctions couple all fibers for rhythmic contraction.
- Cardiac muscle fibers exhibit **autorhythmicity**.

Applied Anatomy

- When the blood supply to cardiac muscle becomes insufficient as in the coronary artery block, the patient experiences chest pain called angina pectoris. If this ischemia prolongs, then it results in the necrosis (death) of cardiac muscle called myocardial infarction (MI).
- Cardiac muscle cells do not regenerate. Thus after MI, they are replaced by fibrotic tissue.
- In brown atrophy of heart there will be accumulation of yellowish brown lipid pigment called lipofuscin in the myocardial fibers (lipofuscin—wear and tear pigment).

Viva voce

Q. What is the position of the nuclei in cardiac muscle cells?
Ans. Central.
Q. Do the myofibrils pass through intercalated discs?
Ans. No.
Q. How can you distinguish cross sections of cardiac muscle fibers from those of skeletal muscle fibers?
Ans. Central nuclei, intercalated discs, branching fibers.

BLOOD VESSELS

GENERAL ASPECTS

- Blood vessel wall is histologically divided into three tunics or coats.
    1. **Tunica intima**
    2. **Tunica media**
    3. **Tunica adventitia**
- **Tunica intima** is the Innermost layer. It is lined by endothelium with underlying subendothelial connective tissue.
- **Internal elastic lamina** separates tunica intima from tunica media.
- **Tunica media** is the middle layer. It contains smooth muscle, elastic and reticular fibers. Autonomic nervous system supplies the smooth muscles. In the artery, it is the thickest layer.
- **External elastic lamina** separates tunica media and adventitia.
- **Tunica adventitia** is the outermost layer. It contains collagen and elastic fibers. In large-sized blood vessels, **vasavasorum** (vessels that supply the vessels) is present in this layer which helps in nutrition. It is the thickest and best developed layer in veins (most contrasting feature of vein with artery).

ARTERIES

- Arterial system is divided into:
    1. **Large/elastic arteries**
    2. **Medium-sized/muscular arteries**
    3. **Arterioles**
    4. **Capillaries**.
- Arterial wall made of three layers, i.e., tunica intima, tunica media and tunica adventitia.
- **Tunica intima** consists of the endothelium and subendothelial connective tissue and internal elastic lamina.
- **Tunica media** is the thickest layer.
- Tunica media is made of mainly **elastic fibers** with few smooth muscle fibers.
- The presence of elastic fibers facilitate distention of the vessel wall and thereby helps in maintaining blood pressure.
- Vasovasorum present in **tunica adventitia**. "Example: **Aorta, common carotid artery, etc.**"

LARGE ARTERY OR ELASTIC ARTERY

- *Large arteries* are also called **elastic arteries**.
- Their tunica media has more elastic fibers and less smooth muscles as compared to medium-sized arteries.
- This feature of elastic arteries helps in damping the fluctuation in blood pressure during the cardiac cycle, known as Windkessel effect.
- Tunica media is thicker than adventitia.
- Vasovasorum present in tunica adventitia.
- Example: **Aorta, common carotid artery, subclavian artery, etc**.

LARGE ARTERY

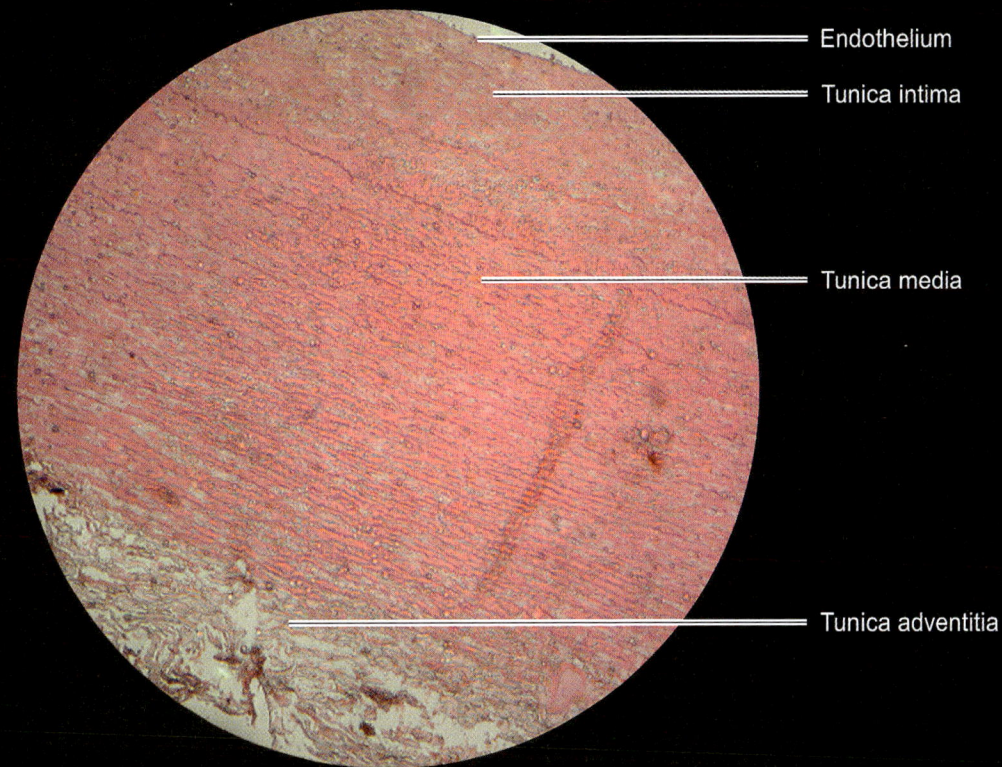

- Endothelium
- Tunica intima
- Tunica media
- Tunica adventitia

SP:
- Presence of three layers: Tunica intima, tunica media and tunica adventitia.
- Tunica media more prominent with more elastic fiber and few smooth muscle fibers.

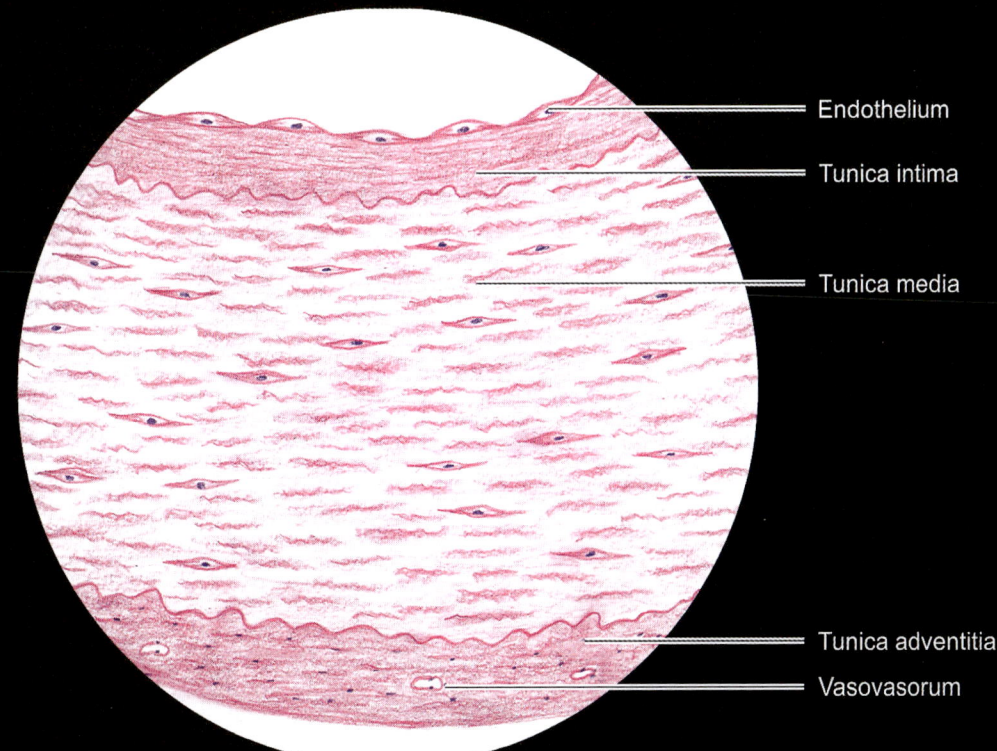

- Endothelium
- Tunica intima
- Tunica media
- Tunica adventitia
- Vasovasorum

MEDIUM-SIZED ARTERY

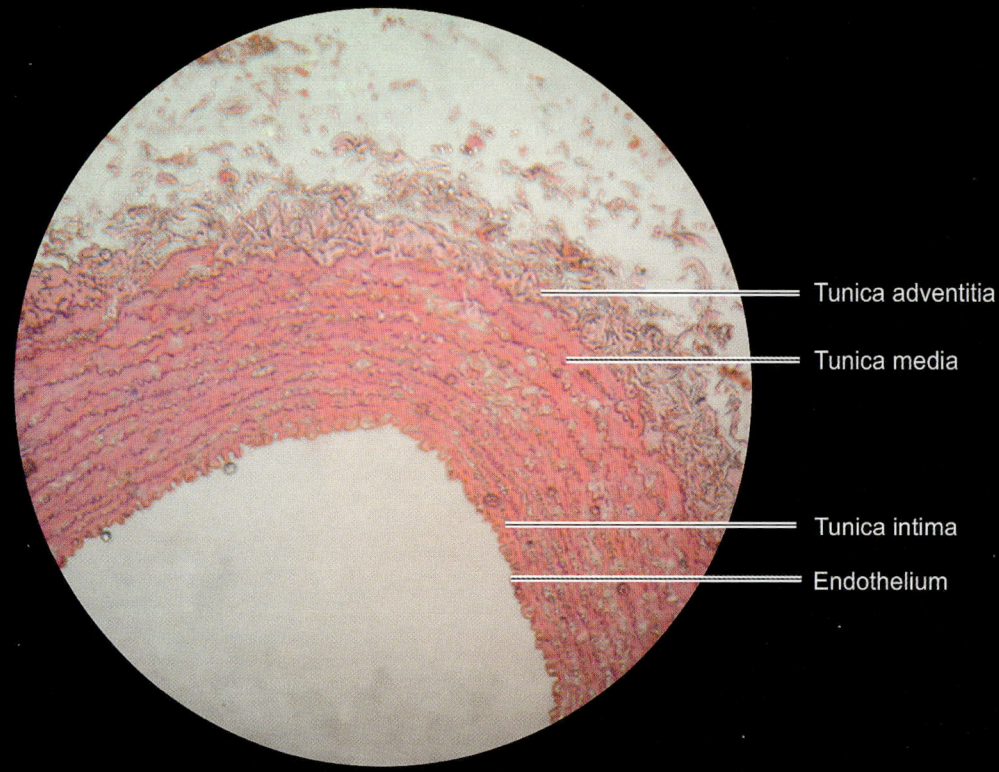

SP:
- Thick tunica media with numerous smooth muscle fibers.
- Presence of internal elastic lamina thrown into folds.

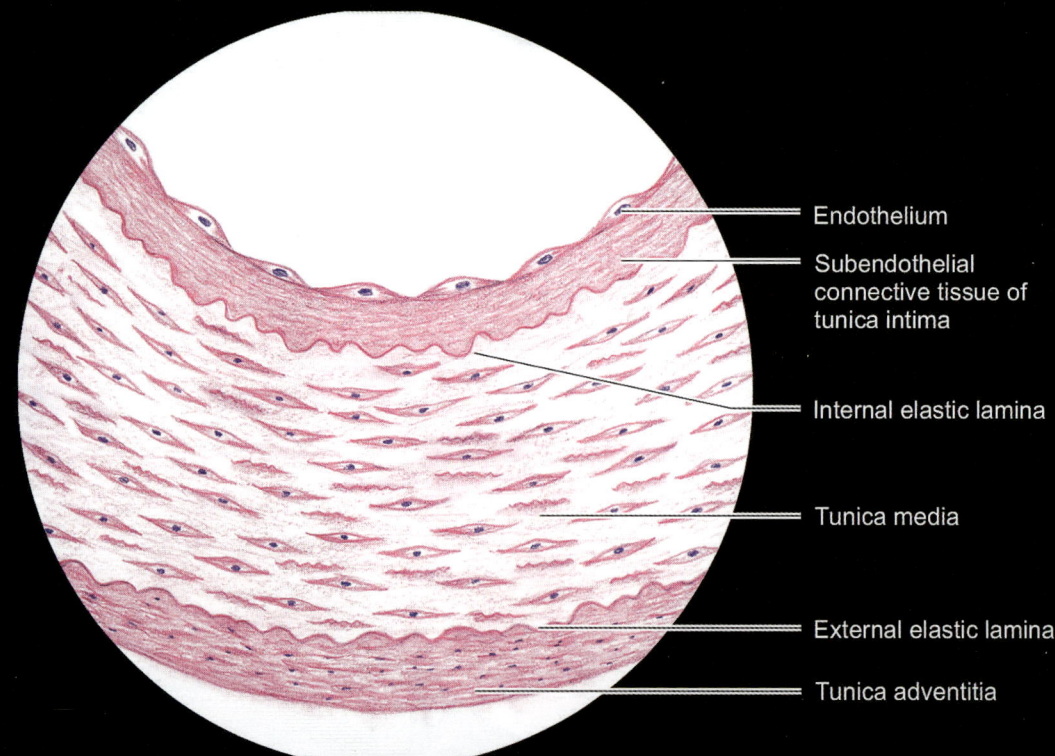

MEDIUM-SIZED ARTERY

- *Medium-sized arteries* are also called muscular arteries.
- Their tunica media has more smooth muscles and less elastic fibers.
- This gives medium sized arteries the ability to do vasoconstriction and relaxation according to the need of different organs.
- Tunica media is thicker than adventitia.
- Example: **Radial artery, ulnar artery, brachial artery.**

Applied Anatomy

- In old age the arteries become stiff. This phenomenon is called arteriosclerosis.
- In atherosclerosis usually large and medium-sized arteries are affected, where smooth muscles and macrophages within the tunica intima are filled with lipid vacuoles with cholesterol esters which crystallizes to form needle-like structures and produce clefts in intimal tissue.
- Inflammation of an artery is known as arteritis.
- Thromboangiitis obliterans is inflammation of peripheral arteries of the legs, seen in smokers.
- The ability of medium-sized arteries to decrease their diameter (to vasoconstrict) regulates the flow of blood to different parts of the body as required.
- The maintenance of blood pressure in the arterial system between contractions of the heart results from the elasticity of large arteries. This quality allows them to expand when the heart contracts and to return to normal between cardiac contractions.

Viva voce

Q. What is a pulse?
Ans. Pulse is a pressure wave transmitted along the artery as a result of the ejection of the blood by the ventricles.
Q. What is blood pressure?
Ans. Blood pressure is the measure of the force that the circulating blood exerts against the artery wall.

VEINS

- Venous system is divided into:
  1. **Large-sized veins**
  2. **Medium-sized veins**
  3. **Venules.**
- Compared to arteries, they have relatively thin walls and bigger lumen.
- *Large veins* have tunica media with thin circular arrangement of smooth muscle fibers. Internal elastic lamina is poorly defined.
- Compared to arteries, tunica adventitia is largely developed where smooth muscles are arranged in longitudinal bundles.
- Vasovasorum is present.
- For example: **Superior and inferior vena cava.**
- *In medium-sized veins*, the lumen is often collapsed and all three layers are thinner than the corresponding layers in a large vein.
- Internal and external elastic lamina are not distinguishable.
- Tunica media is less muscular. However, tunica adventitia is well developed.
- Example: **Saphenous vein, median cubital vein, cephalic vein**

LARGE VEIN

- Tubular organ having relatively thin wall and bigger lumen.
- Thin wall comprises the following: tunica intima, tunica media, tunica adventitia.
- **Tunica intima**—consisting of **endothelium**, small amounts of **subendothelial connective tissue**, and **internal elastic lamina**.
- **Tunica media**—thin circular arrangement of smooth muscle fibers.
- **Tunica adventitia**—largely developed, smooth muscles in longitudinal arrangement as bundles, surrounded by connective tissue containing **vasovasorum**.
- In large vein tunica media and intima is distinguished by the presence of **internal elastic lamina**.
- Longitudinal bundles of smooth muscles are seen as **muscular patches** in the cross section.
- Examples: **Superior and inferior vena cava.**

Viva voce

Q. How will you identify longitudinal smooth muscle bundles in a histology slide under a microscope?
Ans. The longitudinal smooth muscle fibers bundle are seen as muscular patches on cross section when viewed under microscope.
Q. What is aortocaval compression syndrome?
Ans. Aortocaval compression syndrome, is compression of the abdominal aorta and inferior vena cava by the gravid uterus when a pregnant woman lies on her back, and is a frequent cause of maternal hypotension, which can result in loss of consciousness.

LARGE VEIN

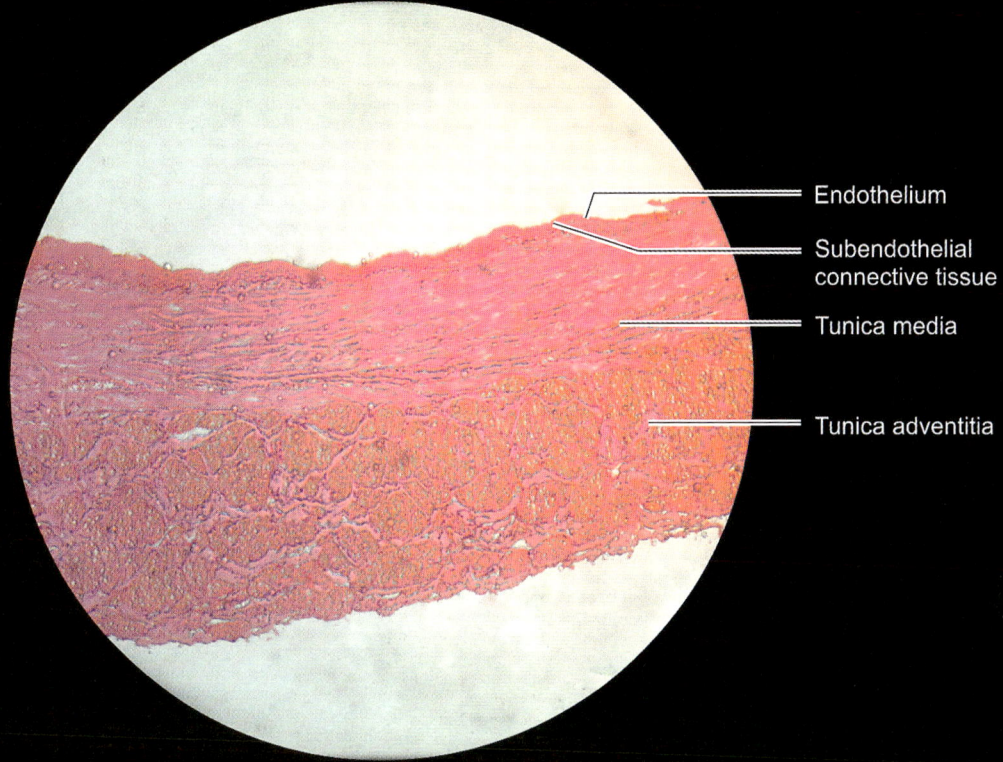

SP:
- Presence of three layers: Tunica intima, tunica media and tunica adventitia.
- Tunica adventitia more prominent with muscular patches seen.

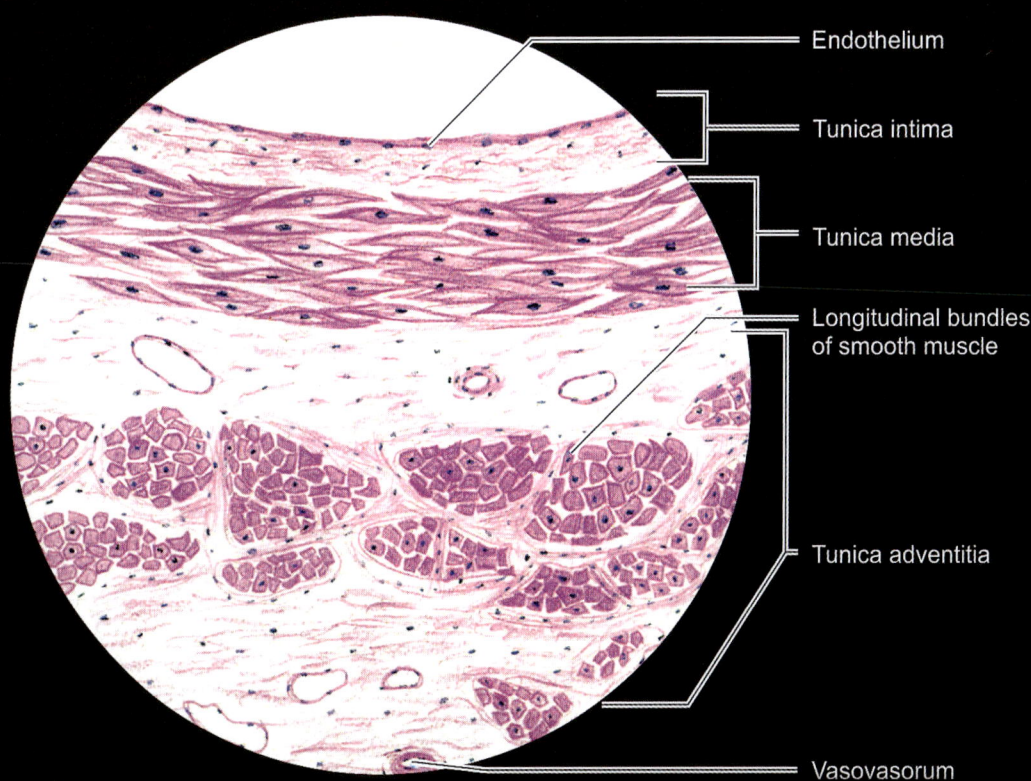

MEDIUM-SIZED VEIN

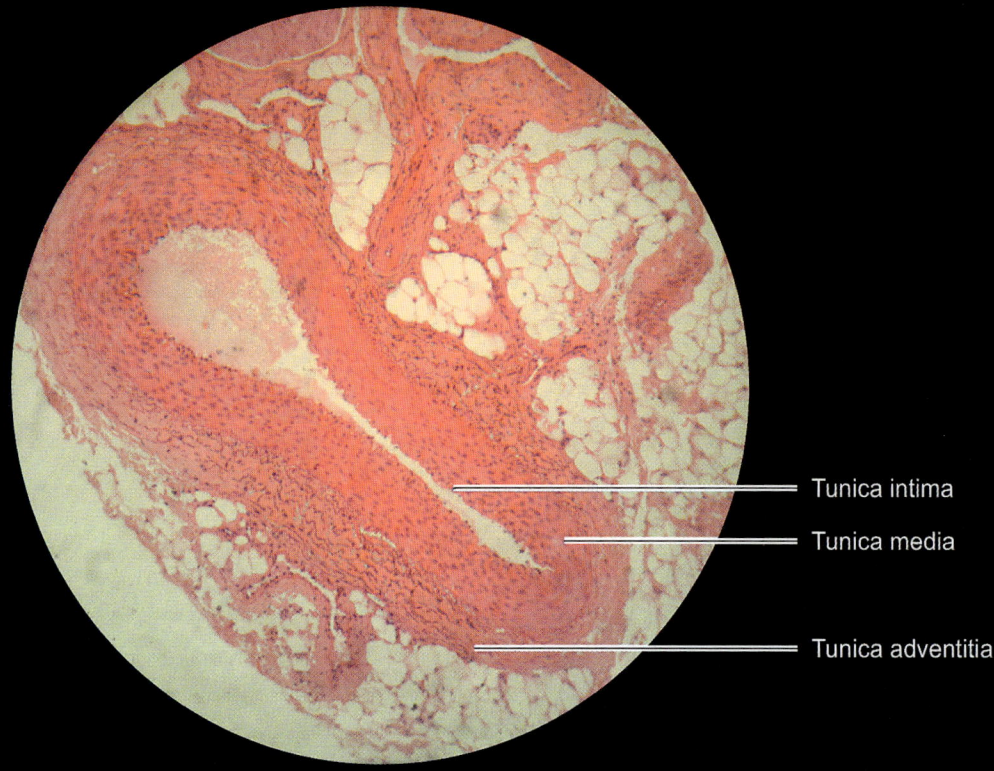

SP:
- Presence of three layers: Tunica intima, tunica media and tunica adventitia.
- Thin tunica intima with collapsed lumen.

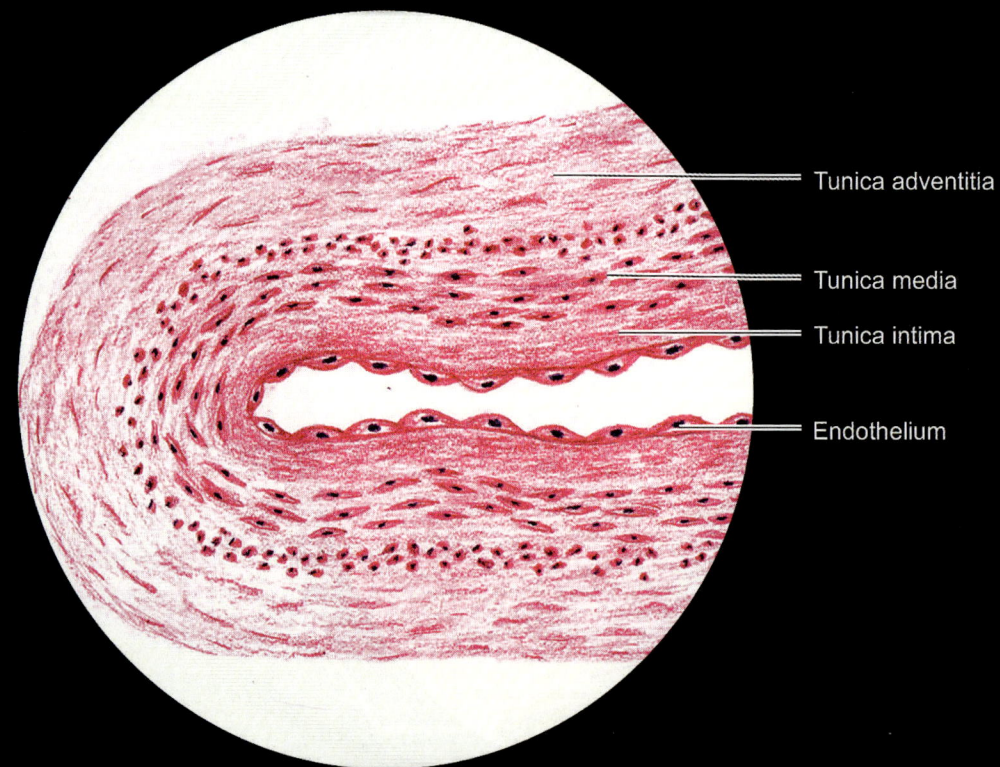

MEDIUM-SIZED VEIN

- It is made up of three layers.
- Tunica intima, tunica media, tunica adventitia.
- Internal and external elastic lamina is **poorly defined**.
- **Tunica media** consists of a few smooth muscle fibers and elastic fibers, in collagen fibers.
- **Tunica adventitia** consists of loose connective tissue.
- **Vasovasorum** and nerve fibers are also present in this layer.
- **Lumen** is collapsed.
- Examples: **Saphenous vein, median cubital vein, cephalic vein.**

Applied Anatomy

- Endothelial cells and the basal lamina can act as selective filters between the blood and the tissue surrounding the blood vessel.
- Venous insufficiency is one of the most common disorders of the venous system, and is usually manifested as spider veins or varicose veins.
- Deepvein thrombosis is a condition in which a blood clot forms in a deep vein, which can lead to pulmonary embolism.
- Valves are present in veins to prevent the backflow of blood. But in cases of large veins like superior vena cava and inferior vena cava, the valves are absent.
- Communicating veins (or perforator veins) are veins that directly connect superficial veins to deep veins which are usually medium-sized veins.
- In neurogenic and hypovolemic shock the smooth muscles surrounding the veins become slack and the veins are filled with the majority of the blood in the body, keeping blood away from the brain and causing unconsciousness.
- Inflammation of a vein is known as phlebitis.

Viva voce

Q. Are there medium-sized veins without valves? If so, name any one vein.
Ans. Yes, emissary veins present in the head and neck region and the besian veins within the myocardium of heart.
Q. How will you distinguish a medium sized artery and vein of same size lying close to each other?
Ans. The medium-sized vein on compression will collapse easily due to less number of smooth muscle fibers, but a medium-sized artery due to its thick muscle coat is difficult to compress.

LYMPHORETICULAR SYSTEM

LYMPH NODE

- It is an oval shaped discrete structure.
- Consist of capsule, outer cortex, inner/paracortex and medulla.
- **Capsule** consist of connective tissue with arterioles, venules and afferent lymphatic vessels. It is separated from cortex by **subcapsular sinus or marginal sinus** to which the afferent lymph vessels empty its contents. Capsule sends numerous **trabeculae** to the substance of the node.
- **Cortex** is made predominantly with lymphocytes. Plasma cells and macrophages are also present.
- For convenience, the cortex is divided into the outer cortex which lies underneath the capsule, and inner/paracortex which lies underneath the outer cortex and surrounds the medulla.
- In the **outer cortex**, the B lymphocytes are arranged as spherical **lymphoid nodules**. The centers of such nodules are often lighter and work as sites of B lymphocyte proliferation known as **germinal centers**. The darker zone surrounding the germinal center, which is made up of smaller mature B lymphocytes is known as the **mantle zone**. Outer cortex is incompletely separated by trabeculae.
- The **inner/paracortex** usually doesn't have lymphoid nodules and predominantly consists of T lymphocytes.
- The **medulla** is the central part of the lymph node and is lighter.
- It consists of medullary cords (anastomosing cords of lymphatic tissues with plasma cells, macrophages and lymphocytes) and **medullary sinus** (capillary channels that drain lymph through different lymph vessels).

Applied Anatomy

- In chronic lymphocytic lymphoma the lymph node architecture is diffusely effaced by tumor cells.
- Lymph node is a site of antigenic recognition and antigenic activation.
- Lymphocytes are relatively small in the medullary sinus than in lymphatic nodules helping to distinguish each other.
- From the primary cancer sites, cancer cells metastases through the lymphatics and get lodged at the lymph nodes draining the corresponding primary site.

Viva voce

Q. What are medullary cords?
Ans. These are anastomosing cords of lymphatic tissues present in the medulla.

LYMPH NODE

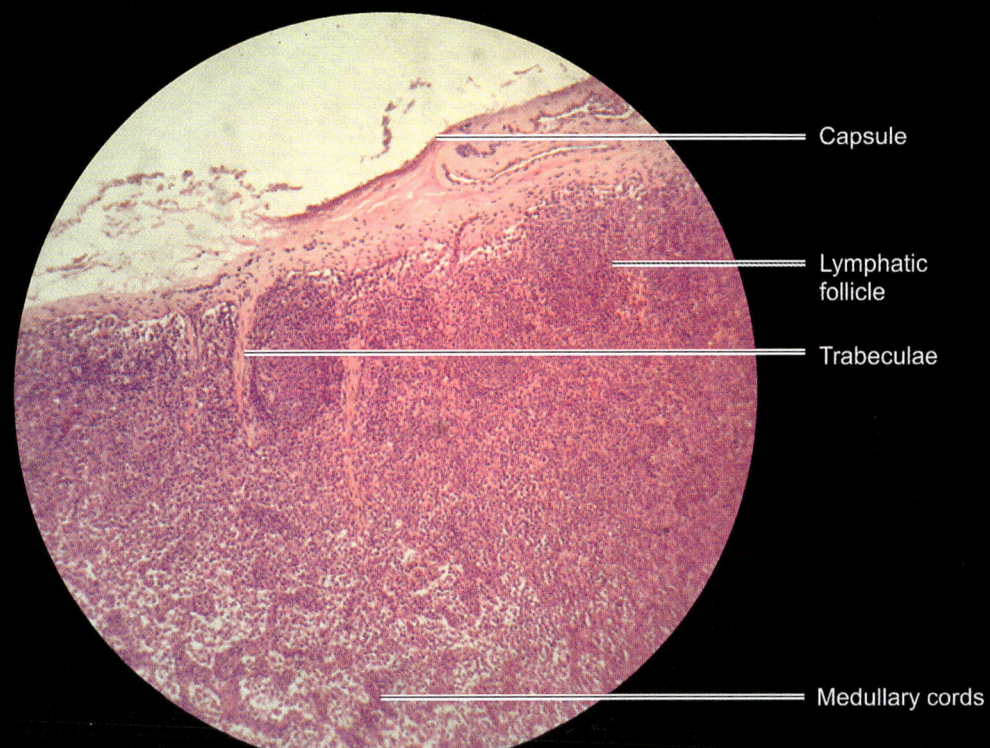

SP:
- Presence of lymphatic nodules in cortex.
- Presence of medullary cords and sinuses in the medulla.

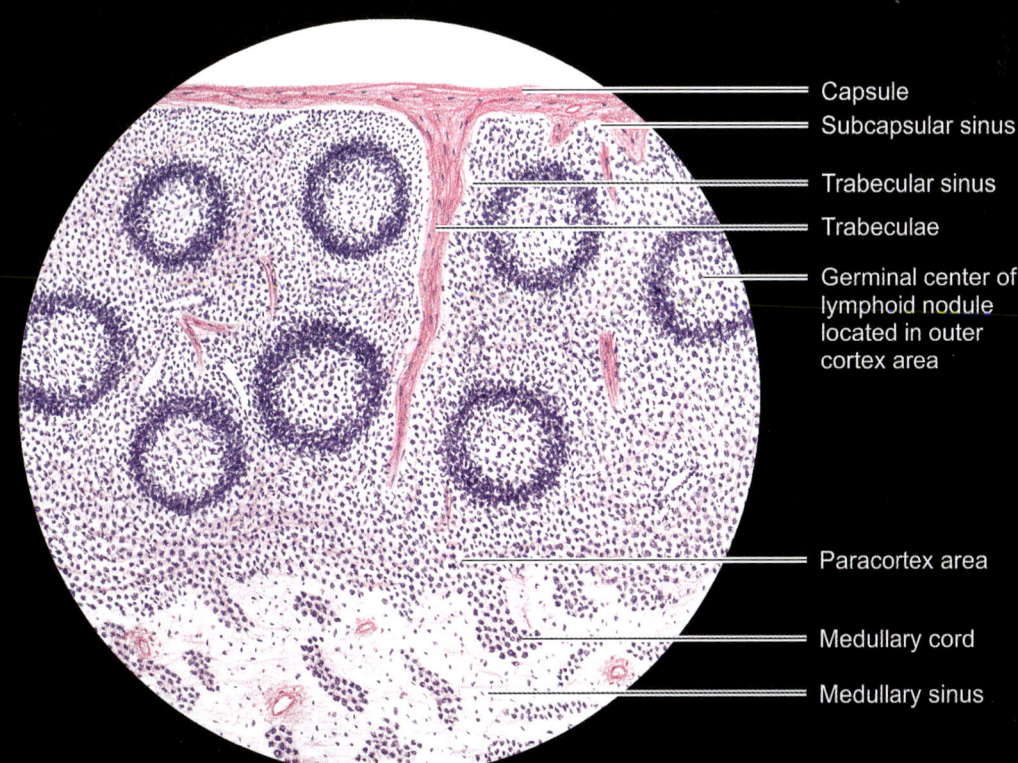

PALATINE TONSIL

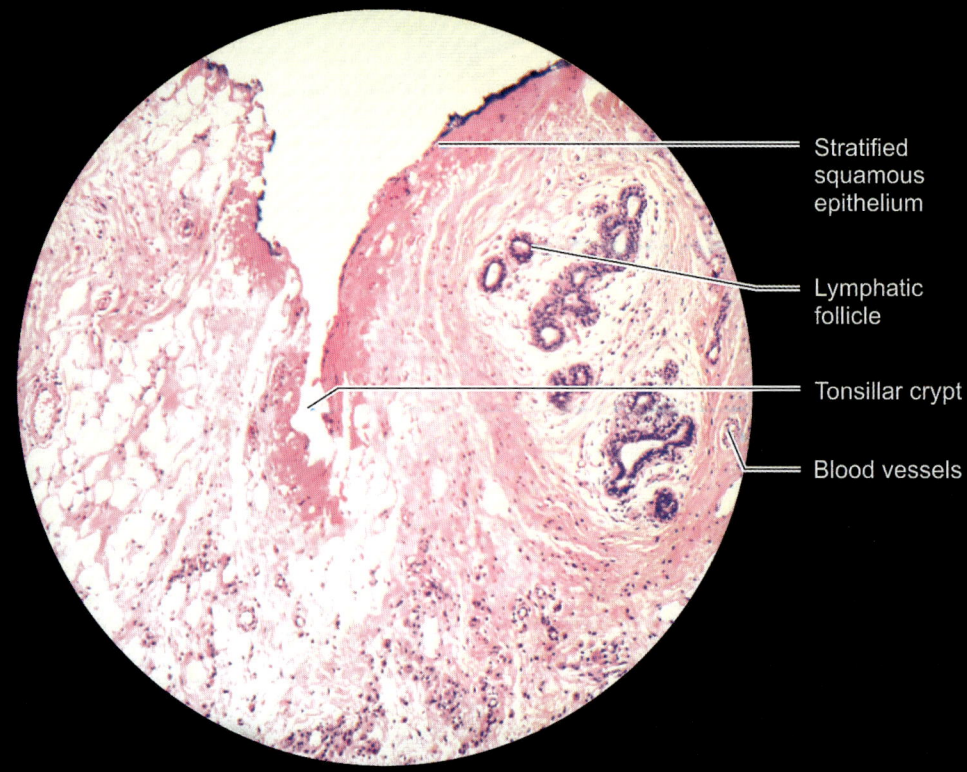

SP:
- Presence of crypts.
- Presence of subepithelial lymphoid nodule.

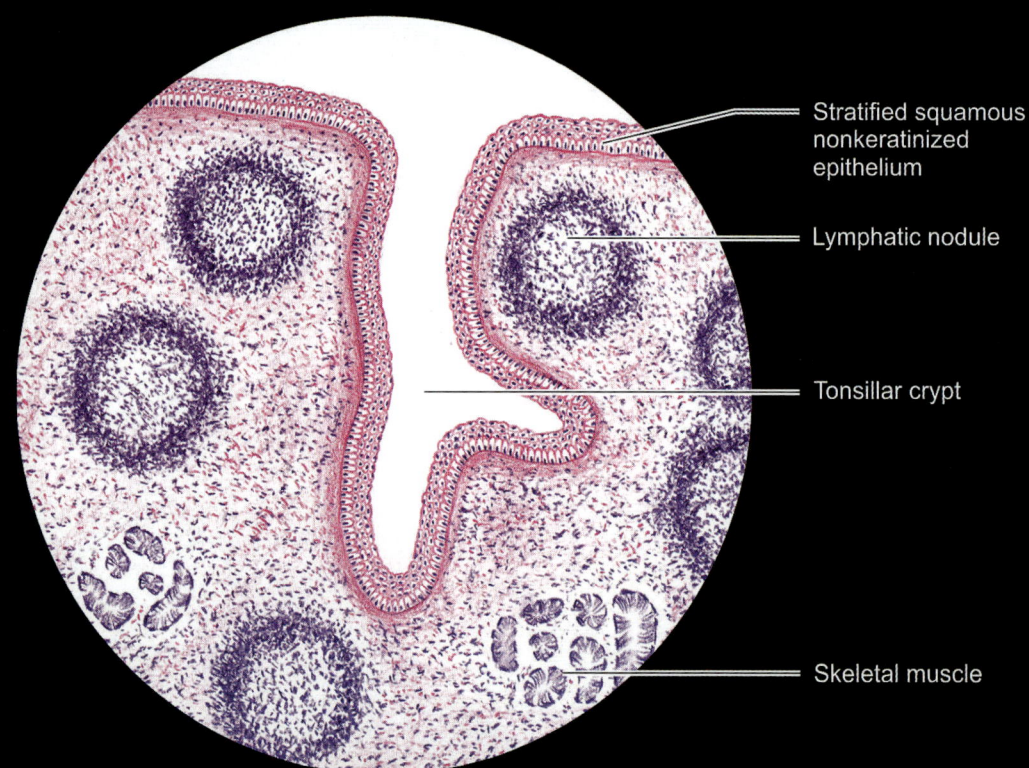

PALATINE TONSIL

- It is a part of the lymphoid tissue located in the lateral wall of pharynx.
- Palatine tonsil has medial and lateral surfaces. The **medial surface** is protected by the continuation of oral mucosa and the **lateral surface** by hemicapsule.
- The mucosa is of **stratified squamous nonkeratinized epithelium** and is invaginated by deep grooves called **crypts**. The tonsillar crypts usually contain the dead antigen, broken debris, disarmed bacteria, etc.
- Below the epithelium, numerous lymphatic nodules are distributed and they merge frequently with each other and exhibits lighter staining **germinal centers**.
- A dense connective tissue underlies the tonsil and forms its **capsule** consisting of some blood vessels.

Applied Anatomy
- In case of secondary infections, the tonsil is one the lymphoid organ where inflammation is distinctly visible.
- Mouth of crypts appear as purulent spots in tonsillitis due to infection and pus formation.

Viva voce
Q. What kind of epithelium lines the tonsil?
Ans. Tonsil is lined by stratified squamous nonkeratinized epithelium.
Q. What are crypts?
Ans. The surface of the tonsil is invaginated by deep grooves. These grooves are known as tonsillar crypts.
Q. What does tonsillar crypts contain?
Ans. The tonsilar crypts usually consist of dead antigen, broken debris, disarmed bacteria, etc.
Q. What does the germinal center contain?
Ans. Germinal center consist of new and mature lymphocytes. The former is present in the inner aspect and the latter is present in the outer aspect of the germinal center.

SPLEEN

- It is the largest lymphoid organ in the body.
- Consists of a **dense connective tissue capsule** from which **trabeculae** arise and contains **trabecular arteries** and **veins**.
- Does not exhibit cortex and medulla, instead it has **white pulp** and **red pulp**.
- Like other lymphoid organs, the spleen also has a network of reticular fibers to provide structural support to the cells of lymphoid tissue.
- **Splenic parenchyma** has sheaths of lymphoid tissue surrounding the central arteries called **periarterial lymphatic sheaths (PALS)**. PALS is the thymus-dependent zone of the spleen because it mainly contains T lymphocytes. But at some places, PALS expands and forms lymphoid nodules called **splenic nodules or Malpighian corpuscles**. In these splenic nodules, the central artery is peripherally located. T cells and B cells are present within the nodules. These PALS and splenic nodules together form the **white pulp**. White pulp is the site of immune response to blood borne antigens.
- **Red pulp** is formed by the diffuse cellular meshwork around the white pulp and acts as a single unit. It contains **venous sinuses** and **splenic cords (cords of Billroth)**. Spleen consists of venous sinuses in contrast to the lymphatic sinuses in lymph nodes. Splenic cords contain macrophages, lymphocytes, plasma cells and different blood cells.

Applied Anatomy

- In spleen lymphatic nodules are found throughout the structure.
- Spleen does not exhibit subcapsular or subtrabecular sinuses.
- The capsule and trabeculae in the spleen are thicker than those in the lymph node.
- In conditions like liver cirrhosis, back pressure develops in the veins and leads to congestive splenomegaly.

Viva voce

Q. Where do the blood vessels directly open in the spleen?
Ans. The blood vessels open into the red pulp giving the characteristic red color.
Q. What are the contents of splenic cords?
Ans. Splenic cords consist of macrophages, lymphocytes, plasma cells and different blood cells.
Q. What are splenic pulps?
Ans. Splenic pulps are the different compartments of the spleen formed by the passage of a capsule into the organ.

SPLEEN

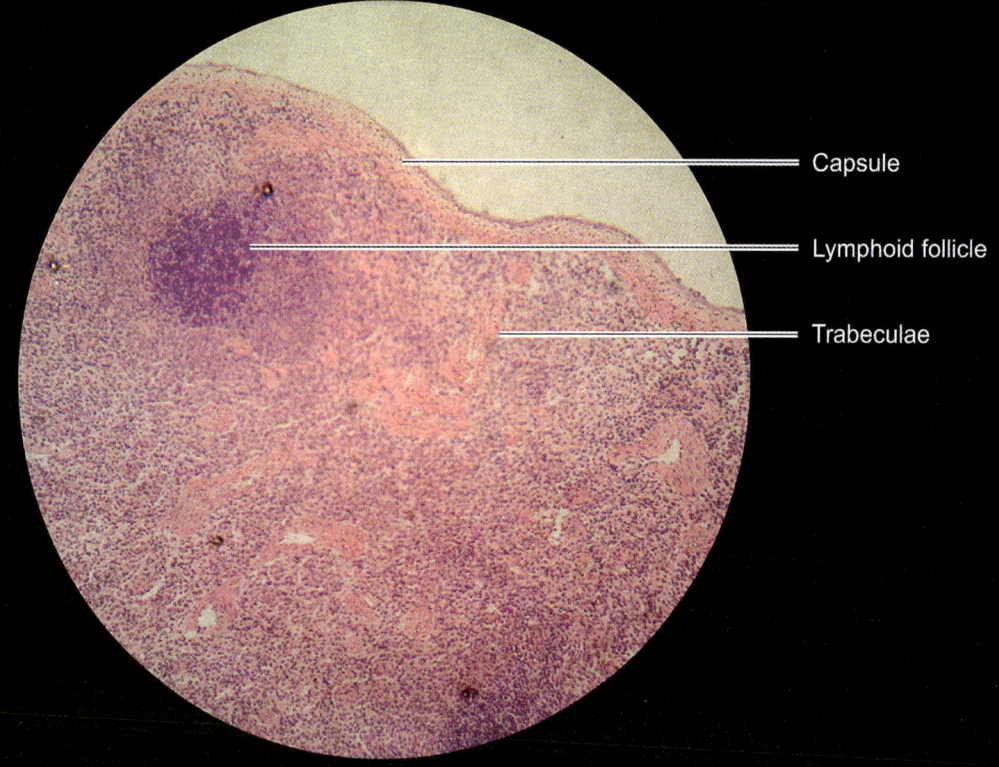

SP:
- Presence of thick capsule and trabeculae.
- Red pulp containing splenic cords and sinusoids and white pulp present.

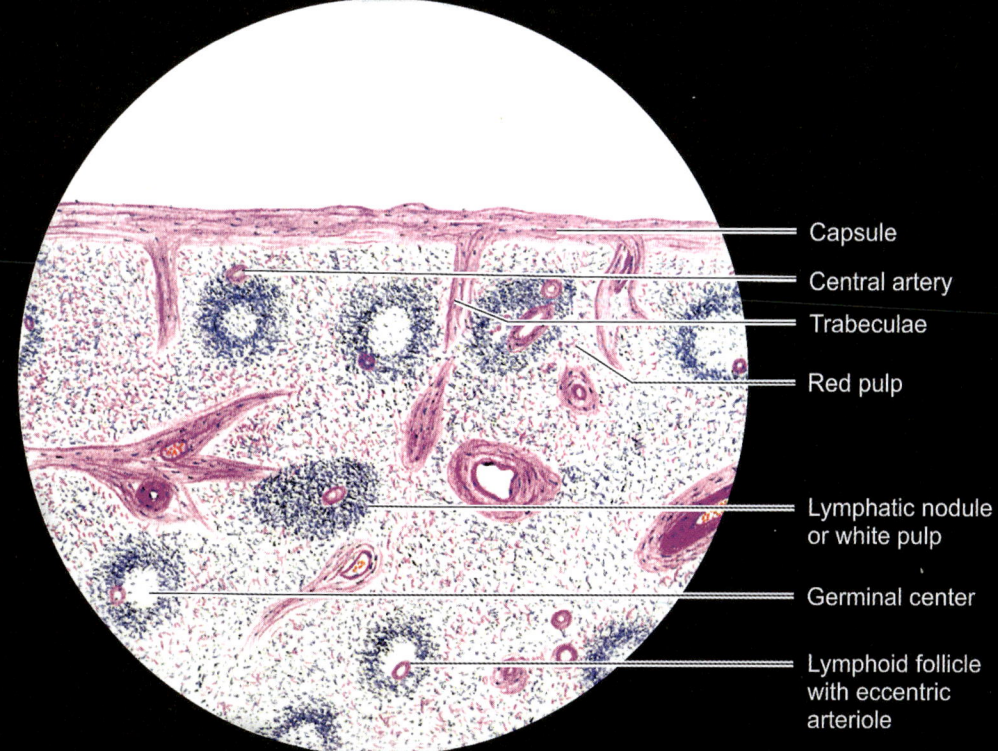

THYMUS

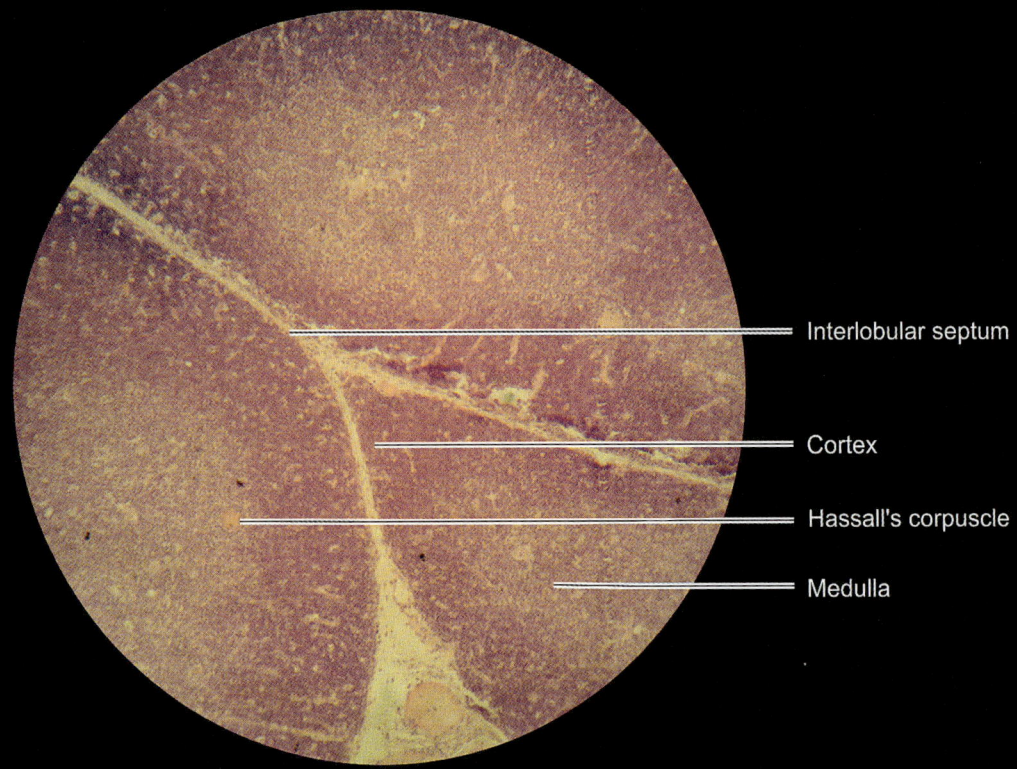

SP:
- Presence of lobules with lymphoid tissue.
- Presence of Hassall's corpuscles in the medulla.

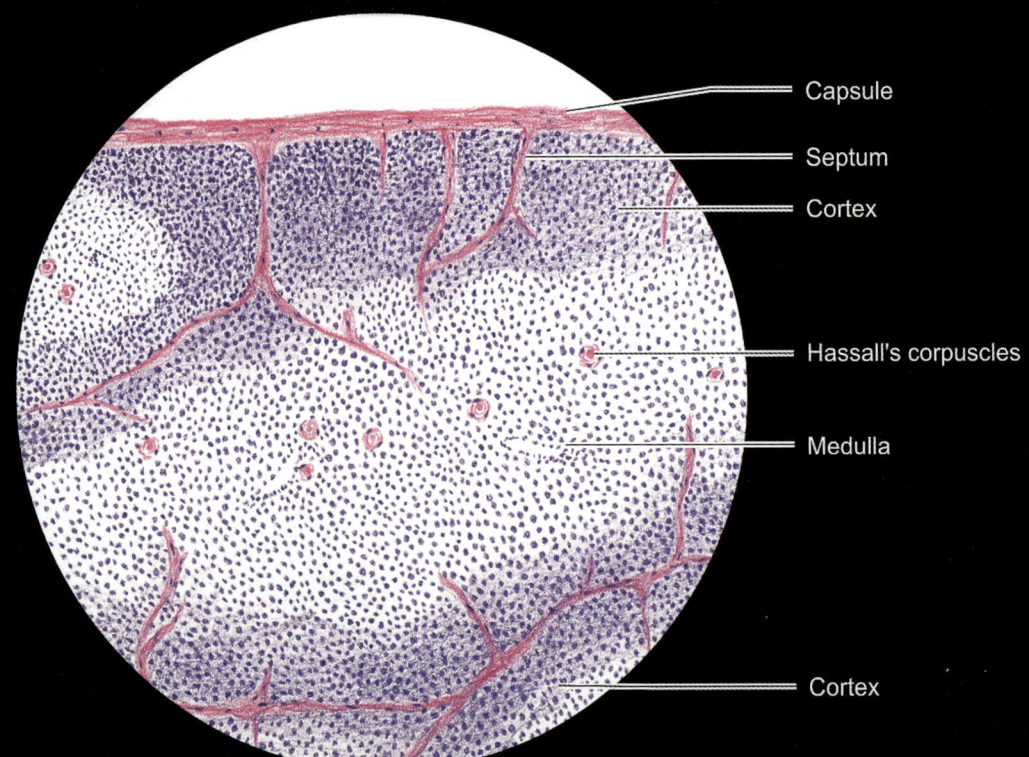

Histology

THYMUS

- Thymus is an important site for T lymphocyte maturation and starts to degenerate as age of a person advances.
- **Lobes** of the thymus gland are covered with coonective tissue capsule.
- **Trabeculae** arise from this capsule and extend into the interior, dividing the gland into numerous incomplete **lobules**. Through this trabeculae, blood vessels pass to the gland.
- Each lobule consists of **dark staining outer cortex** and **lighter staining inner medulla.**
- **Cortex** consists of densely packed lymphocytes, hence look darker.
- **Medulla** contains few lymphocytes, more epithelial reticular cells and appears lighter.
- These epithelial reticular cells form **Hassall's corpuscle or thymic corpuscle.**
- Hassall's corpuscles are oval structures consisting of aggregations or whorls of flattened epithelial cells which later undergo degeneration.
- Since the trabeculae are incomplete, the medulla of each lobule is continuous with the medulla of the adjacent lobules.
- Lymphocytes proliferate in the cortex and migrate to medulla. Later, they enter the systemic circulation and reach the various lymphoid organs.

Applied Anatomy

- In thymic follicular hyperplasia, there is the appearance of numerous B cell germinal centers within the thymus. Usually this is seen in myasthenia gravis and rheumatoid arthritis.
- Di George syndrome is a congenital disease that occurs due to the absence of thymus, as a result T lymphocytes are reduced and there is abnormal cell-mediated immunity.

Viva voce

Q. What are Hassall's corpuscles?
Ans. These are whorls or aggregations of flattened epithelial reticular cells which later undergo degeneration.
Q. Why is there a medullary continuity?
Ans. Since the lobules are incompletely separated there is medullary continuity between the adjacent lobules.
Q. How do blood vessels and other lymphatic vessels enter the organ?
Ans. The blood vessels and lymphatics enter the capsule and then pass through the trabeculae to enter the thymus.

NERVOUS TISSUE

- The nervous system regulates and controls bodily functions and activities.
- It has two parts: the **central nervous system(CNS)** (brain and spinal cord) and the **peripheral nervous system (PNS).**
- The nervous tissue basically has two types of cells: (1) Neurons which transmit impulses. (2) Glial cells which are supporting cells.

NERVE FIBER

- An **axon** or **nerve fiber** carries electrical impulse away from the nerve cell body to different sites.
- Nerve fiber can be myelinated or nonmeylinated.
- **Myelin sheath** is formed by **glial cells**. In the CNS, they are called **oligodendrocytes** and in the PNS, these glial cells are called **Schwann cells**.
- In histology, the nerve fiber consists of a **central axon** appearing as a slender thread which stains lightly, surrounded by myelin sheath.
- Myelin sheath is not continuous throughout the length of the axon, forming interruption called **nodes of Ranvier** and occurs between adjacent Schwann cells.
- At the node of Ranvier, the Schwann cell membrane is seen as a thin peripheral boundary that descends towards the axon.
- Around some of the axons a **connective tissue layer** is also present.
- A possible Schwann cell nucleus and a fibrocyte is usually associated with it.
- Outside the axons a capillary with blood cells is also found.
- Nodes of Ranvier are responsible for **saltatory conduction** in large myelinated neurons resulting in more efficient and faster conduction.
- Usually the surrounding myelin sheath will be dissolved by chemicals during preparation and are seen as empty spaces.

Applied Anatomy

- Inflammation of the nerve is known as neuritis.
- Neuropathy is damage or disease of nerves which may affect sensation, movement, gland or organ function or other health aspects depending on the nerve involved.
- Neuropraxia is a temporary interruption or physiological block of conduction without loss of axon continuity.
- Axonotmesis is the loss of relative continuity of the axon and its myelin, but connective tissue framework is preserved.
- Neurotmesis is the total destruction of the entire nerve fiber.

Viva voce

Q. What are the nodes of Ranvier?
Ans. These are interruptions or discontinuities in the myelin sheath surrounding the axon.
Q. Which structure helps to maintain the appropriate microenvironment for peripheral nerve fibers?
Ans. Perineurium.
Q. Which cell type forms the myelin sheath around myelinated axons in the central nervous system?
Ans. Oligodendrocyte.

NERVE FIBER

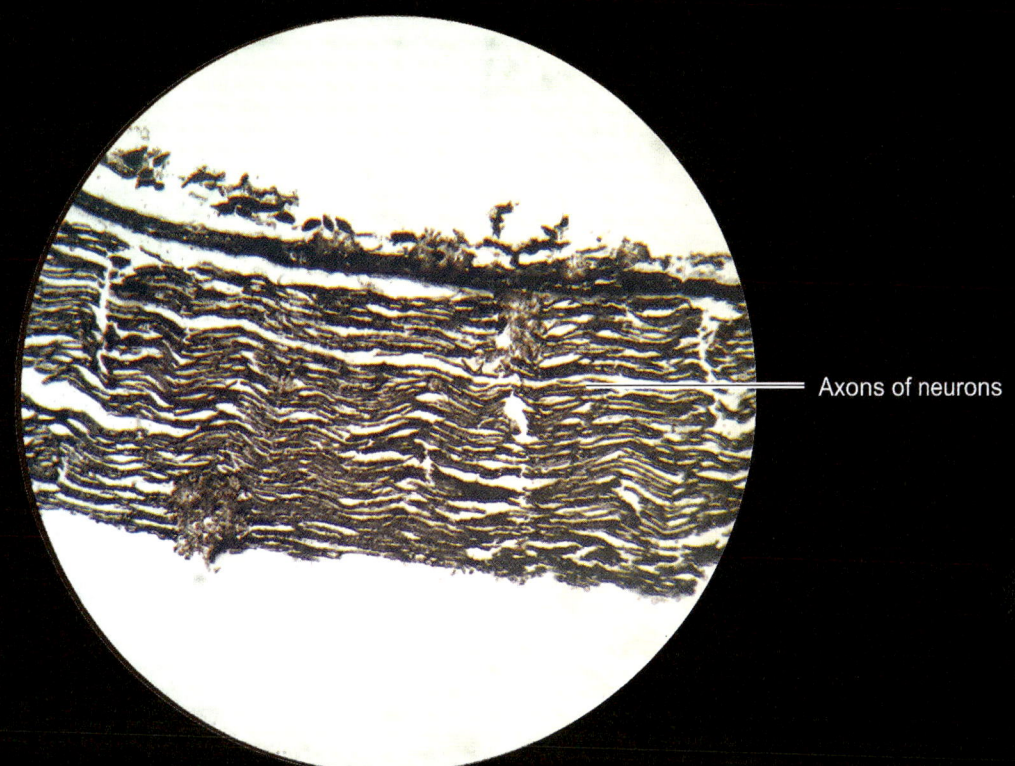

SP:
- Axon cylinder seen at the center.
- Nodes of Ranvier present.

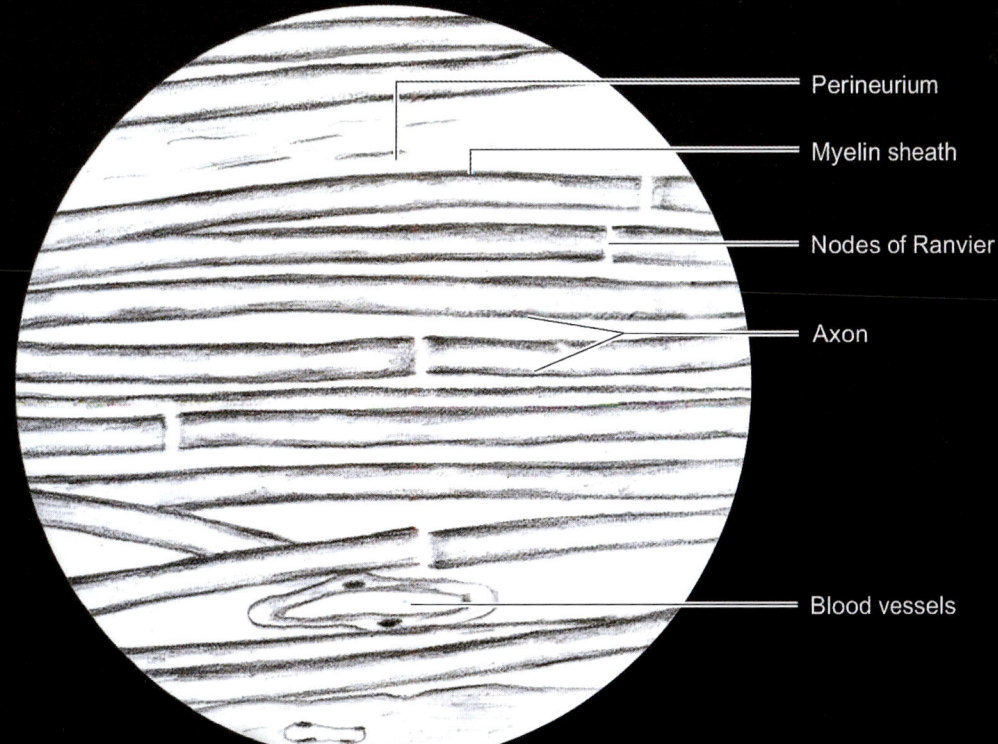

SPINAL GANGLION

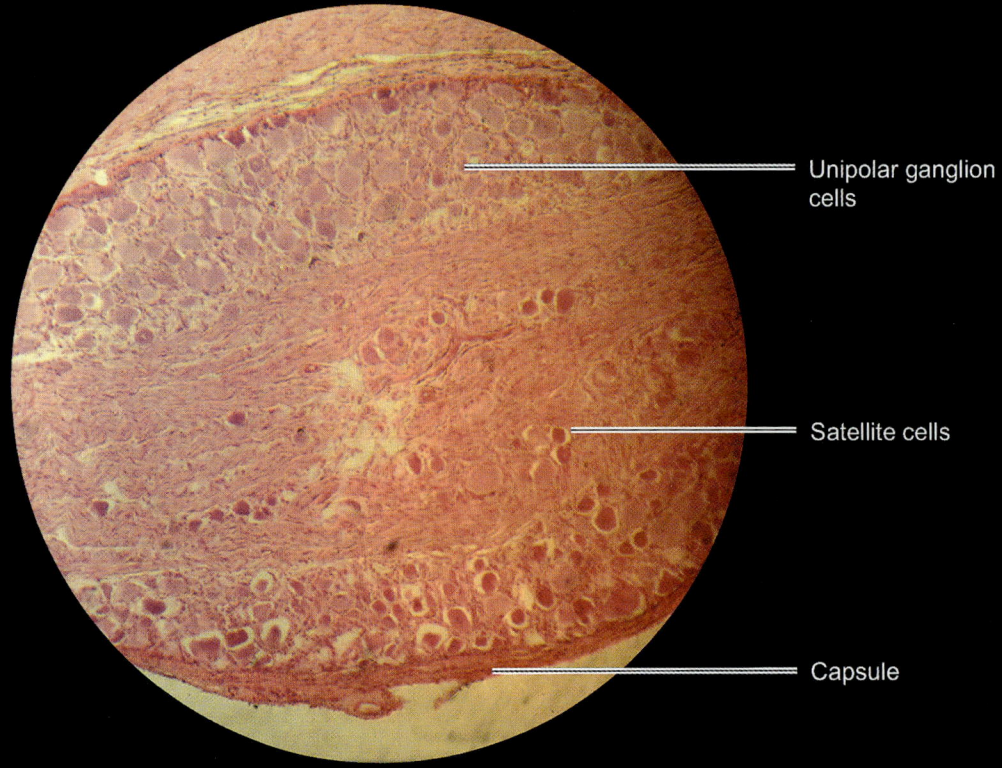

- Unipolar ganglion cells
- Satellite cells
- Capsule

SP:
- Presence of round pseudounipolar neurons in groups.
- Presence of nerve fibers in the form of bundles in between ganglion cells.

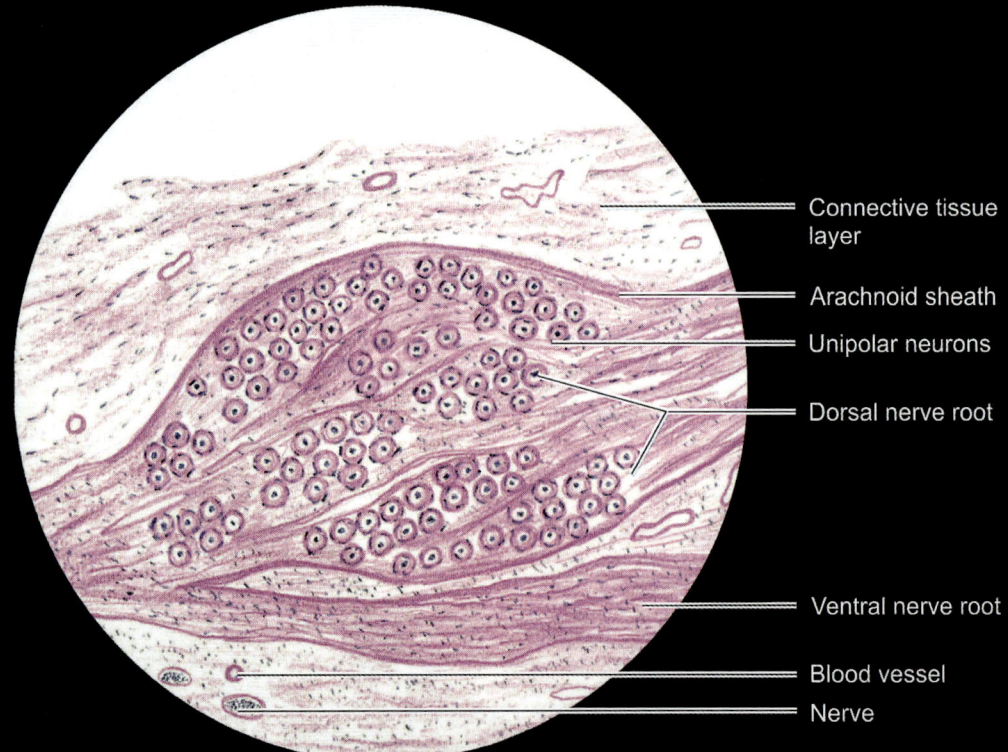

- Connective tissue layer
- Arachnoid sheath
- Unipolar neurons
- Dorsal nerve root
- Ventral nerve root
- Blood vessel
- Nerve

SPINAL GANGLION

- Each ganglion is enclosed by an irregular **connective tissue** layer that contains **adipose cells, nerves** and **blood vessels**.
- Consists of mainly numerous round **pseudounipolar neurons** in groups with **central nucleus**.
- Numerous **fascicles** of nerve fibers pass between the neurons. These nerve fibers represent the nerve process formed by bifurcation of a single axon.
- Regularly arranged nerve fibers enter and leave the ganglion.
- Contain well-defined **satellite cells** which are small flat cells that surround the neurons of the ganglia of the peripheral nervous system and provide structural support for **neuronal bodies**, insulate them and regulate exchange of different metabolic substances.
- They are enclosed in a well-defined **connective tissue capsule** and capsular cells.

Applied Anatomy

- Develops from the neural crest cells and not from the neural tube.
- The nerve endings of dorsal root ganglion neurons have a variety of sensory receptors that are activated by mechanical, thermal, chemical, and noxious stimuli.
- Unlike the majority of neurons found in the central nervous system, an action potential in dorsal root ganglion neuron may initiate in the distal process in the periphery, bypass the cell body, and continue to propagate along the proximal process until reaching the synaptic terminal in the dorsal horn of the spinal cord.

Viva voce

Q. What kind of neurons are mainly present in spinal ganglion?
Ans. Pseudounipolar neurons.
Q. What are the supportive cells present in spinal ganglion?
Ans. Satellite cells which are small flat cells that surround the neurons of ganglia.
Q. Does spinal ganglion have a capsule?
Ans. Yes, spinal ganglion consists of a well-defined connective tissue capsule.

SYMPATHETIC GANGLION

- Neurons are **multipolar** and more uniform in size due to which their outlines and their dendritic process appear irregular.
- Neurons contain **eccentric nuclei** and may be **binucleate** and in older individuals a brownish lipofuscin pigment accumulates in cytoplasm.
- **Satellite cells** surround multipolar neurons but are less in number compared to spinal ganglion and the **connective tissue capsule** and cells are not well-defined around the neurons but fibrocytes and venules are usually present.
- Nerve fibers are not arranged in groups and the nerve fibers are seen irregularly or scattered.
- The flattened nuclei on the periphery are the **Schwann cells**.
- These nerve fibers represent both preganglionic and postganglionic axons.

Applied Anatomy

- Responsible for fight or flight response in stress and in impending danger.
- Neuroblastoma tumor arises from the sympathetic ganglial tissue.
- If the sympathetic nervous system takes control for long durations, it may release the cortisol hormone instead of the adrenaline, which can harm the brain and can cause anxiety, mood swings, hypertension and palpitation of the heart.

Viva voce

Q. What kind of neurons are mainly present in sympathetic ganglion?
Ans. Multipolar neurons.
Q. What are the suppportive cells present in sympathetic ganglion?
Ans. Satellite cells which are small flat cells that surround the neurons of ganglia and fibrocytes.
Q. Does spinal ganglion have a capsule?
Ans. Yes, spinal ganglion consists of a connective tissue capsule which is not so well-defined when compared to that of the spinal ganglion.

SYMPATHETIC GANGLION

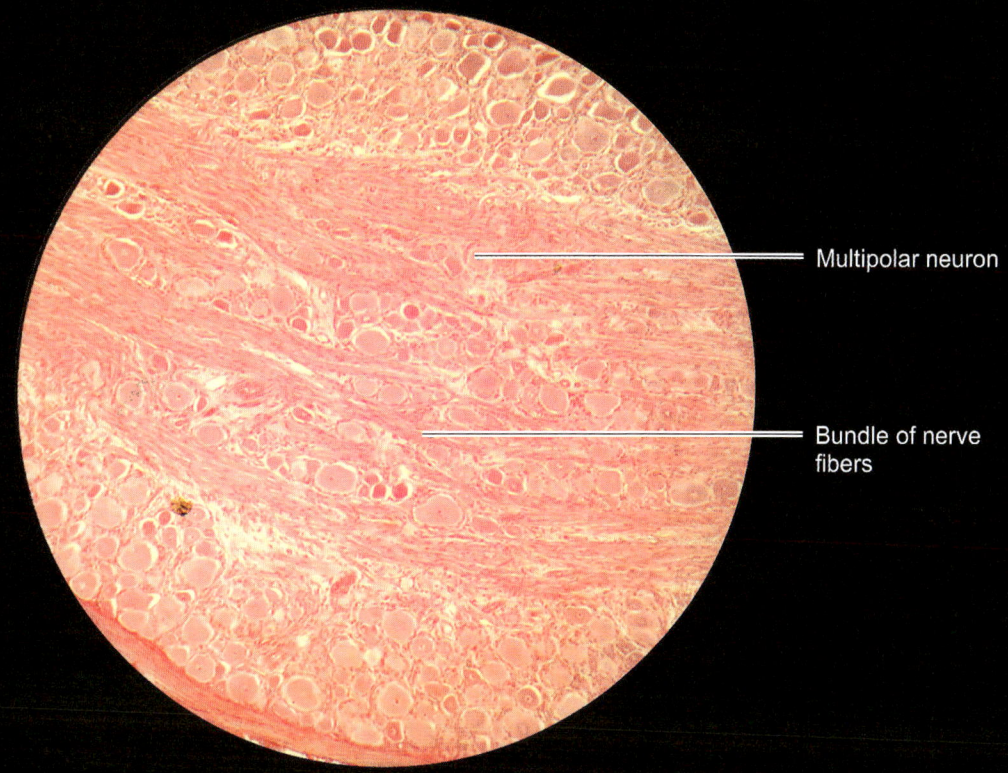

- Multipolar neuron
- Bundle of nerve fibers

SP:
- Presence of small and scattered multipolar neurons with eccentric nucleus.
- Presence of satellite cells.

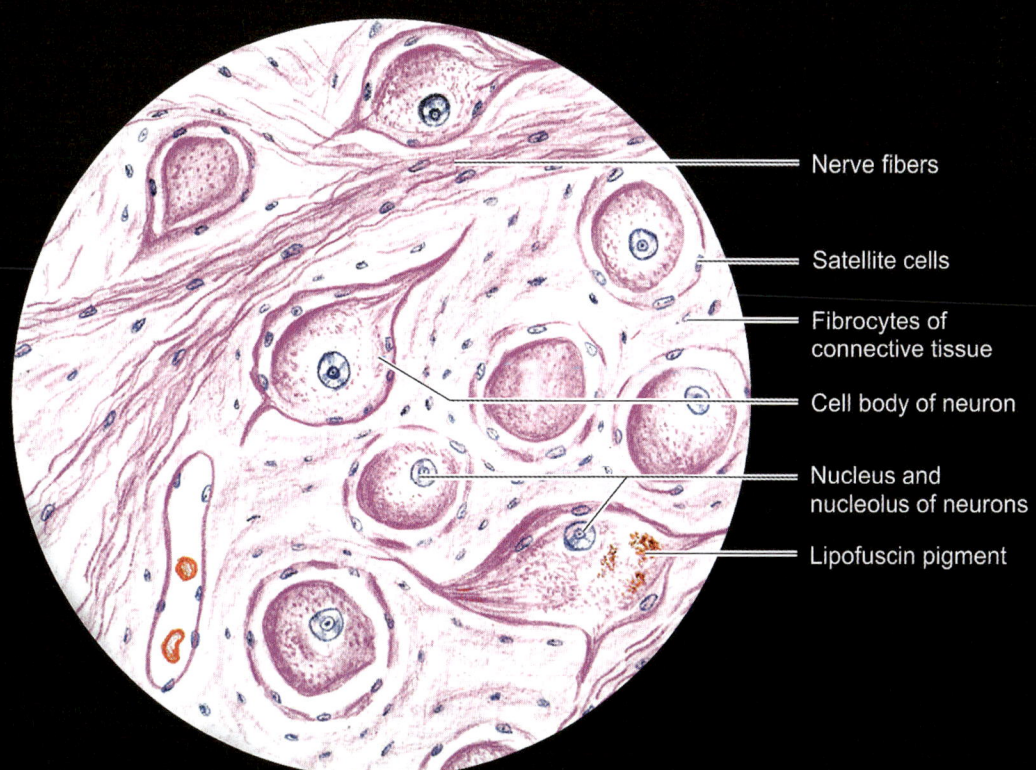

- Nerve fibers
- Satellite cells
- Fibrocytes of connective tissue
- Cell body of neuron
- Nucleus and nucleolus of neurons
- Lipofuscin pigment

SEROUS SALIVARY GLAND

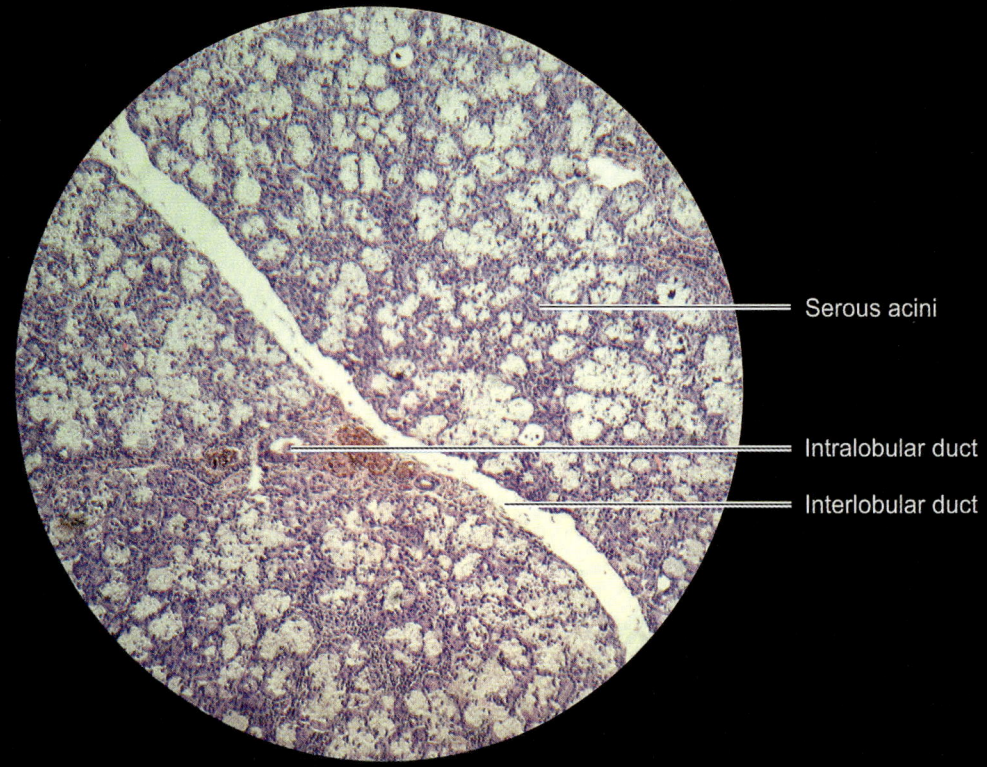

SP:
- Presence of serous acini with round basal nuclei and small lumen.
- Presence of lobar and interlobular ducts.

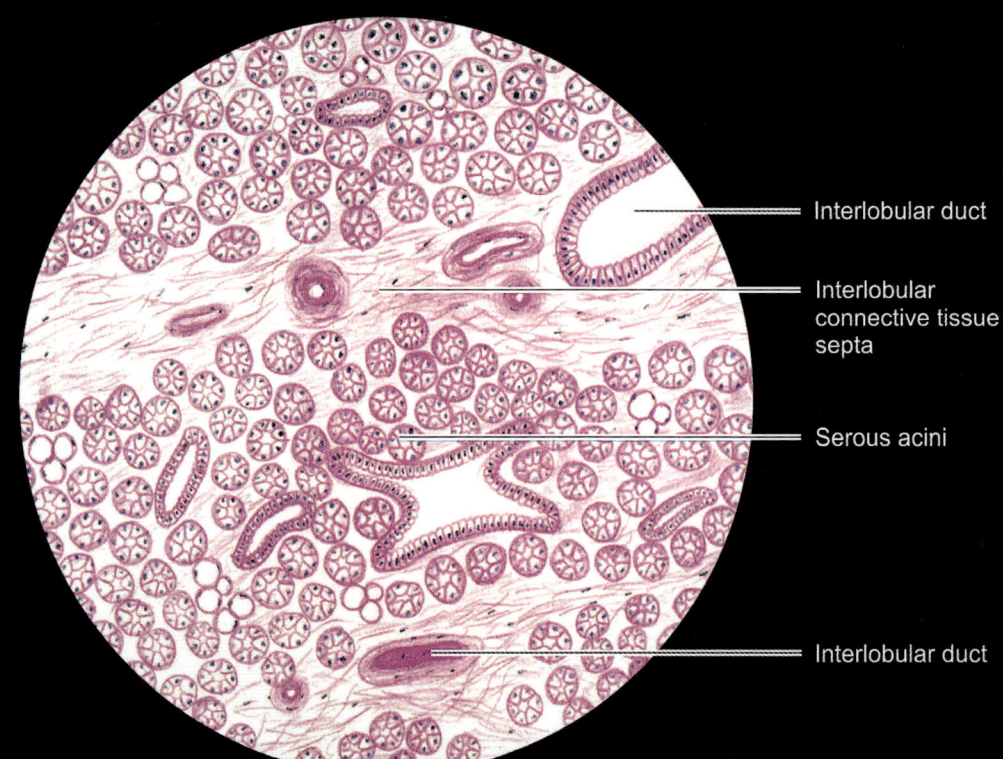

ORAL CAVITY

SEROUS SALIVARY GLAND

- Example: **Parotid gland**.
- The gland is surrounded by **dense connective tissue capsule** from which **septa** arise and subdivide gland into lobes and lobules.
- Each lobule consists of pyramidal shaped serous cells (secretory cells) with round basal nuclei that form the **serous acini**.
- Serous acini are surrounded by thin **contractile myoepithelial** cells.
- Small secretory granules are visible in the cell apices of serous cells (at high power).
- In between the lobules, in the connective tissue septa arterioles, venules, and **interlobular excretory ducts** are located.
- Some lobules may also contain numerous **adipose cells**.
- Secretory acini empty their product into the **intercalated ducts.** The secretory product from intercalated ducts drains into **striated ducts** and then to **intralobular ducts**.

Applied Anatomy

- Lymphoid infiltrates of the salivary glands is a common finding in varieties of pathologic conditions including autoimmune disorders, malignant lymphomas, and immunoregulatory responses to parenchymal neoplasms.
- Mumps affects the parotid gland.
- Adenoma is one of the benign epithelial tumor that affect the parotid gland.
- Sialadenitis is the inflammation of the salivary gland.
- A sialocele is a localized, subcutaneous cavity containing saliva. It is caused by trauma (e.g., surgical trauma) or infection. They are relatively common complication following surgery to the salivary glands, commonly the parotid gland.

Viva voce

Q. What is Frey syndrome?
Ans. After parotidectomy, at times there may be regeneration of secretomotor fibers of the auriculotemporal nerve which joins the great auricular nerve. This causes stimulation of sweat glands and hyperemia in the area of its distribution, thus producing redness and sweating in the area of skin supplied by the nerve.

MUCOUS SALIVARY GLAND

- Example: **Sublingual gland**.
- Predominantly, they have mucous acini. but very few serous acini are also present.
- **Mucous acini** are formed by mucous cells with flat, single, basally located nuclei. Their cytoplasm is filled with mucus.
- **Contractile myoepithelial cells** are seen around individual mucous acini.
- Arteriole, venule, nerve fibers and interlobular excretory ducts are seen in the septa.
- Oval shaped **adipose tissues** are found scattered in connective tissue of the gland.
- **Saliva** is produced after autonomic stimulation.

Applied Anatomy

- Salivary duct calculus may cause blockage of the ducts, causing pain and swelling of the gland because of cysts.
- Ranula is the name used when a mucocele occurs in the floor of the mouth (underneath the tongue) and may grow to a larger size than mucoceles at other sites, and they are usually associated with the sublingual gland.
- Sialadenosis (sialosis) is an uncommon, non-inflammatory, non-neoplastic, recurrent swelling of the salivary glands. The cause is hypothesized to be abnormalities of neurosecretory control and may be associated with alcoholism.

Viva voce

Q. What percentage of the total salivary volume does the sublingual gland contribute?
Ans. Only 10% of total salivary volume.
Q. From what structure does sublingual gland develop from?
Ans. They develop from epithelial buds in the sulcus surrounding the sublingual folds on the floor of the mouth, lateral to the developing submandibular gland.

MUCOUS SALIVARY GLAND

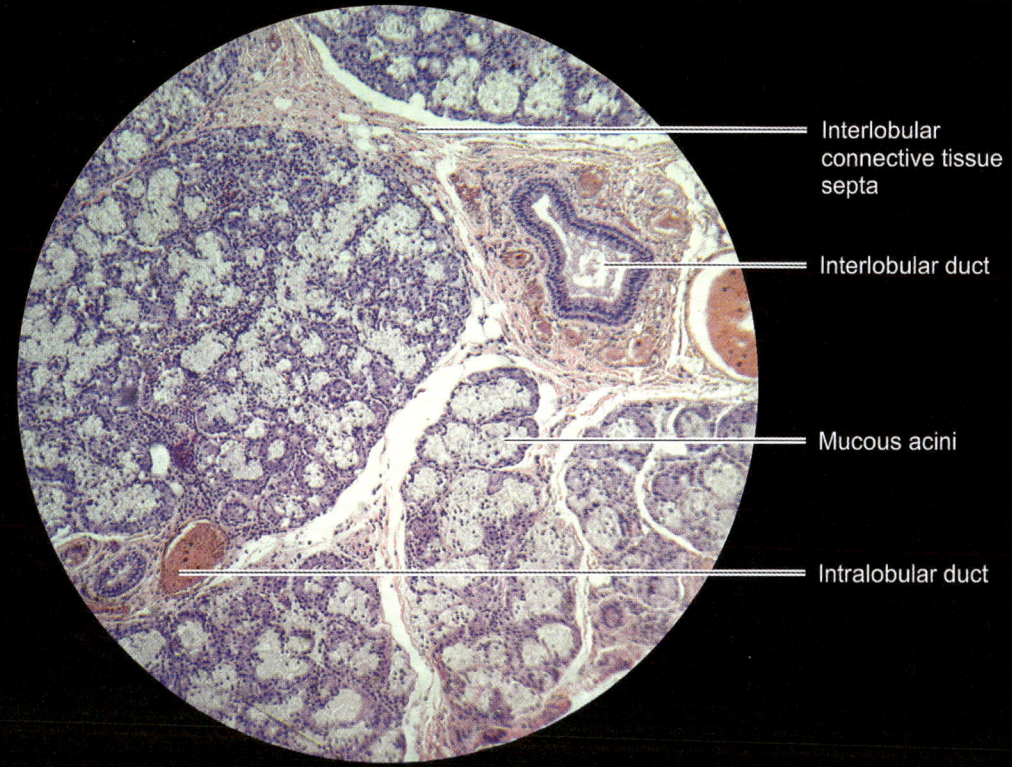

SP:
- Presence of mucous acini with flattened basal nucleus.
- Presence of interlobular and intralobular ducts.

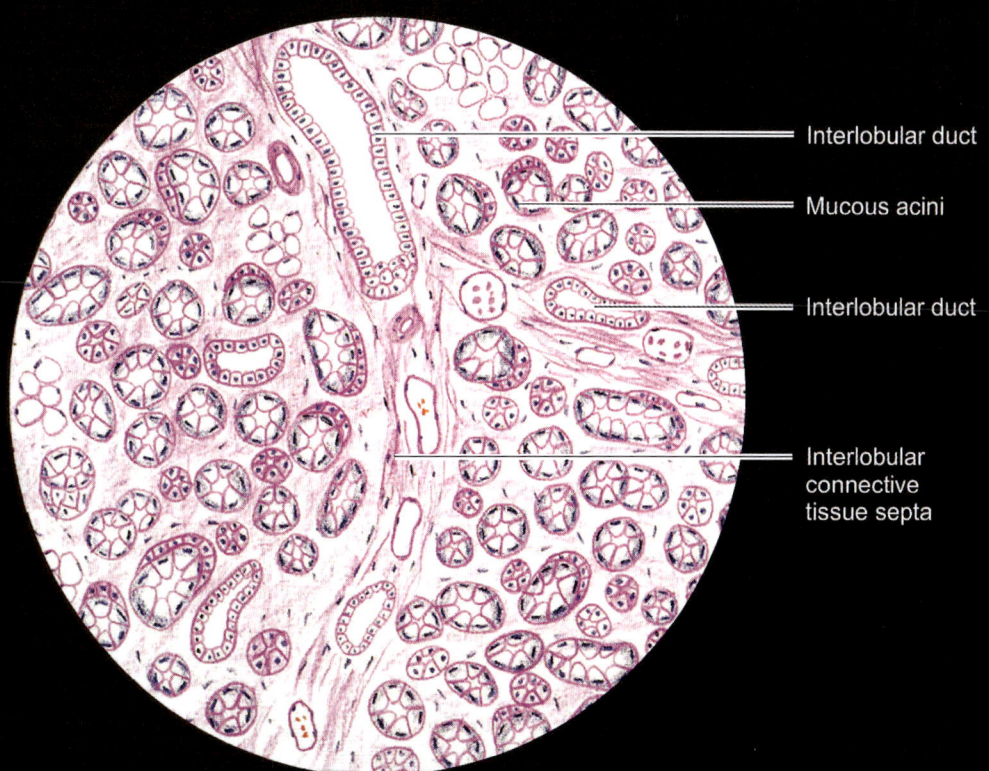

MIXED SALIVARY GLAND

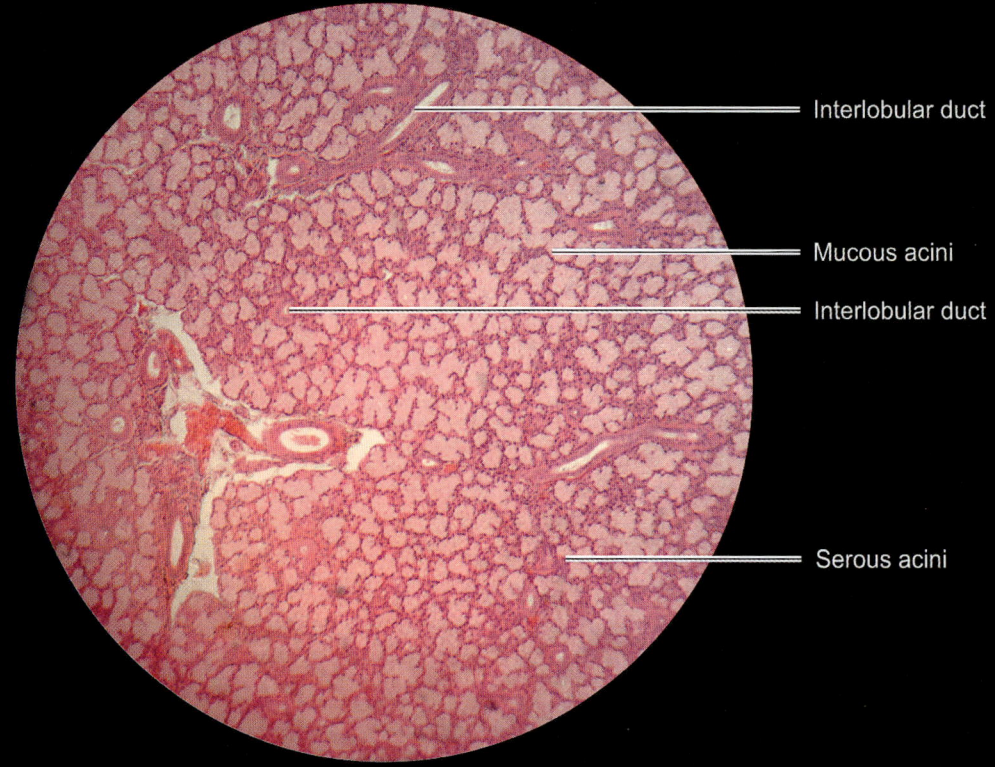

SP:
- Presence of mucous and serous acini with serous demilunes.
- Presence of lobar and interlobar ducts.

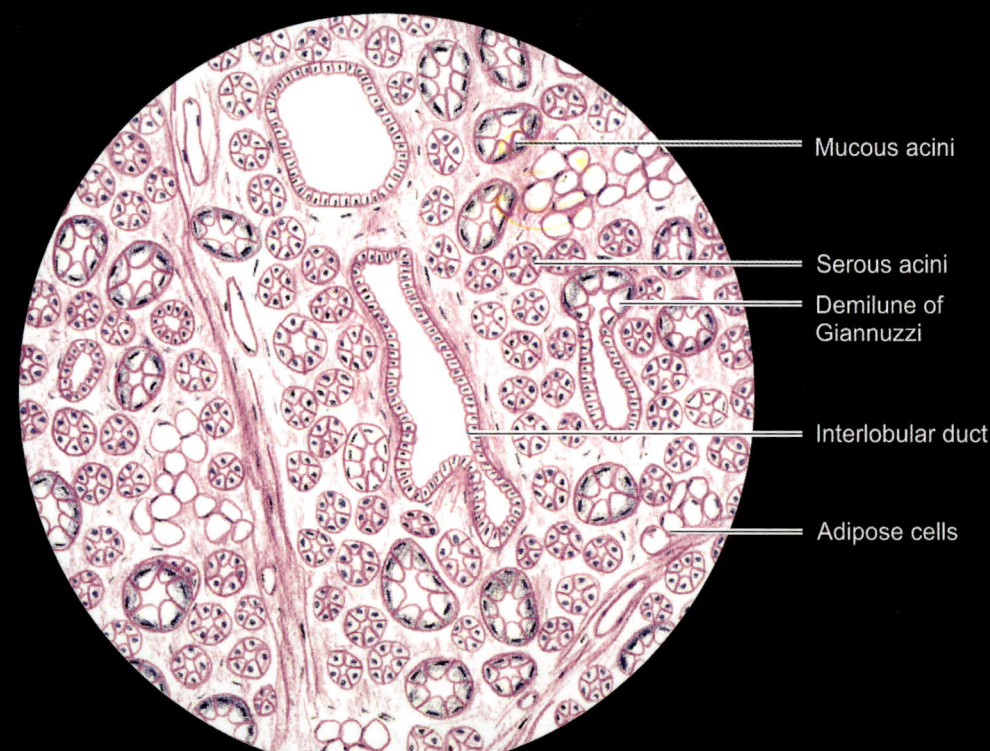

MIXED SALIVARY GLAND

- Example: **Submandibular gland**.
- It consists of both **serous** and **mucous acini** but mucous acini predominating.
- Serous cells form a crescent shaped cap over the mucous acini and are known as serous demilunes or demilunes of Giannuzzi.
- Both the serous and mucous acini are covered by the contractile myoepithelial cells along with **intercalated ducts**.
- **Interlobular connective tissue septa** divides the glands into lobules.
- Located in the connective tissue septa are nerves, arteriole, venule and adipose cells.
- The duct system of the submandibular gland is similar to that of the parotid gland.

Applied Anatomy

- Sialolithiasis is a condition where a calcified mass forms within a salivary gland, usually in the duct of the submandibular gland.
- Sialolithiasis can result in chronic obstructive type of sialadenitis (inflammation).
- Chronic sclerosing sialadenitis is a chronic (long-lasting) inflammatory condition affecting the salivary gland. It is benign, but presents as hard, indurated and enlarged masses that are clinically indistinguishable from salivary gland neoplasms or tumors.
- The chorda tympani nerve supplying the secretomotor fibers to the submandibular gland lies medial to spine of sphenoid. Any injury to the spine may involve the nerve and can result in loss of secretion of saliva.

Viva voce

Q. Which muscle divides the submandibular gland?
Ans. Mylohyoid muscle.
Q. Why does the submandibular gland have a greater chance of getting calculi or small stones?
Ans. Due to the presence of both serous and mucous acini, the secretions from the gland is more viscous as a result there are more chances of getting calculi.

TONGUE

- Consists of **intercalated skeletal muscle fibers**.
- Surface covered by surface elevations called **filiform, fungiform, foliate and circumvallate papillae**.
- **Filiform papillae** are the most numerous and smallest that cover the tongue, lack taste buds and help to hold food.
- **Circumvallate papillae** are the largest, are in the back of the tongue and have furrows, underlying serous glands and taste buds.
- **Fungiform papillae** are dispersed along filiform papillae in the anterior 2/3rd of the tongue and have taste buds.
- **Foliate papillae** are rudimentary in humans and are present over the lateral aspect of the tongue.
- **Posterior lingual glands** in the connective tissue open onto the dorsal surface of the tongue.
- **Skeletal muscle fibers** are arranged both longitudinally and transversely.

Applied Anatomy

- The loss of taste sensations in the anterior 2/3rd of the dorsum is mainly due to lesions in facial nerves.
- The loss of taste from vallate papillae is seen most likely due to lesion of the glossopharyngeal nerve or its nucleus. In routine clinical practice, inspection of tongue gives idea in diagnosis of various diseases like:
    - Reddish tongue in glossitis, excessive furrowing in prolonged fever, black hairy tongue in AIDS, oral lichen planus, geographical tongue, vitamin deficiencies, etc.

Viva voce

Q. What are papillae?
Ans. These are surface elevations present on the surface of the tongue.
Q. What are the types of papillae present on the tongue?
Ans. Filiform, fungiform and circumvallate papillae.
Q. Which papillae contain taste buds?
Ans. Circumvallate papillae.
Q. Which papillae lack taste buds?
Ans. Filiform papillae.
Q. Where do the posterior lingual glands open into?
Ans. The posterior lingual glands open into the dorsal surface of the tongue.

TONGUE

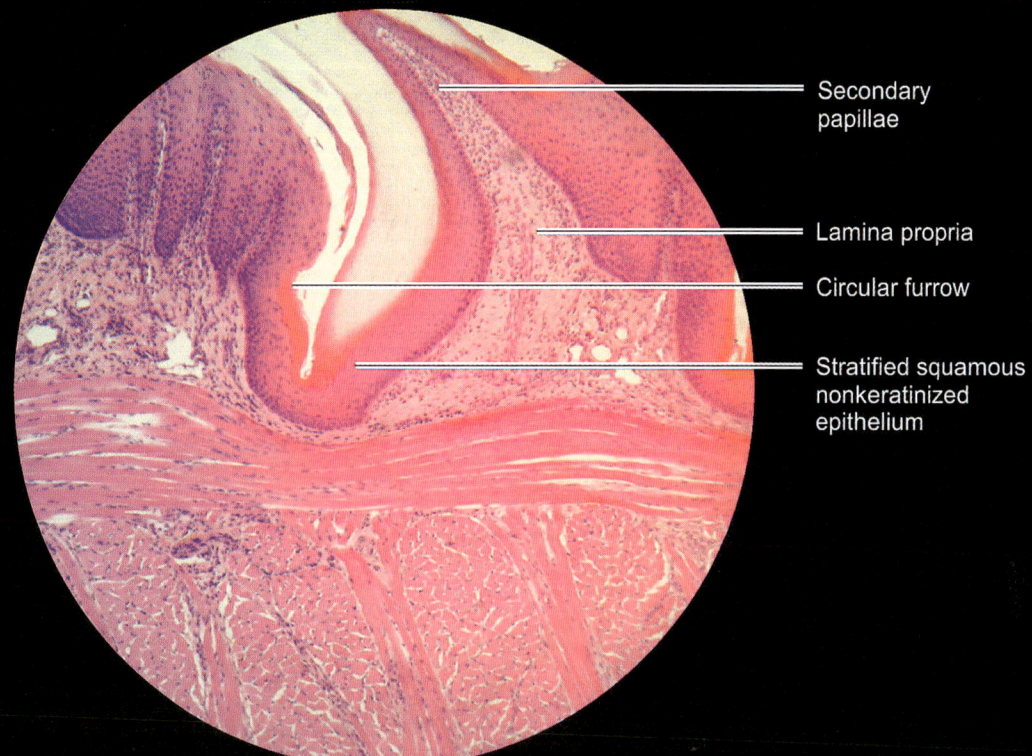

SP:
- Presence of different kinds of papillae with skeletal muscle fibers.
- Presence of glands and stratified nonkeratinized squamous cell lining.

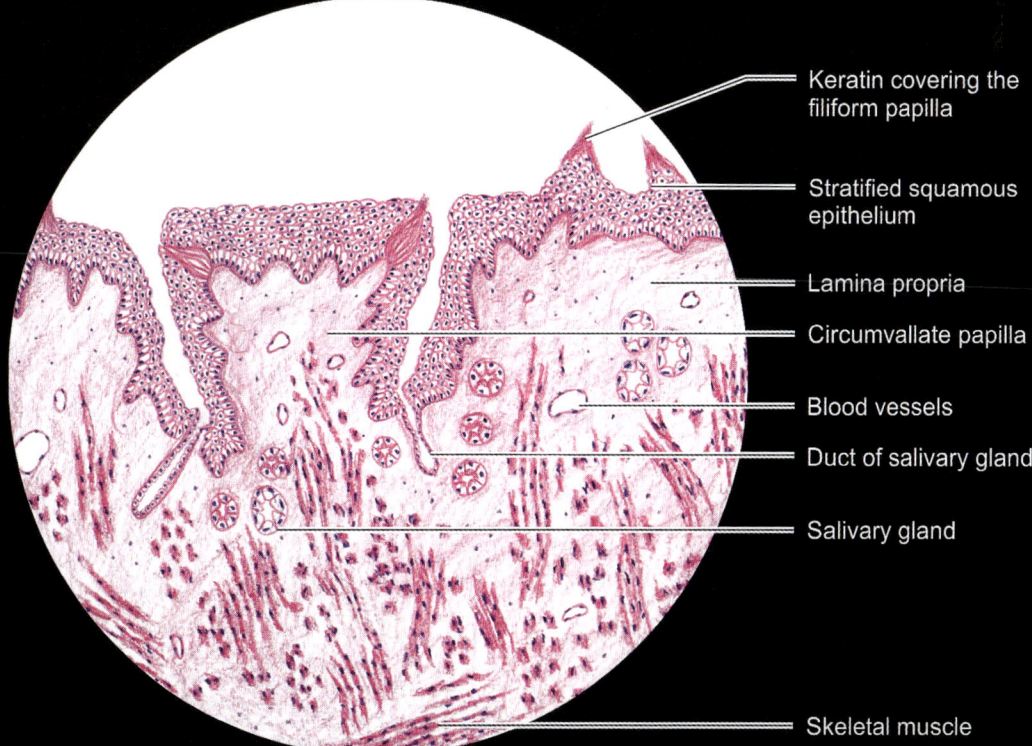

ESOPHAGUS

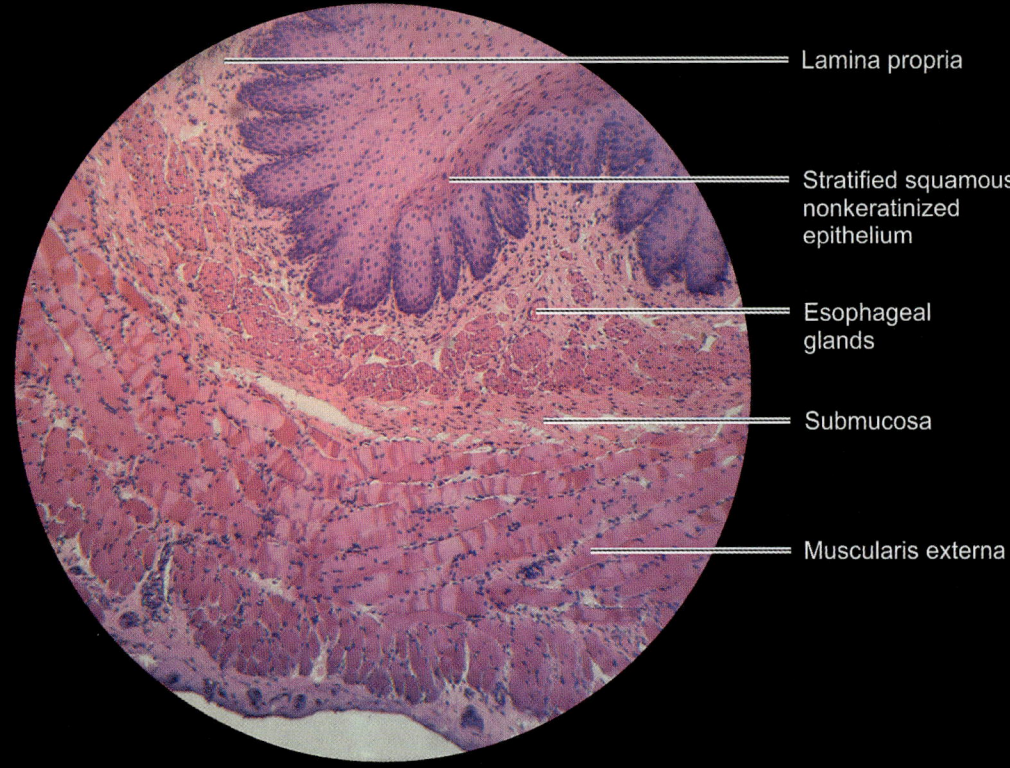

SP:
- Presence of four layers of gastrointestinal tract (GIT).
- Presence of esophageal glands in submucosa.

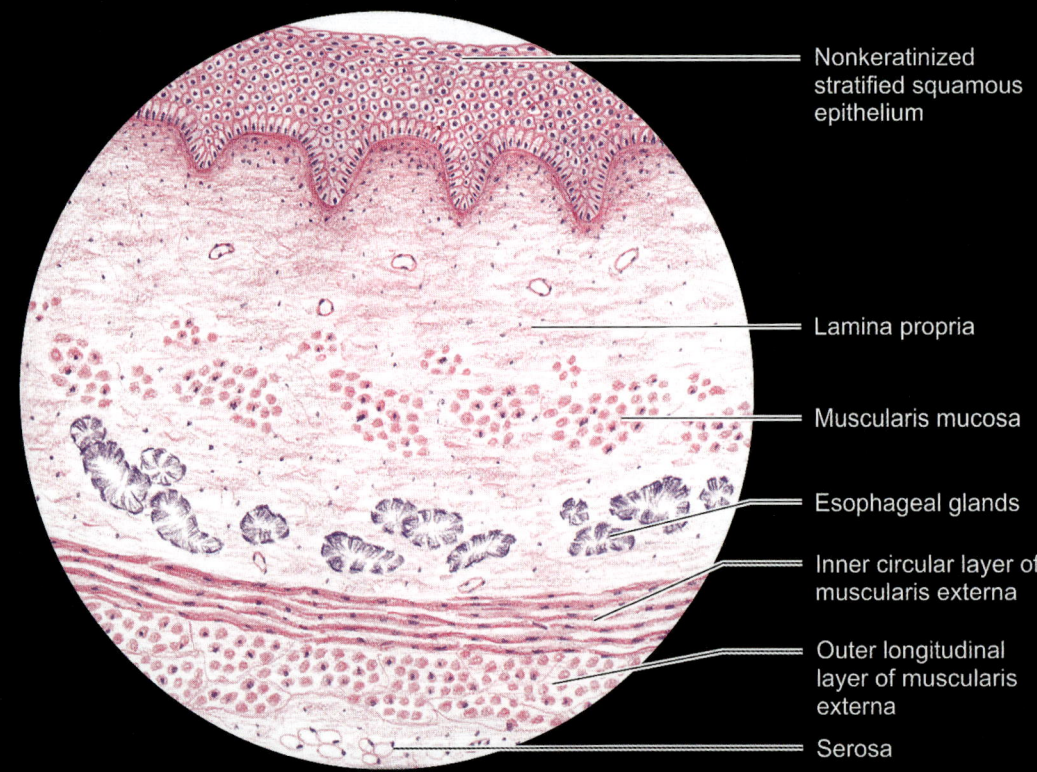

ALIMENTARY SYSTEM

GENERAL ASPECTS

- Wall of gastrointestinal tract or the GIT has four basic layers:
  1. Mucosa
  2. Submucosa
  3. Muscularis externa
  4. Serosa or adventitia
- These layers exhibit variations at different sites due to the functional differences of these sites.
  1. **Mucosa** consists of:
     - Lining epithelium
     - Lamina propria
     - **Muscularis mucosa** with **inner circular** and **outer longitudinal** smooth muscle layers.
  2. **Submucosa:**
     - Located below mucosa
     - Made up of dense irregular connective tissue with numerous blood vessels and lymphatic vessels.
     - Consists of submucosal or **Meissner's nerve plexus** containing postganglionic parasympathetic neurons controlling the motility of the mucosa as well as secretory activities of associated mucosal glands.
     - In the duodenal region, numerous branched mucous glands are present.
  3. **Muscularis externa:**
     - Thick smooth muscle layer situated inferior to the submucosa.
     - Consists of **inner circular** and **outer longitudinal** layers of smooth muscle except at the site of the large intestine.
     - **Myentric nerve plexus or Auerbach's plexus** is located in between these two smooth muscle layers.
     - This plexus contains some **postganglionic parasympathetic neurons** and controls the motility of the intestine.
  4. **Serosa and adventitia:**
     - The visceral organs may or may not be covered by a thin outer layer of squamous epithelium called **mesothelium**.
     - If the mesothelium covers the visceral organs, the organs will be within the abdominal or pelvic cavity (intraperitoneal) and now the outer layer is called **serosa**.
     - When the visceral organs are not covered by mesothelium, then they will lie outside the visceral cavity (retroperitoneal) and now, the outer layer is called **adventitia**.

ESOPHAGUS

- Inner lining mucosa made up of **stratified nonkeratinized squamous epithelium**.
- Underlying thin layer of connective tissue—**lamina propria** and layer of longitudinal smooth muscle fiber—**muscularis mucosae**.
- **Submucosa** is wider and consists of adipose tissue, mucous acini of esophageal glands proper and numerous blood vessels such as veins, arteries, etc.
- The **muscularis externa** consists of an inner circular and outer longitudinal muscle layer separated by a thin layer of connective tissue.
- The **adventitia** consists of a loose connective tissue layer that blends with the adventitia of trachea and surrounding structures.
- Adipose tissue, blood vessels, arteries, veins and nerve fibers are numerous in adventitia.
- In the upper 1/3rd muscularis externa contains skeletal muscle fibers. Middle 1/3rd consists of both skeletal and smooth muscle and the lower 1/3rd entirely of smooth muscle fibers.

STOMACH FUNDUS

- Possess four layers.
- **Mucosa** consists of:
  - **Surface epithelium** formed by the simple columnar epithelial cells extends into maina propria to form **gastric pits** and lines it. They produce mucus and protect the stomach lining from gastric acid.
  - **Lamina propria** contains **gastric glands**, loose connective tissue, lymphoid tissue, blood vessels and lymphatics. The gastric glands open into gastric pits.
  - **Muscularis mucosa** extends into lamina propria.
- **Gastric glands** consists of five types of cells mainly—**parietal (oxyntic)** cells producing HCl, **chief (zymogenic)** cells producing pepsinogen and other digestive enzymes, **mucous neck cells** producing mucus, **endocrine cells**—secrete gastrin and serotonin, and **undifferentiated (stem) cells**—replace other cells when there is a damage.
- The subglandular region of lamina propria consists of either lymphatic tissue or small lymphatic nodules.
- **Submucosa** forms rugae and consists of capillaries, arterioles, venules and **Meissner's nerve plexus**.
- **Muscularis externa** consists of inner oblique, middle circular and outer longitudinal layers of smooth muscle along with **myenteric nerve plexus**.
- **Serosa** is covered by simple squamous mesothelium of the visceral peritoneum and may contain adipose cells.

STOMACH FUNDUS

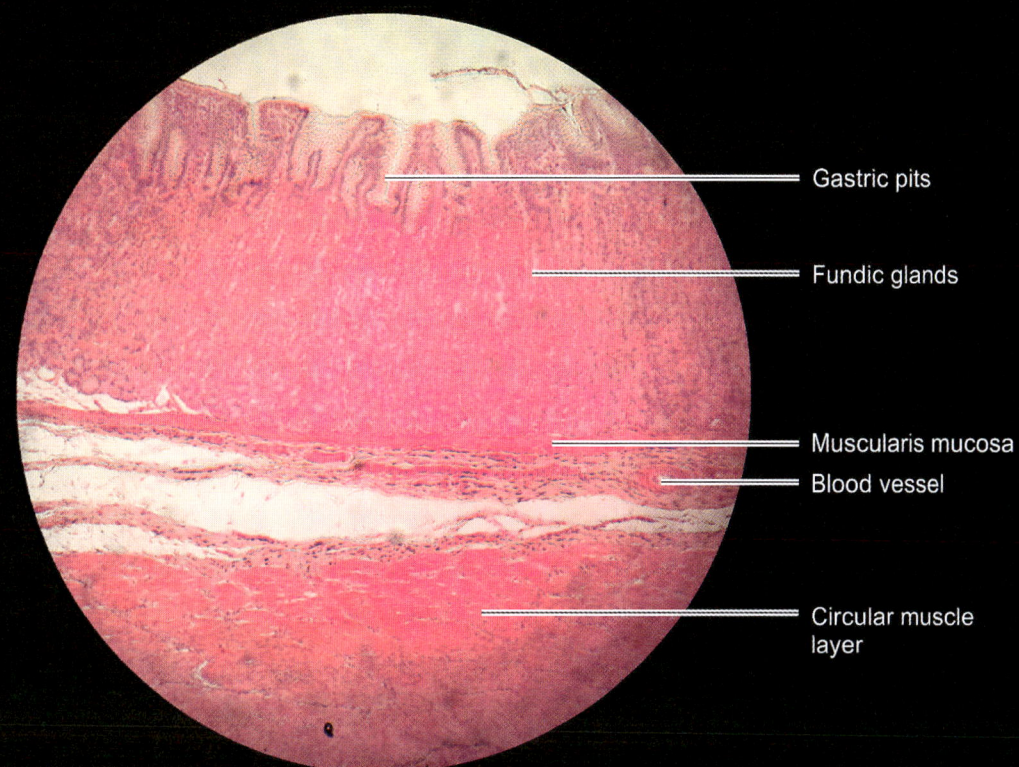

SP:
- Presence of four layers of GIT.
- Presence of fundic glands, gastric pits and mucosal folds.

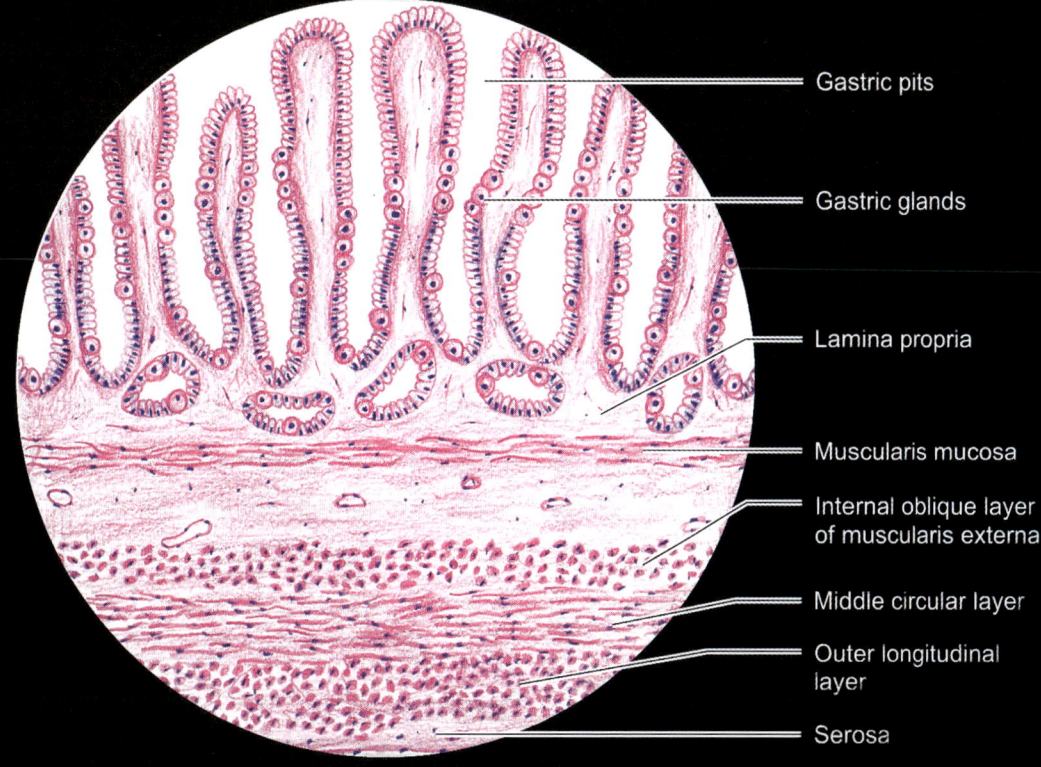

STOMACH PYLORUS

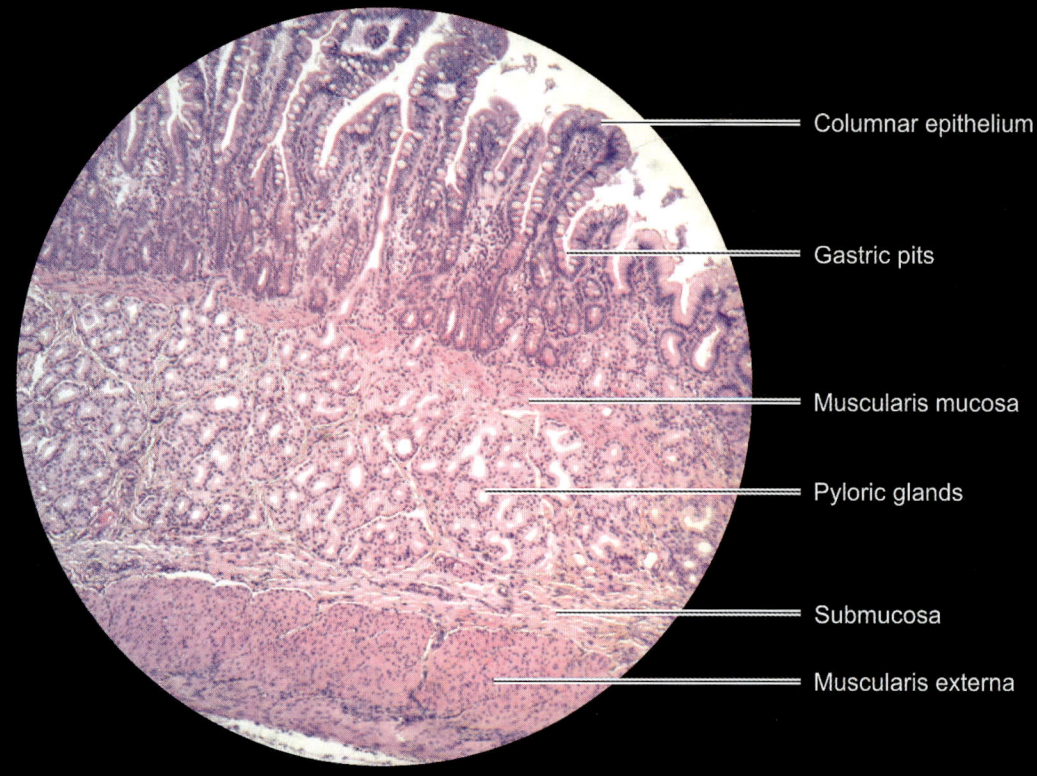

SP:
- Presence of four layers of GIT.
- Presence of pyloric glands, and abundant mucous neck cells.

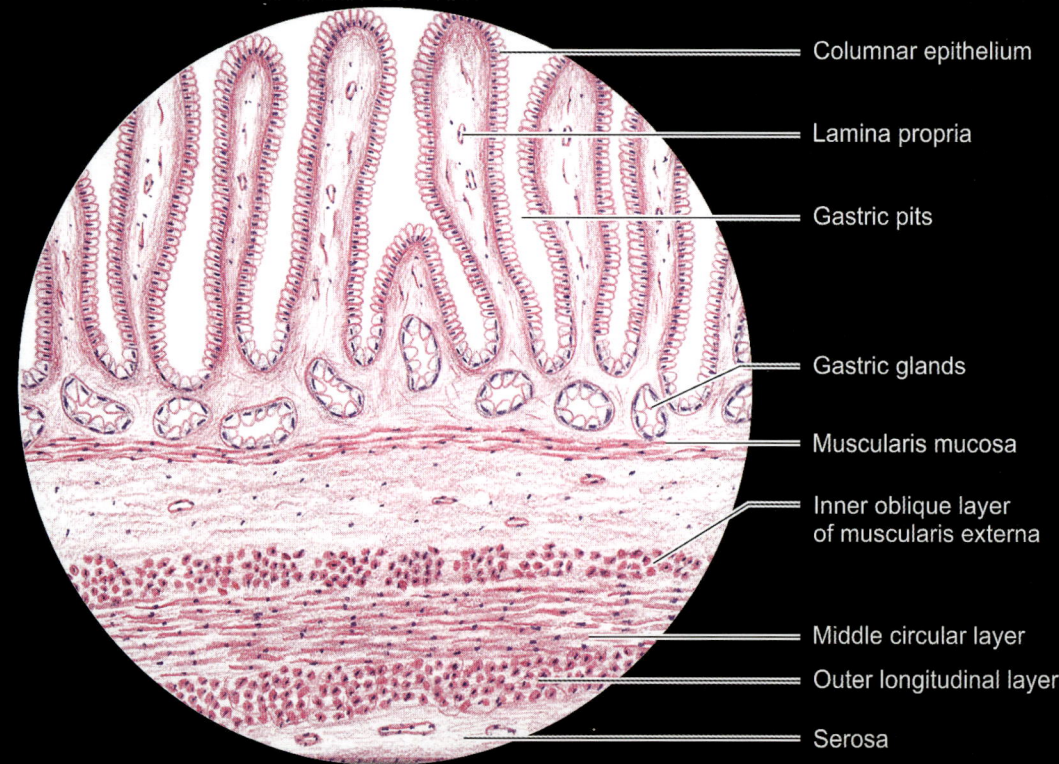

STOMACH PYLORUS

Stomach pylorus consists of four layers.
1. **Mucosa:**
   - The surface is lined by **simple columnar epithelium** which extends into and lines all the deeply located **gastric pits**.
   - Gastric pits are deeper compared to the fundus part.
   - **Gastric glands** are opened into the gastric pits. Here, mucous secreting cells are predominant. Enteroendocrine cells (G cells) producing gastrin are also present. Although very few parietal cells are seen in the pylorus, chief cells are almost absent in this part of the stomach.
   - Unlike the stomach fundus, pyloric portion have more coling of the base of the glands.
   - **Lamina propria** contains diffuse lymphatic tissue and an occasional lymphatic nodule.
   - Individual smooth muscle fibers from the circular layer of muscularis mucosa pass upwards into lamina propria.
2. **Submucosa** contain blood vessels (arteriole and venule) of different sizes.
3. **Muscularis externa** consists of **inner oblique, middle circular** and **outer longitudinal layers** of smooth muscles of which the middle layer is more thickened to form the **pyloric sphincter**.
4. **Serosa** is covered by simple squamous mesothelium of the visceral peritoneum and may contain adipose cells.

Applied Anatomy

- In achalasia cardia, the tone of lower esophageal sphincter is increased due to impaired smooth muscle relaxation, causing esophageal obstruction.
- **GERD (gastroesophageal reflux disease) and Barret esophagus:**
  - Reflux of gastric contents into the lower part of the esophagus leads to esophagitis.
  - Long standing gastroesophageal reflux may cause replacement of distal squamous mucosa by metaplastic columnar epithelium known as Barret esophagus and esophageal adenocarcinoma.
- **Peptic ulcer:** It is a chronic, most often solitary lesion that occurs in any part of the GI tract exposed to aggressive action of acid/peptic juices.
- Gastric leiomyosarcoma is rare among gastric malignancies, and only 20% of the cases are located in the gastric cardia or fundus.
- In pyloric stenosis, there is narrowing of the opening from the stomach to the first part of the small intestine known as the duodenum, due to enlargement (hypertrophy) of the muscle surrounding this opening, which spasms when the stomach empties.

SMALL INTESTINE

General Aspects
- Extends from junction with stomach to join with large intestine or colon.
- Divided into:
    - **Duodenum**
    - **Jejunum**
    - **Ileum**
- **Mucosa shows plica circularis:** The permanent spiral folds, villi—permanent finger like projections of lamina propria that extend into intestinal lumen, microvilli—the cytoplasmic extensions that cover the apices of intestinal absorptive cells—all these aids the absorption better.
- **Intestinal glands (crypts of Lieberkuhn)** are located between the villi at the base throughout the small intestine. **Stem cells, absorptive cells, goblet cells, paneth cells** and some **enteroendocrine cells** are also present.
    - **Enterocytes (absorptive cells)** are involved in the absorption process.
    - **Goblet cells** are present in between enterocytes and produce mucous secretions.
    - **Paneth (zymogen)** cells produce lysozymes and defensins which provide some protection against intestinal infections.
    - **Enteroendocrine (enterochromaffin)** cells are associated with endocrine function.
- **Brunner's gland** are present in duodenal submucosa. Their alkaline mucus protects intestinal mucosa from gastric acid and activates pancreatic enzymes.
- **Peyer's patches** are present in lamina propria of ileum.
    - **M-cells** are present along the epithelium above lymphatic follicles.

DUODENUM
- Shortest segment of the small intestine and consists of four layers.
- **Mucosa** lined by **simple columnar epithelium with brush a border, lamina propria**, and **muscularis mucosae** with connective tissue cells, lymphatic cells, plasma cells, macrophages, smooth muscle cells, etc.
- **Villi** in this region are **leaf-like**, tall and numerous with fewer goblet cells in the epithelium.
- **Submucosa** consist of mucous duodenal (Brunner's) glands.
- **Muscularis externa** consist of two smooth muscle layers, inner circular and outer longitudinal layers.
- Some parts consist of visceral peritoneum or serosa which is incomplete.

DUODENUM

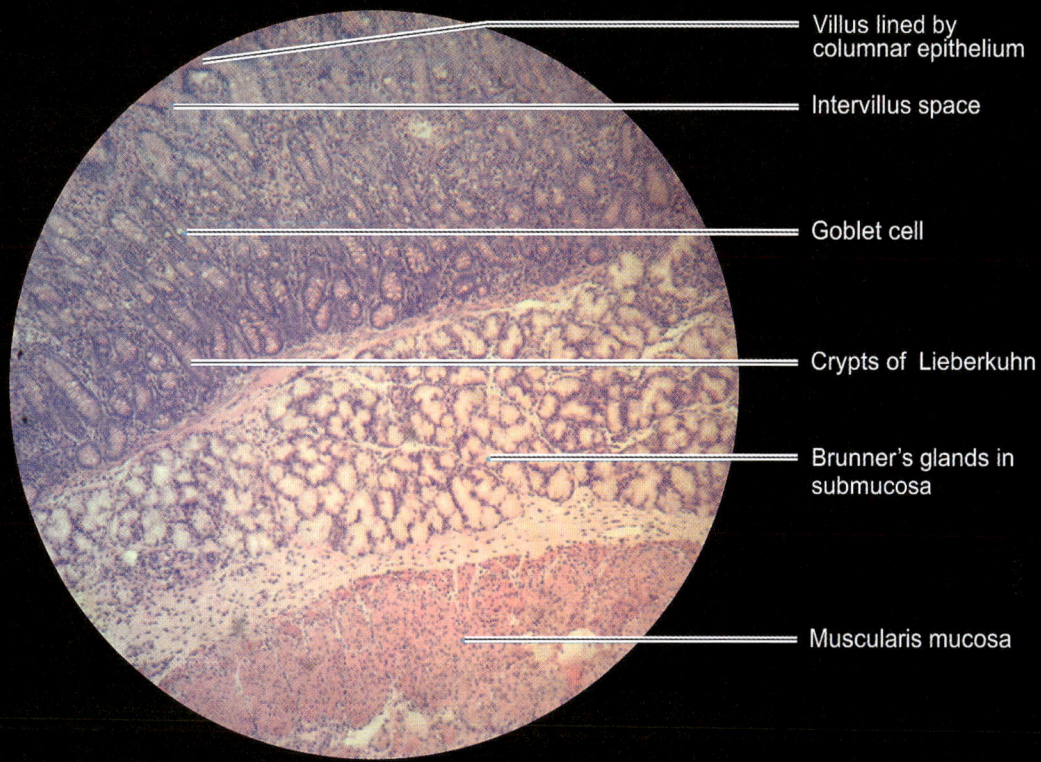

SP:
- Presence of four layers of GIT.
- Presence of Brunner's glands in submucosa and villi on mucous membrane.

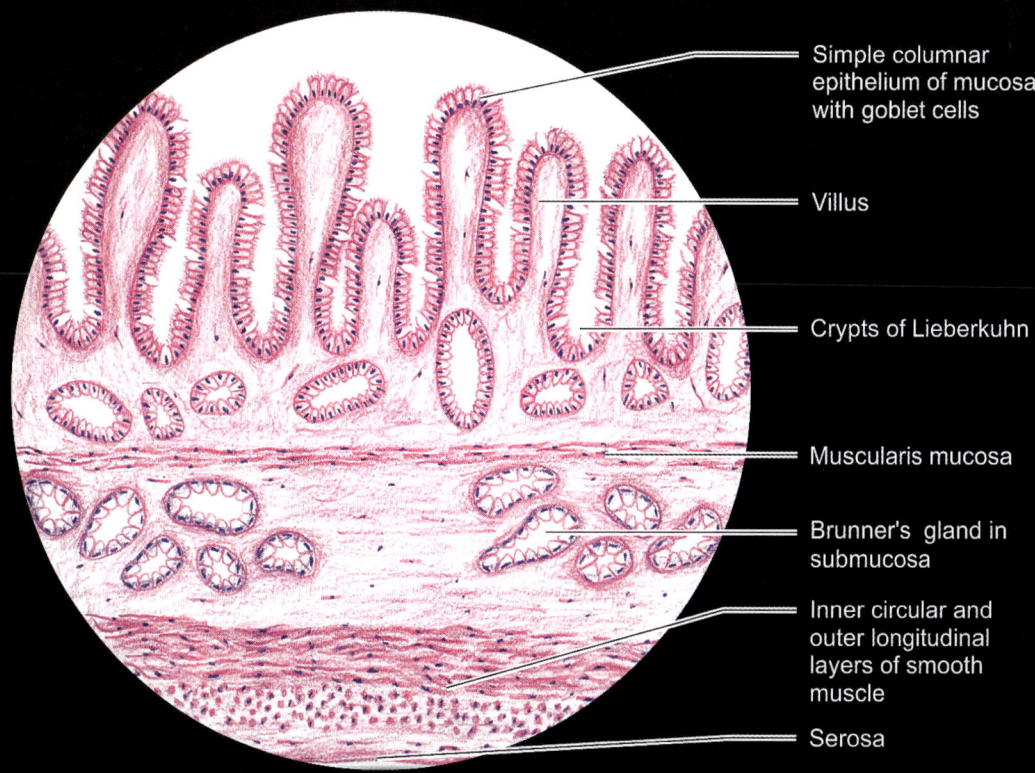

JEJUNUM

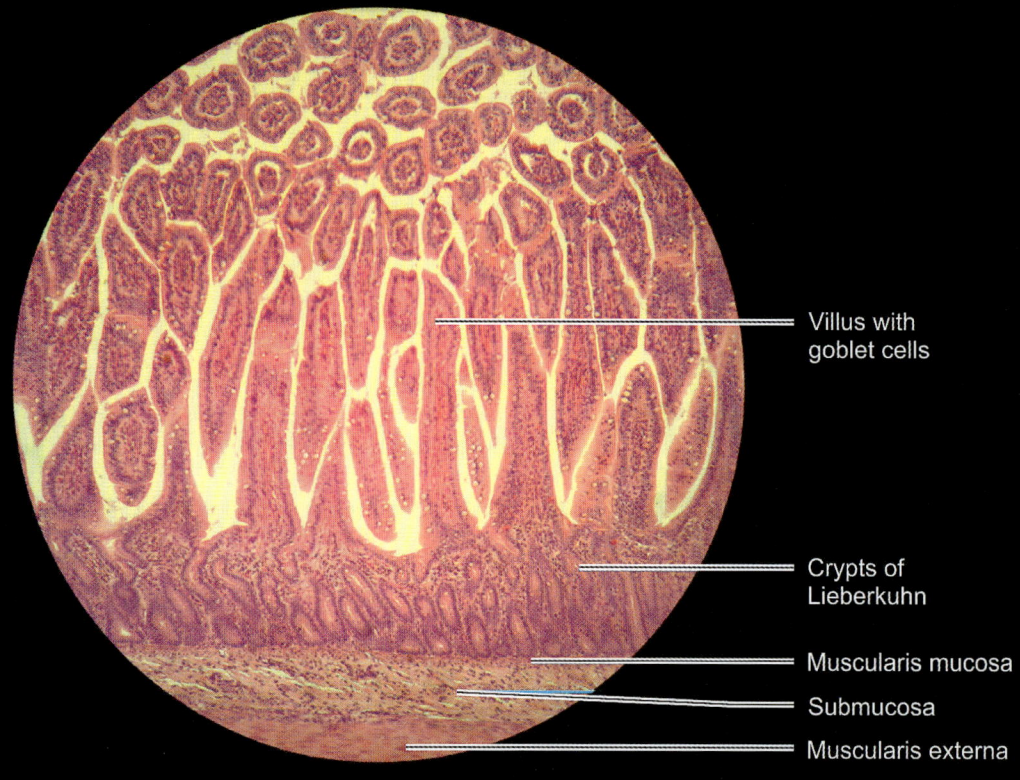

- Villus with goblet cells
- Crypts of Lieberkuhn
- Muscularis mucosa
- Submucosa
- Muscularis externa

SP:
- Presence of four layers of GIT.
- Presence of intestinal crypts and tongue-shaped villi.

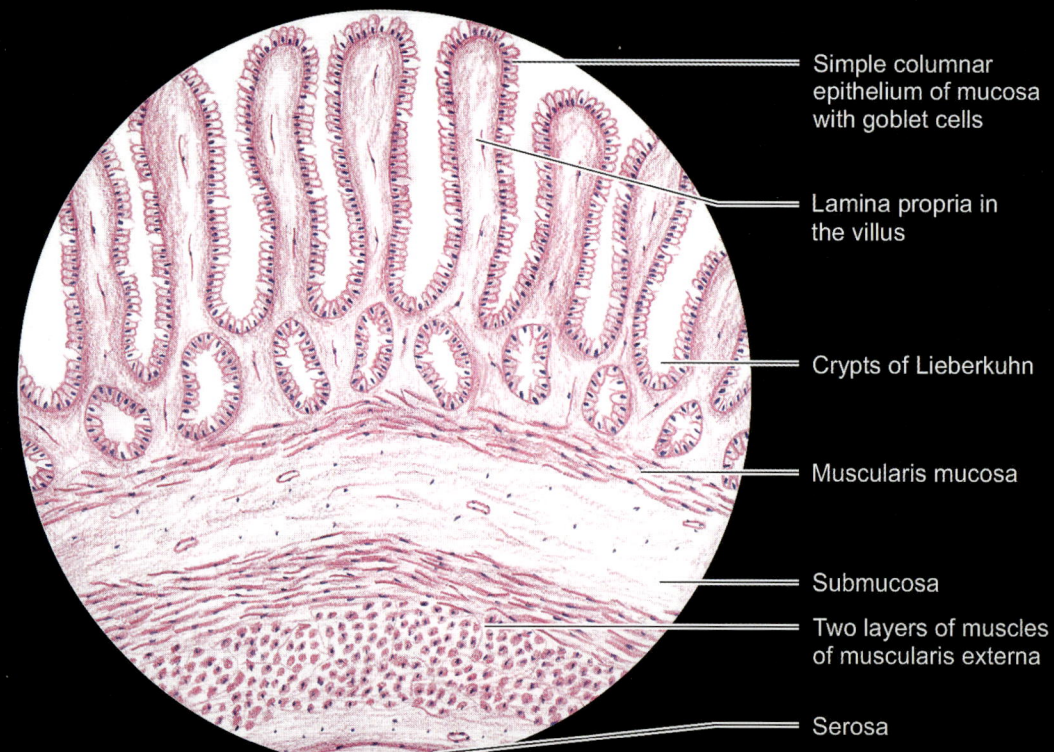

- Simple columnar epithelium of mucosa with goblet cells
- Lamina propria in the villus
- Crypts of Lieberkuhn
- Muscularis mucosa
- Submucosa
- Two layers of muscles of muscularis externa
- Serosa

JEJUNUM

- Consists of four layers.
- **Mucosa** is lined by **simple columnar epithelium with a brush border.**
- The **goblet cells** lie in between columnar cells and are more in number when compared to duodenum.
- **Shorter, narrower** and fewer villi than the duodenum with **tongue shape**.
- **Lamina propria** consists of lymphatic cells, macrophages, smooth muscle cells, blood vessels, etc.
- Intestinal gland ends at muscularis mucosae.
- **Submucosa** lacks Brunner's gland and Peyers, patches.
- **Muscularis externa** has inner circular and outer longitudinal smooth muscle layers with **myenteric plexus** present in between them.
- Visceral peritoneum or **serosa** surrounds the small intestine.

Applied Anatomy (Duodenum and Jejunum)

- The first part of duodenum is overlapped by liver and gallbladder, either of these structures can adhere to the duodenum, and may be eroded by the duodenal ulcer, if present.
- It is in the first part of duodenum where the majority of ulcers are present.
- Even gallstones can be extruded from the fundus of an inflamed gallbladder to duodenum and from duodenum to jejunum as well as ileum.
- In a barium meal procedure, after intake of contrast, the first part of duodenum becomes visible in the radiograph as a triangular shadow called duodenal cap and is emptied to the jejunum every one minute.
- Intestinal atresia (congenital absence of lumen) and stenosis (narrowing of lumen) is most commonly seen in duodenum and jejunum.

Viva voce

Q. Where are myenteric plexus present?
Ans. Myenteric plexus is present in between the inner circular and outer longitudinal smooth muscle layers.
Q. What kind of epithelium lines the mucosa?
Ans. Simple columnar epithelium with brush border.

ILEUM

- Consists of four layers.
- **Mucosa** is lined by **simple columnar epithelium** and with **goblet cells**.
- **Villi are thin and slender, having** lacteals.
- **Lamina propria** contains intestinal glands and aggregation of lymphatic nodules called **Peyer's patches**.
- Usually the lymphatic nodules are seen in close association to each other with indistinct boundaries.
- **Muscularis mucosa** is disrupted by Peyer's patches by extending into the submucosa.
- **Muscularis externa** having inner circular and outer longitudinal layer of smooth muscle fibers.
- **Serosa** having blood vessels and connective tissue.

Applied Anatomy

- Pathogenic microorganisms and other antigens entering the intestinal tract encounter macrophages, dendritic cells, B lymphocytes and T lymphocytes found in Peyer's patches and aids immunity.
- Peyer's patches are present only in ileum throughout the GIT, Brunner's gland is absent in ileum, the villi present are finger shaped.

Viva voce

Q. What are Peyer's patches?
Ans. Lamina propria contains aggregation of lymphatic nodules called Peyer's patches.
Q. What type of epithelium lines the ileal mucosa?
Ans. Mucosa is lined by simple columnar epithelium with goblet cells. Specialized epithelilal cells called M-cells are present over Peyer's patches.

ILEUM

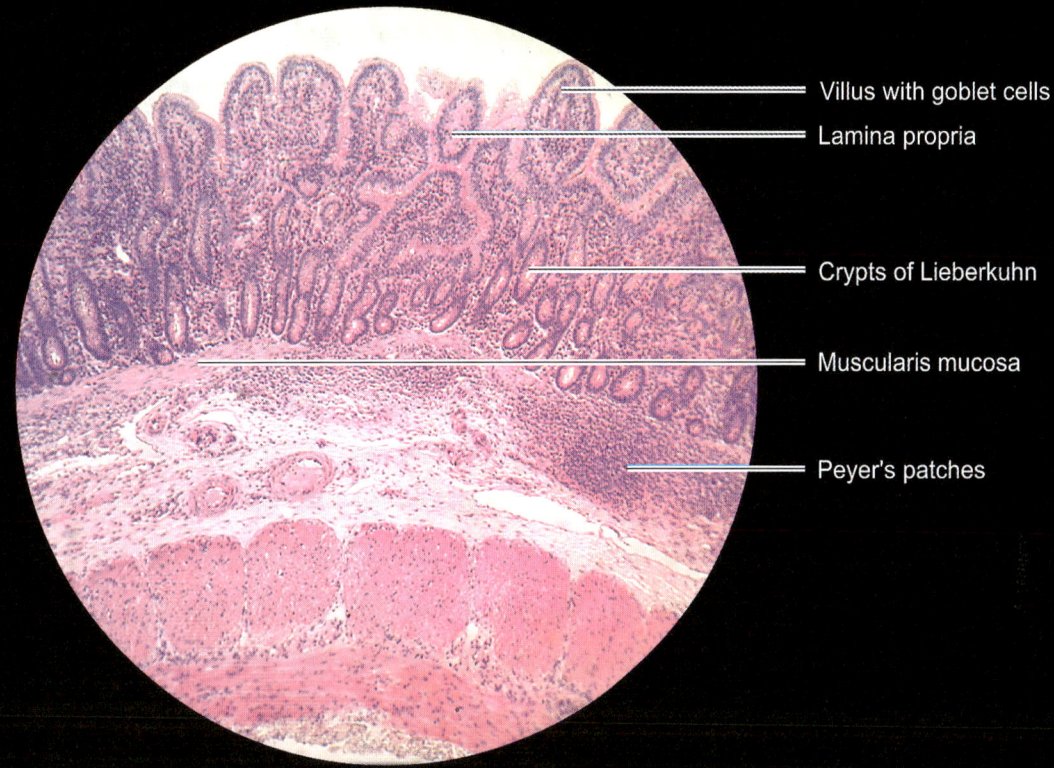

SP:
- Presence of four layers of GIT.
- Presence of Peyer's patches and finger-shaped villi.

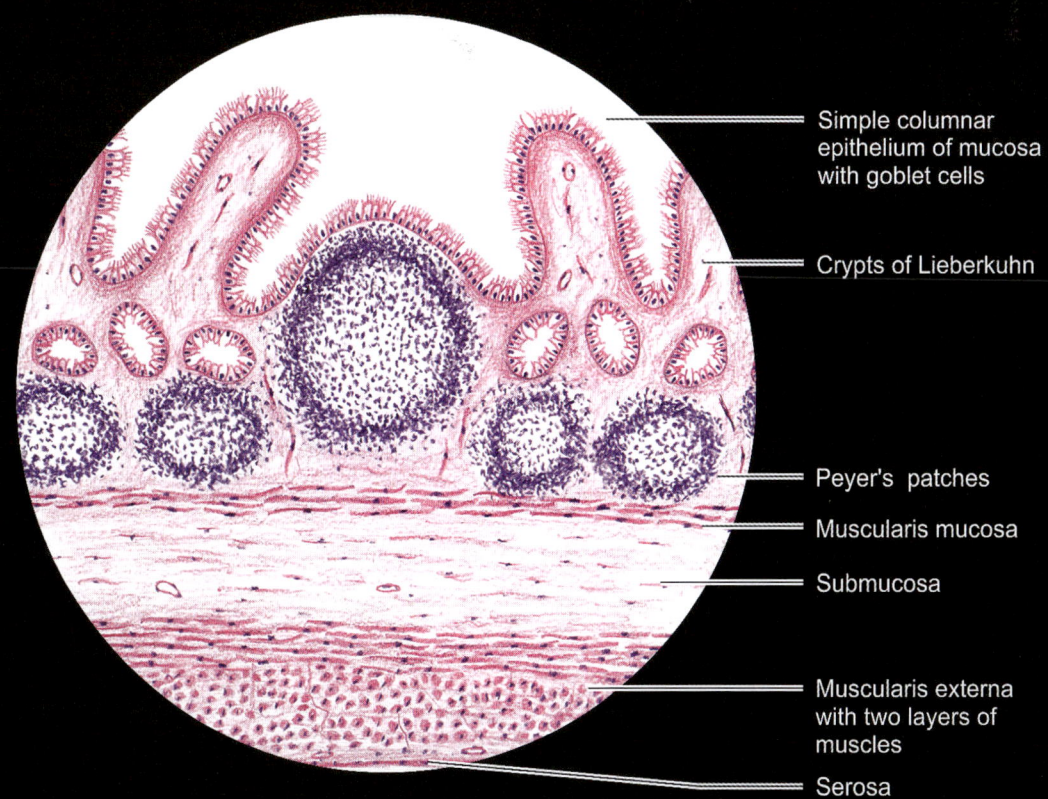

COLON

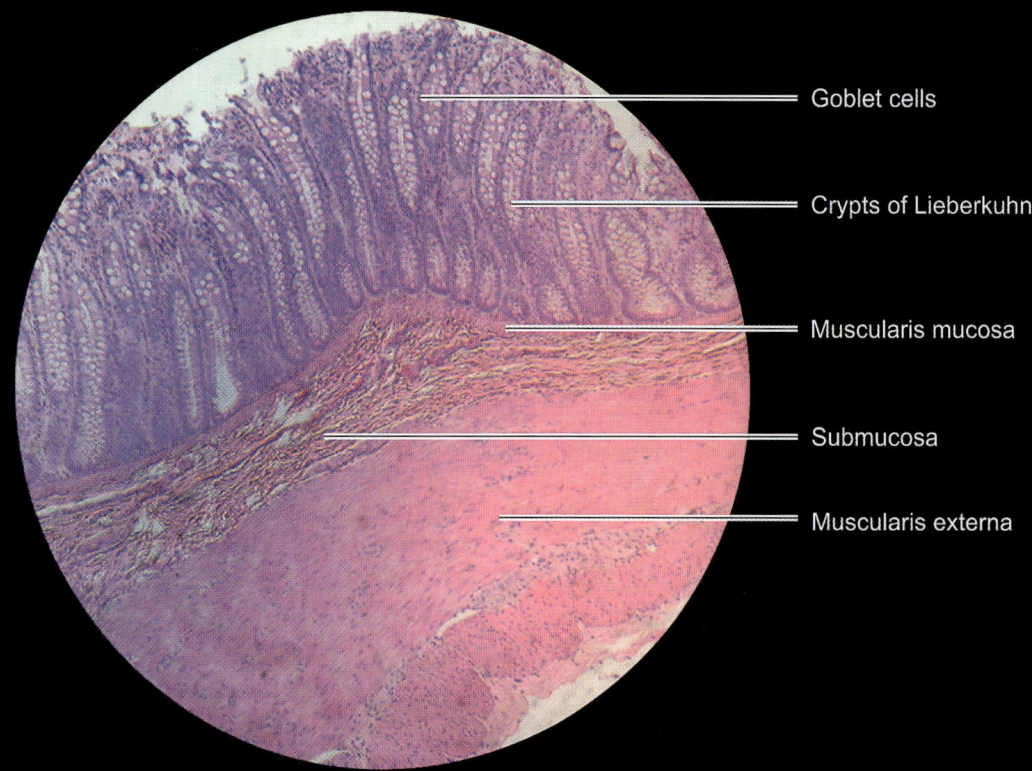

SP:
- Presence of four layers of GIT.
- Presence of taenia coli and tubular glands in folds with goblet cells.

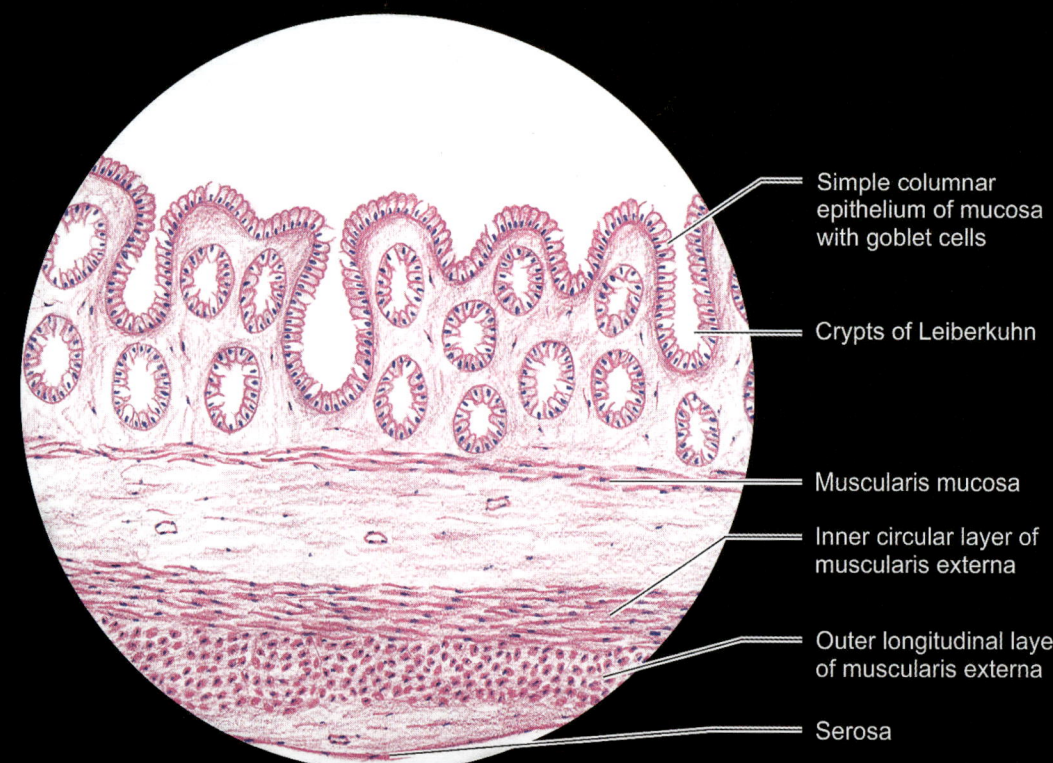

COLON

- Consists of four basic layers.
- Villi is absent. Instead there are tubular glands in folds with goblet cells.
- **Mucosa** is lined by **absorptive simple columnar epithelial cells** and more number of mucous filled goblet cells.
- **Lamina propria** contains intestinal glands.
- **Muscularis mucosae** is well-defined.
- **Submucosa and lamina propria** are filled with aggregations of lymphatic cells and lymphatic nodules.
- **Submucosa** also contains connective tissue cells and fibers, various blood vessels and nerves.
- **Muscularis externa** consists of:
  - **Inner circular** layer throughout the length of colon.
  - **Outer longitudinal** layer is condensed into three broad longitudinal bands called **taeniae coli** whose contraction causes **sacculations** or **haustra**.
  - **Parasympathetic ganglion cells** of the myenteric nerve plexus are found between the circular and longitudinal muscle layers.
  - **Serosa** covers transverse colon and sigmoid colon.
  - Serosa shows fat filled peritoneal pockets called **appendices epiploicae**.

Applied Anatomy

Ulcerative colitis is a recurrent ulceroinflammatory lesion of the colon characterized by diffuse inflammation ulcerations, crypt abscess formation, goblet cell depletion and paneth cell metaplasia.

Viva voce

Q. What is taenia coli?
Ans. Outer longitudinal layer of muscularis externa is condensed into three broad longitudinal bands called taeniae coli and they extend from base of appendix to cecum.
Q. What are the characteristic features of the submucosa of the large intestine?
Ans. Submucosa and lamina propria are filled with aggregations of lymphatic cells and lymphatic nodules. It also contains connective tissue cells and fibers, various blood vessels and nerves.

APPENDIX

- Consist of four basic layers.
- **Mucosa** having epithelium containing numerous goblet cells.
- **Lamina propria** shows intestinal glands (crypts of Lieberkuhn).
- In appendix villi are absent and it has small angular lumen compared to the thick wall.
- **Lymphatic nodules** with a germinal center originate in lamina propria and may extend from the surface epithelium to submucosa.
- **Muscularis mucosae** is disrupted by lymphatic nodules.
- **Submucosa** having numerous blood vessels.
- **Muscularis externa** with inner circular and outer longitudinal layer.
- Parasympathetic ganglia of **myenteric plexus** are located in between the smooth muscle layers.
- Outermost layer is the **serosa** under which adipose cells are seen.

Applied Anatomy

- Appendicitis is the inflammation of the appendix and is a medical emergency.
- The lymphoid tissue in the mucosa and submucosa is similar to the Peyer's patches in the small intestine.

Viva voce

Q. Where are the parasympathetic ganglia of myenteric plexus present?
Ans. Parasympathetic ganglia of myenteric plexus are located in between the smooth muscle layers of muscularis externa.
Q. What are the characteristic features of lamina propria of appendix?
Ans. Lamina propria shows intestinal glands (crypts of Lieberkuhn) and lymphatic nodules with germinal center originate in lamina propria and may extend from the surface epithelium to submucosa.

APPENDIX

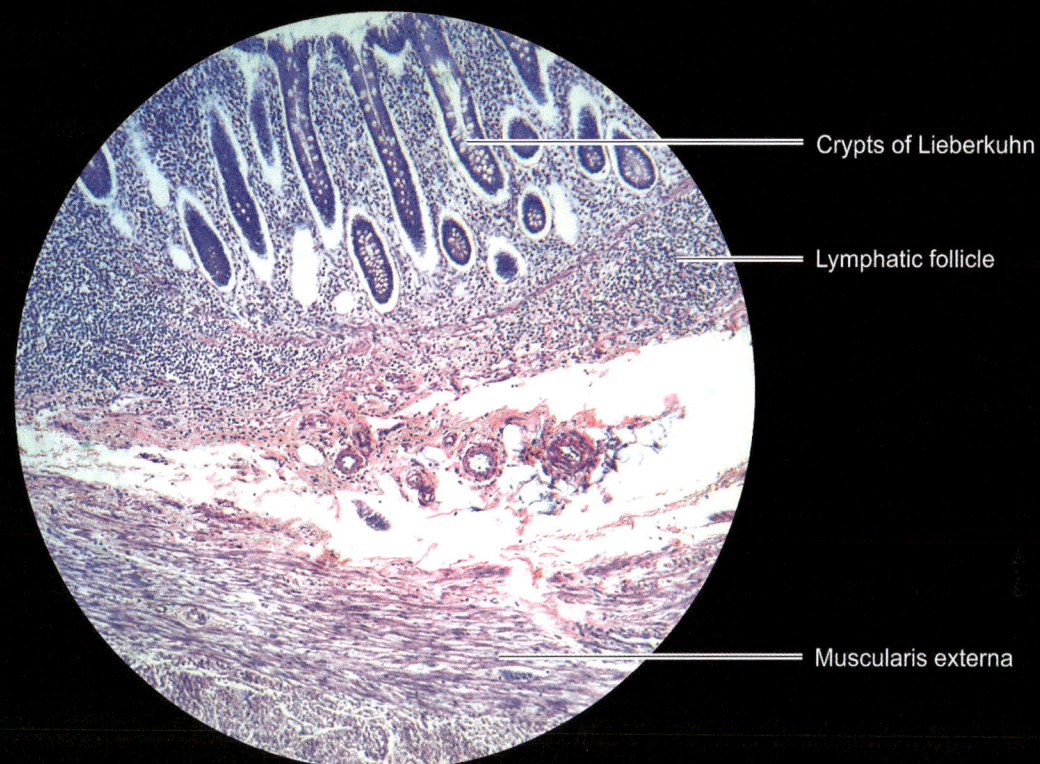

SP:
- Presence of four layers of GIT.
- Lymphatic nodules present in submucosa.

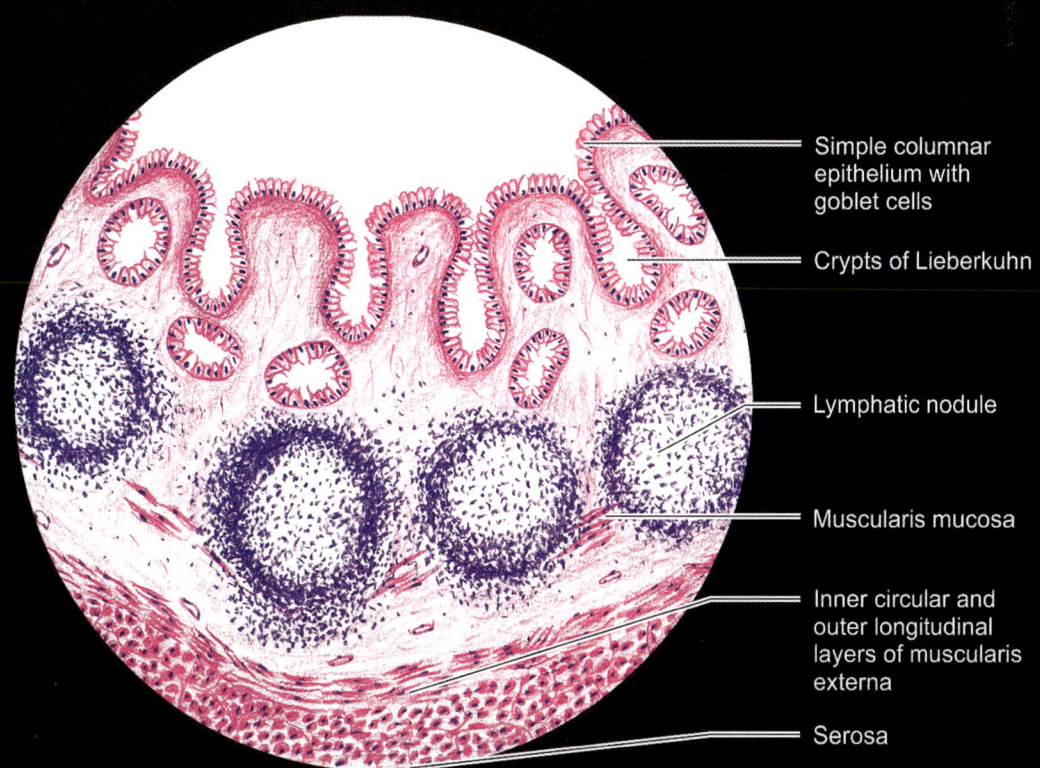

LIVER

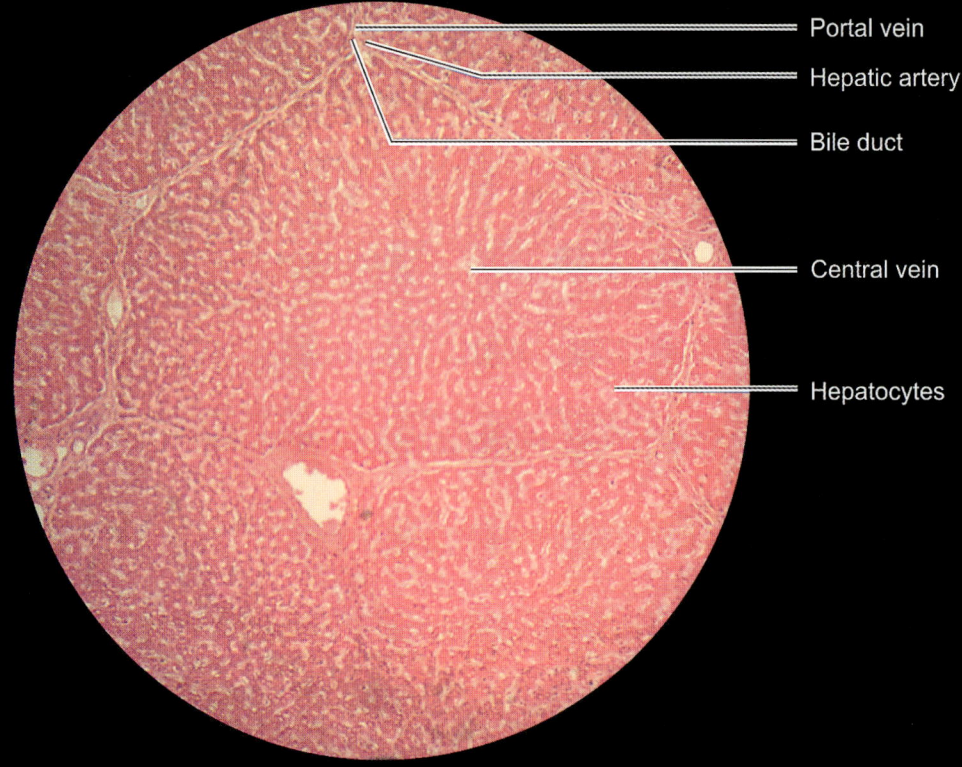

SP:
- Hexagonally arranged hepatocytes with portal triad.
- Presence of central vein.

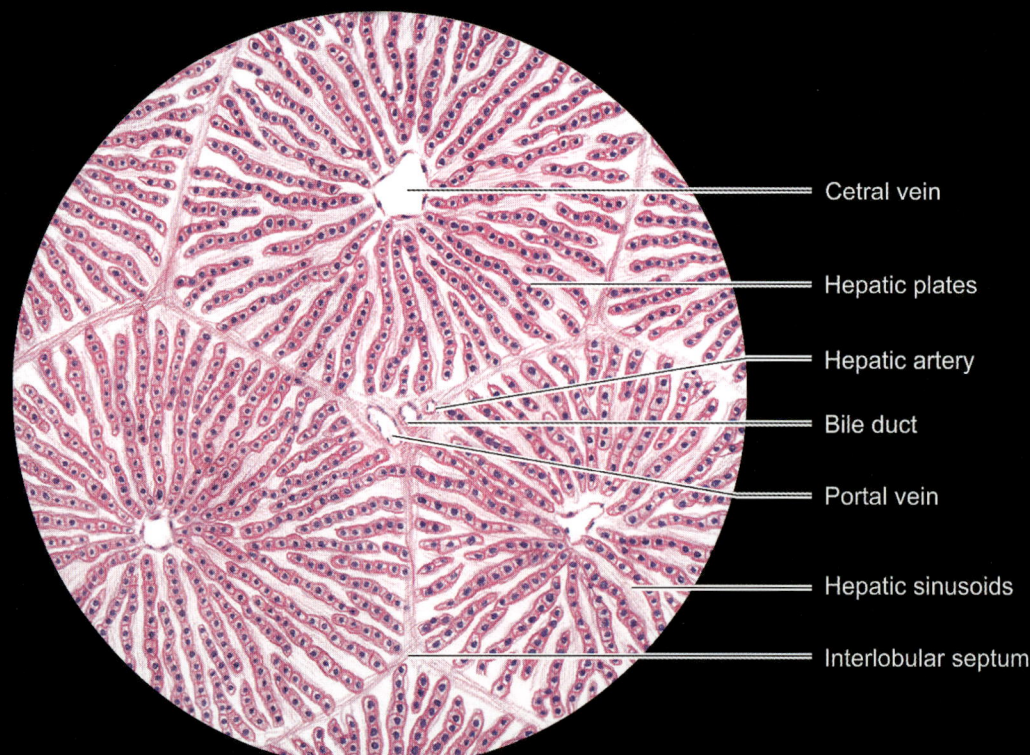

LIVER AND PANCREAS

LIVER

- Accessory digestive organ.
- Covered by Glissons capsule and is made up of connective tissues.
- Microscopic structure consists of hexagonal units called **hepatic lobules**.
- A **central vein** is present in the center of each lobule.
- From the central vein, radiating plates of **hepatocytes and sinusoids** are present towards the periphery.
- **Sinusoids** are located in between plates of hepatocytes and possess **Kupffer cells (macrophagic cells)**.
- **Hepatic sinusoids** are dilated blood channels lined by discontinuous fenestrated endothelial cells.
- Sinusoids and hepatocytes are separated by a subendothelial **perisinusoidal space (space of Disse)**.
- At the periphery of each lobule 3-6 portal areas/canals are present.
- **Portal canal** contains portal triad viz. **hepatic artery, portal vein, bile duct** and also lymph vessels.
- Hepatic artery, portal vein and bile duct are covered by fibrocollagenous tissue.
- Portal area is bounded by a layer of hepatocytes called the limiting plate.
- Arterial and venous blood mix at liver sinusoids and open into the central vein.
- **Bile canaliculi** (tiny channels) are present between hepatocytes which receive the bile secreted by the liver cells, they converge and open into the bile duct.

Applied Anatomy

- In hepatitis, the limiting plate gets destroyed and is known as Piecemeal necrosis.
- The structural features of sinusoids help in efficient exchange of substances between hepatocytes and blood.
- Since bile flow in canaliculi towards bile duct and blood in sinusoids towards central vein, i.e., in the opposite direction, the blood and bile do not mix.

GALLBLADDER

- It is a muscular sac.
- Its walls consist of **mucosa, muscularis and serosa**.
- **Muscularis mucosa** or muscularis interna and submucosa are absent.
- **Mucosa** lined by **simple columnar epithelium** with underlying lamina propria.
- Lymphatics, blood vessels, loose connective tissue, etc., are present in lamina propria.
- **Mucosal folds** are seen in nondistended states.
- **Crypts** are seen between mucosal folds and resemble glands.
- But glands are only present in the neck region of the organ.
- **Muscularis layer** consists of smooth muscle bundles arranged in circular longitudinal and oblique planes.
- This layer also contains lymphatics, nerves and blood vessels.
- **Serosa** contains connective tissue.

Applied Anatomy

- Usually gallbladder is nonpalpable during clinical examination, but it becomes palpable in cases of jaundice, mucocele and empyema.
- In cholelithiasis, stones may be present in gallbladder or in biliary passages and can cause obstructive jaundice and obstructive cholecystitis.
- In cholecystitis the mucosa is ulcerated with areas of necrosis.

Viva voce

Q. What is the distinguishing feature of gallbladder from other parts of the gastrointestinal system?
Ans. Submucosa is absent in gallbladder, whereas present in almost all parts of GIT.
Q. What is the characteristic feature of the muscularis layer?
Ans. Muscularis layer consists of randomly placed bundles of smooth muscles with interlacing elastic fibers.
Q. What is the characteristic feature of lamina propria of gallbladder?
Ans. Lymphatics, blood vessels, loose connective tissue, etc., are present in lamina propria.

GALLBLADDER

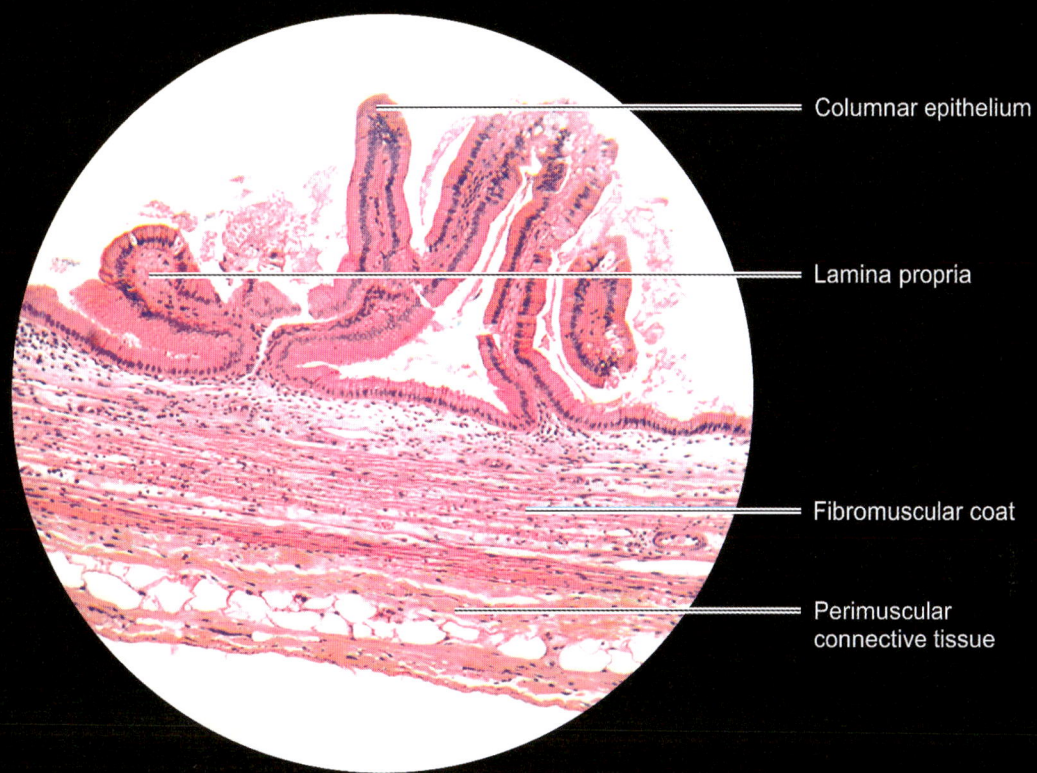

SP:
- Presence of three layers of GIT.
- Absence of submucosa.

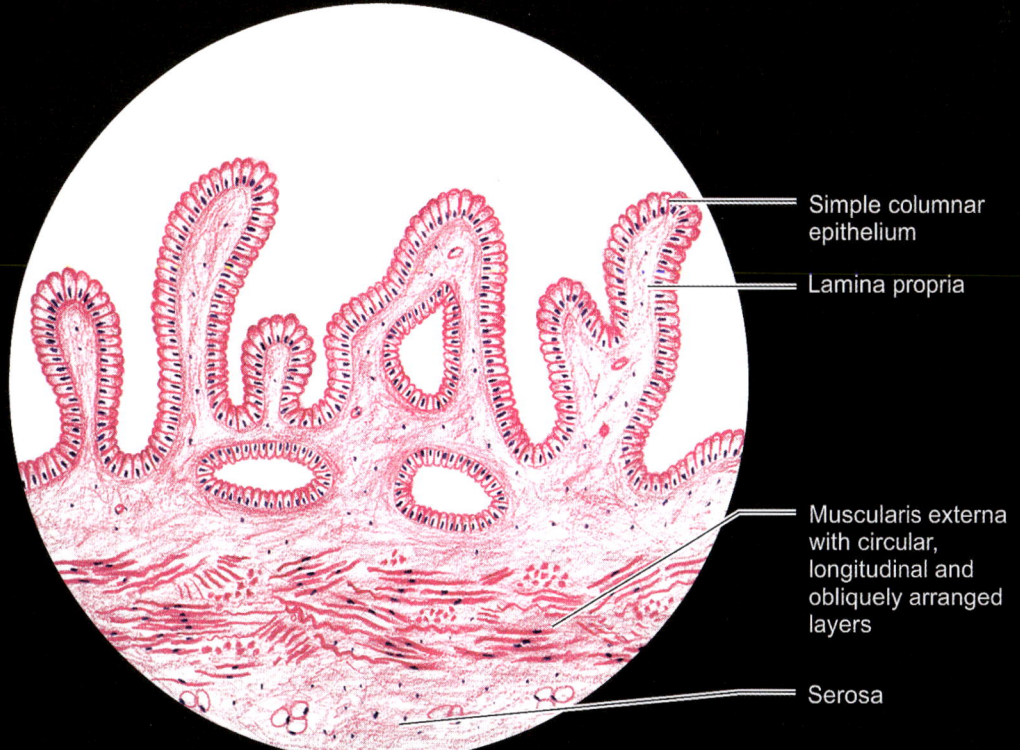

PANCREAS

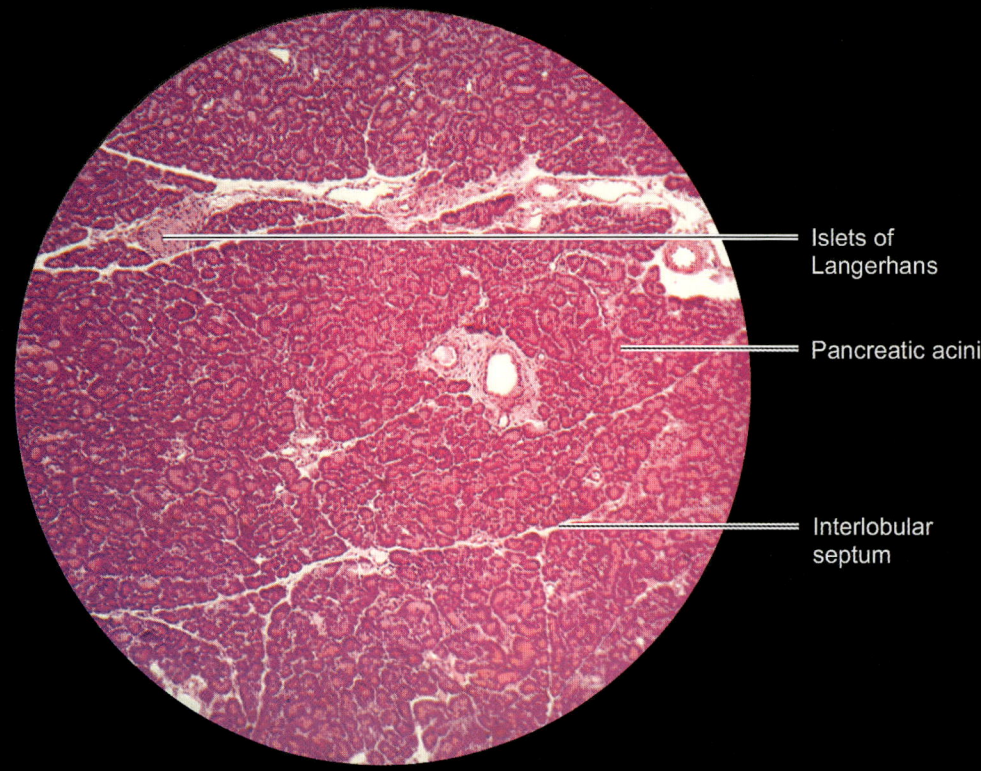

- Islets of Langerhans
- Pancreatic acini
- Interlobular septum

SP:
- Presence of pancreatic acini.
- Presence of islets of Langerhans.

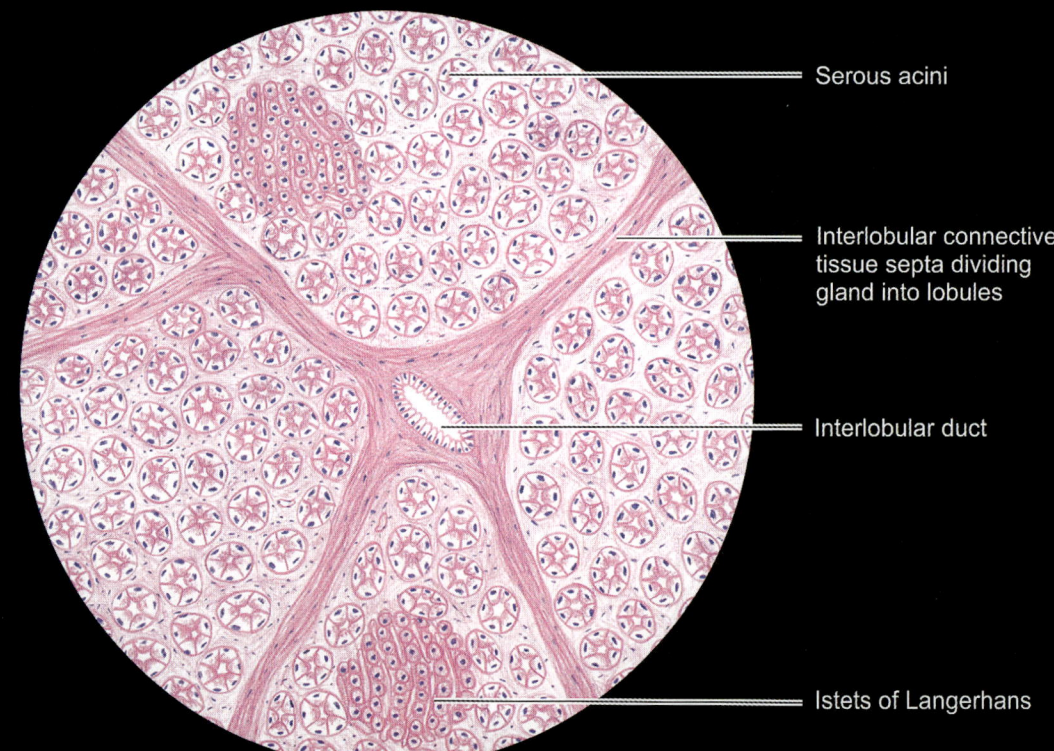

- Serous acini
- Interlobular connective tissue septa dividing gland into lobules
- Interlobular duct
- Istets of Langerhans

PANCREAS

- Consists of endocrine and exocrine parts.
- **Exocrine part** forms the major portion and consists of **secretory serous acini and zymogenic cells**.
- These are arranged into small lobules bounded by **thin intralobular** and **interlobular connective tissue septa** having **interlobular ducts** and blood vessels.
- **Endocrine part** is represented by the isolated **pancreatic islets or islets of Langerhans** present between serous acini.
- Each **acinus** consists of pyramidal shaped protein secreting cells that surround a small lumen. Their ducts are visible as centroacinar cells and the secretions leave via intralobular ducts to interlobular ducts.
- Islets are separated from acini by a thin layer of reticular fibers and are actually compact clusters of epithelial cells permeated by capillaries and have alpha, beta, delta and F-cells.

Applied Anatomy

- The exocrine part of the pancreas is responsible for the production of digestive enzymes like pancreatic amylase, lipase, etc.
- The pancreas secretes digestive enzymes in the form of inactive precursors called zymogens.
- Hormones produced by the islets are as follows:
  - **Alpha cells:** Glucagon
  - **Beta cells:** Insulin
  - **Delta cells:** Somatostatin
  - **F-cells:** Pancreatic polypeptide

Viva voce

Q. What is the characteristic feature of an acini?
Ans. Each acinus consists of pyramidal shaped protein secreting cells that surround a small lumen. Their ducts are visible as centroacinar cells and the secretions leave via intralobular ducts to interlobular ducts.
Q. What is the endocrine part of the pancreas represented by?
Ans. The endocrine part is represented as pancreatic islets or islets of Langerhans.
Q. What is the exocrine part of pancreas formed from?
Ans. Exocrine part consists of secretory serous acini and zymogenic cells.

RESPIRATORY SYSTEM

TRACHEA

- **Tracheal** wall consists of **mucosa, submucosa, hyaline cartilage and adventitia**.
- Tracheal lumen is lined by **pseudostratified ciliated columnar epithelium** with **goblet cells**.
- The underlying **lamina propria** contain fine connective tissue fibers and lymphatic tissue.
- In the deeper part **longitudinal elastic membrane** is present that divides lamina propria from submucosa.
- **Submucosa** consists of connective tissue fibers, tubuloacinar seromucous tracheal gland and ducts opening to tracheal lumen.
- The **'C' shaped hyaline cartilage** is present in incomplete ring which form the frame work and is surrounded by connective tissue perichondrium.
- The **chondrocytes** in the lacunae are larger and become flatter towards perichondrium.
- The gap between the posterior ends of cartilage is filled by **trachealis muscle**.

Applied Anatomy

- Cilia filters out all foreign particles that enter the body during inhalation.
- Smoking destroys cilia allowing bacteria, viruses, etc., to enter the body and produces diseases like pneumonia.
- Tracheostomy consists of making an incision on the anterior aspect of neck and opening a direct airway through a direct incision in the trachea.

Viva voce

Q. What is the distinctive structural component wall of the trachea?
Ans. Cartilage rings.
Q. What type of epithelium lines the tracheal lumen?
Ans. Tracheal lumen is lined by pseudostratified ciliated columnar epithelium with goblet cells.
Q. What is the characteristic feature of submucosa layer in trachea?
Ans. Submucosa consists of connective tissue fibers, tubuloacinar seromucous tracheal gland and ducts opening to tracheal lumen.

TRACHEA

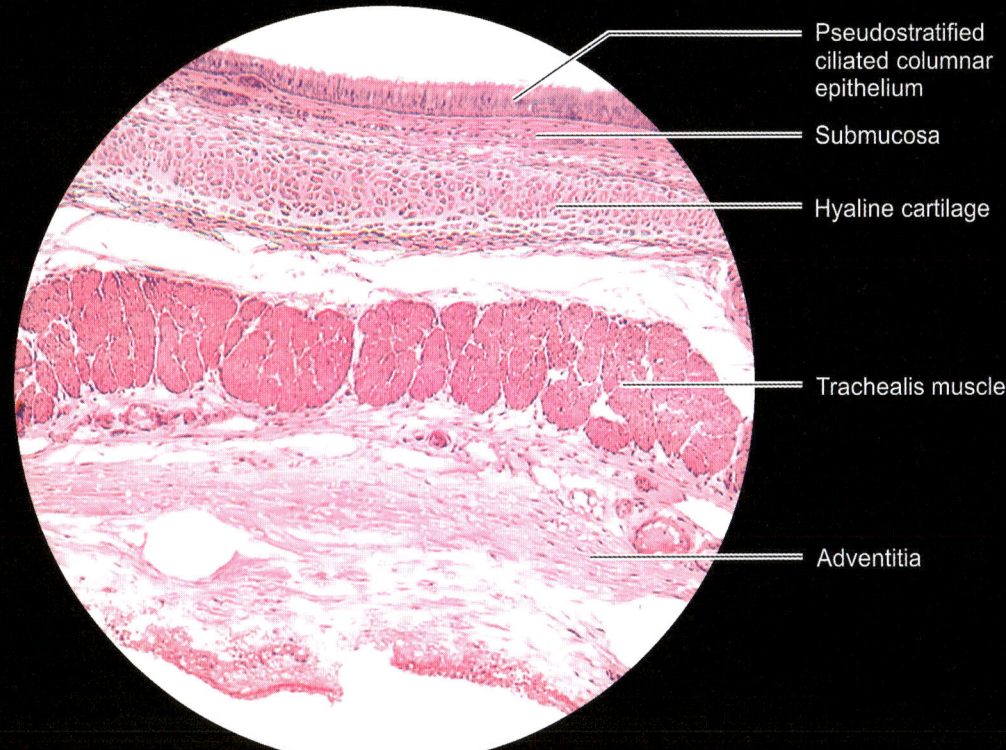

SP:
- Presence of hyaline cartilaginous plates.
- Presence of mucous and serous glands in lamina propria.

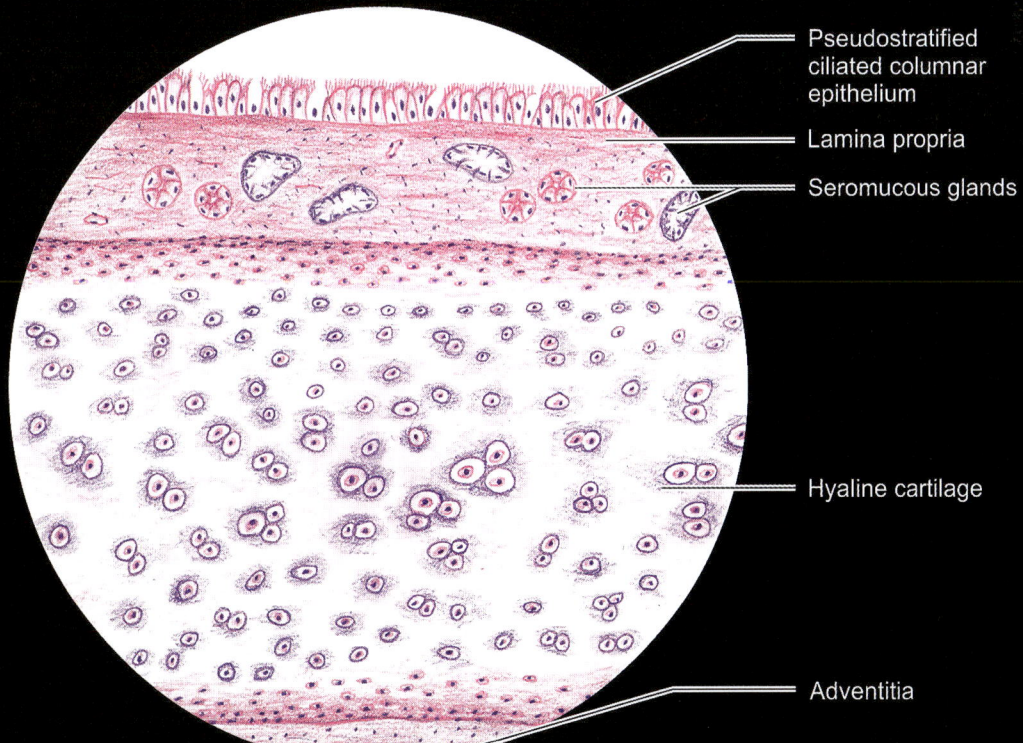

LUNG

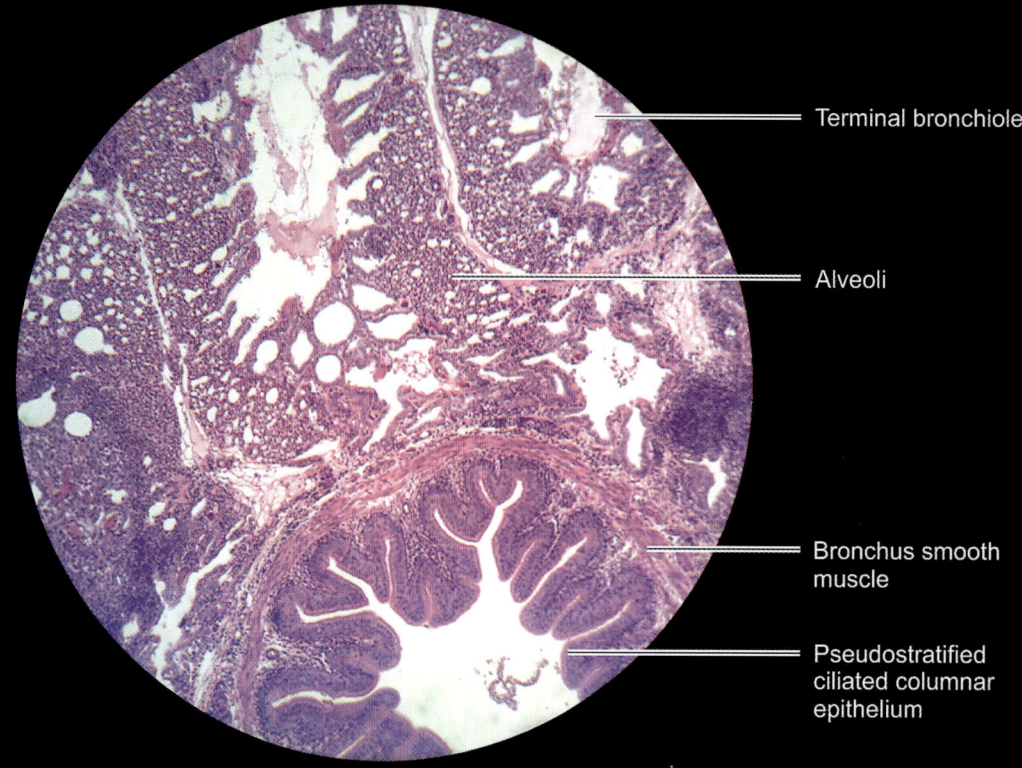

SP:
- Presence of various bronchioles.
- Presence of alveoli lined by simple squamous epithelium.

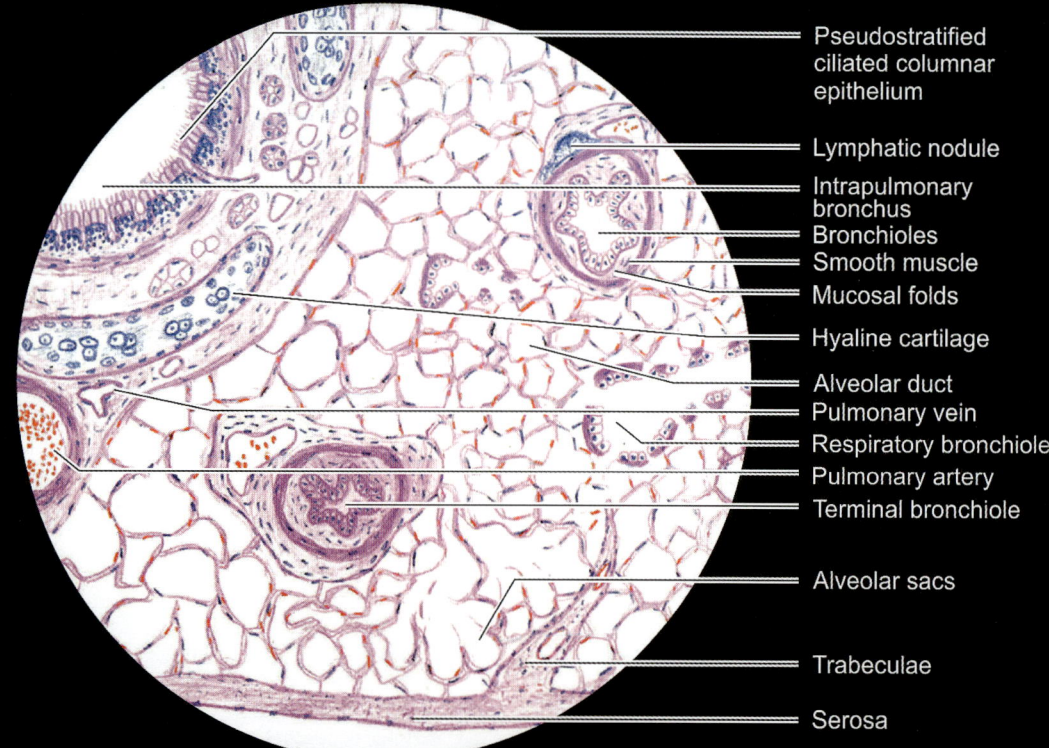

LUNG

- Consists of intrapulmonary bronchus (2° or 3° bronchi), bronchiole, terminal bronchiole, respiratory bronchiole and parenchyma.
- **Parenchyma** is composed of alveolar duct and alveoli.
- **Intrapulmonary bronchus** is identified by surrounding hyaline cartilage plates, lined by pseudostratified ciliated epithelium.
- Consists of thin **lamina propria**, small layer of **smooth muscle, submucosa with bronchial glands, hyaline cartilage and adventitia**.
- **Bronchiole** lined by **pseudostratified columnar ciliated epithelium**, lumen shows mucosal folds, smooth muscle present, adventitia present, glands and cartilage are absent.
- **Terminal bronchiole** is lined by **ciliated low columnar epithelium**, characterized by irregular lumen, smooth muscle layer and adventitia present.
- **Respiratory bronchiole** is lined by columnar or cuboidal cells with cilia, thin connective tissue cells with smooth muscle and elastic fibers seen in association with alveoli.
- **Alveolar duct** formed from respiratory bronchiole, smooth muscle bundles are present in the rim of the duct.
- **Alveoli** lined by thin simple squamous cells, share a common interalveolar septum numerous capillaries are present in these septa, at the free ends of the septa and open end of alveoli narrow band of smooth muscle is present.

Applied Anatomy

- In interstitial lung disease like pulmonary eosinophilia, there will be thickening of alveolar septa with infiltration of eosinophils.
- In bronchioalveolar carcinoma, the tumor cells lines the alveolar septa and thus giving an alveolar appearance to the tumor.

Viva voce

Q. What is the importance of elastin in the respiratory system?
Ans. Allows for expandability and return to original volume during expiration.
Q. Which cells are responsible from keeping the lungs free from obstructing particulate matter? How do they carry out this function?
Ans. Macrophages (dust cells). By means of phagocytosis.

RENAL SYSTEM

KIDNEY

- Consists of an outermost capsule, i.e., **the renal capsule**. Beneath it is the outer dark cortex and inner lighter medulla.
- **Cortex** consists of both **proximal convoluted tubule (PCT)** and **distal convoluted tubule (DCT)**, renal corpuscle, interlobular arteries and veins, and medullary rays (formed by straight portions of nephrons blood vessels, and collecting tubules that join in medulla to form collecting ducts) and these do not extend to capsule.
- **Medulla** consists of **renal pyramids** and base of each pyramid is adjacent to cortex and apex forms the renal papilla which projects to minor calyx which is the dilated portion of ureter and they joins to form major calyx which then join to form the renal pelvis.
- The renal **corpuscle** consists of **Bowman's capsule and glomerulus**. Bowman's capsule is made of an outer parietal layer and inner visceral layer. Outer layer is made by simple squamous epithelium and inner layer by specialized cells called **podocytes**.
- **Glomerulus** is made of tuft of anastomosing capillaries lined by fenestrated epithelium.
- **PCT** is lined by simple cuboidal epithelium with microvilli giving **brush bordered appearance**.
- The thin segment of **loop of Henle** is lined by simple squamous epithelium and is permeable to water and sodium whereas thick segment is lined by cuboidal epithelium and is impermeable to water.
- **DCT** is lined by simple cuboidal epithelium and is not brush bordered.
- The **collecting tubules** are lined by simple cuboidal epithelium whereas collecting ducts are by simple columnar epithelium.

Applied Anatomy

In membranous glomerulonephritis there is diffuse thickening of glomerular basement membrane with subepithelial deposit of immunoglobulins.

Viva voce

Q. What is the functional significance of the occurrence of a brush border in the proximal tubule?
Ans. The brush border increases the surface area, facilitating the reabsorption that occurs in the proximal tubule.

KIDNEY

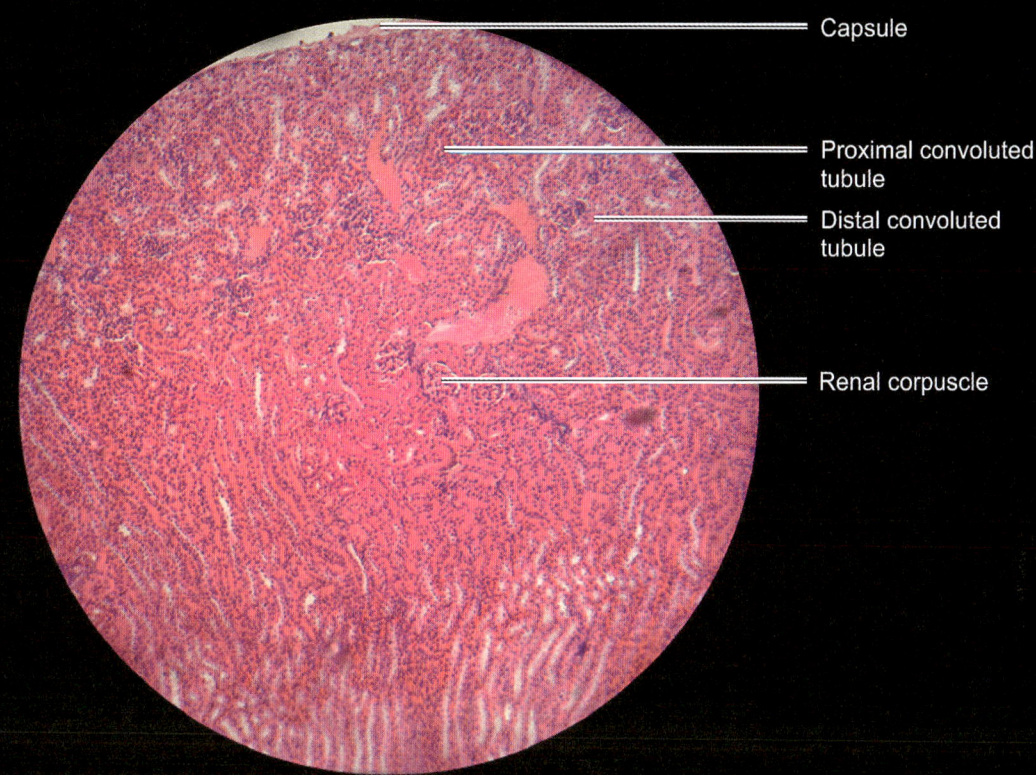

SP:
- Presence of cortex and medulla with cut sections of PCT, DCT, etc.
- Presence of medullary rays and renal corpuscles.

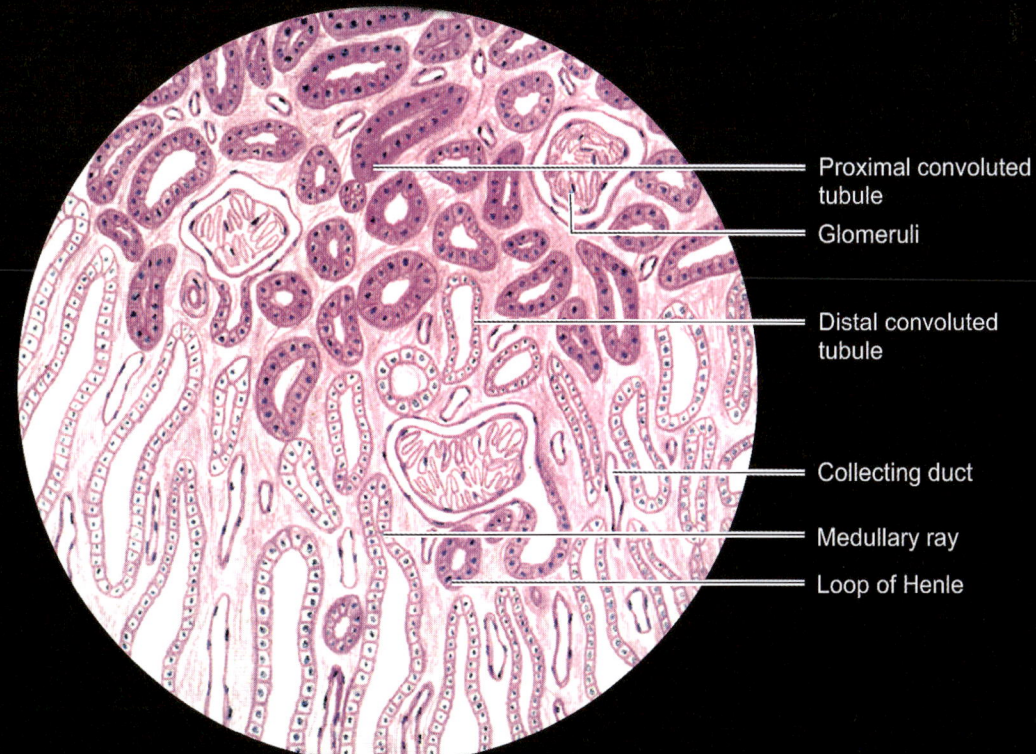

URETER

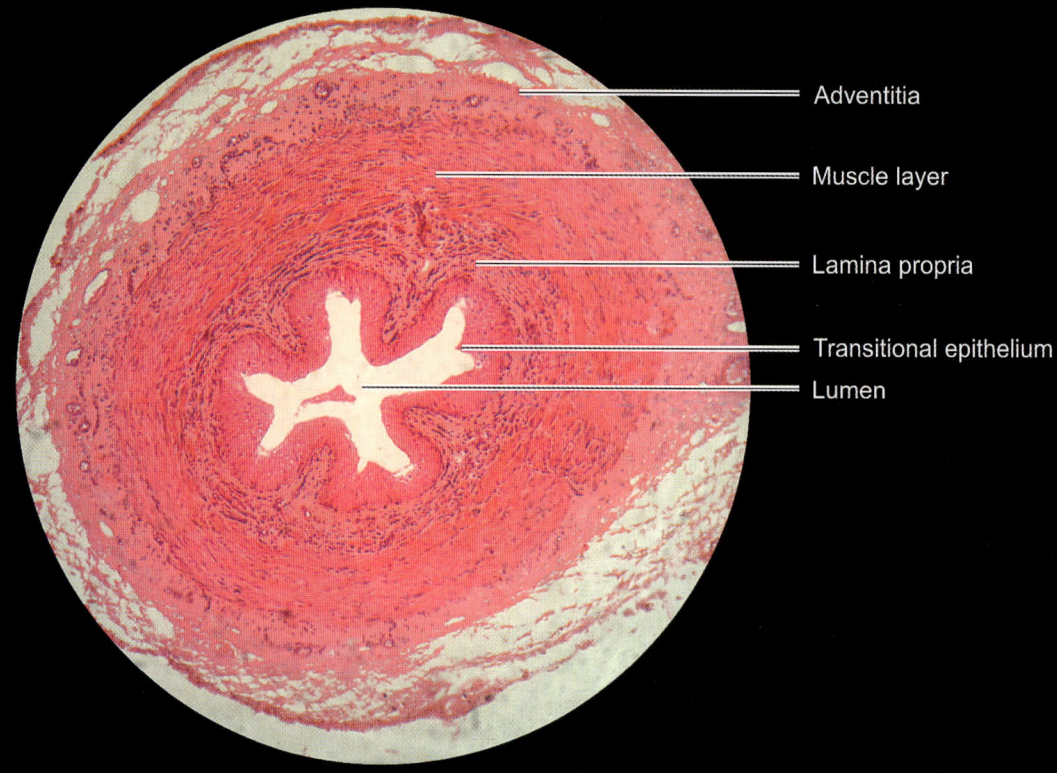

SP:
- Presence of star-shaped lumen lined by transitional epithelium.
- Presence of three muscle coats.

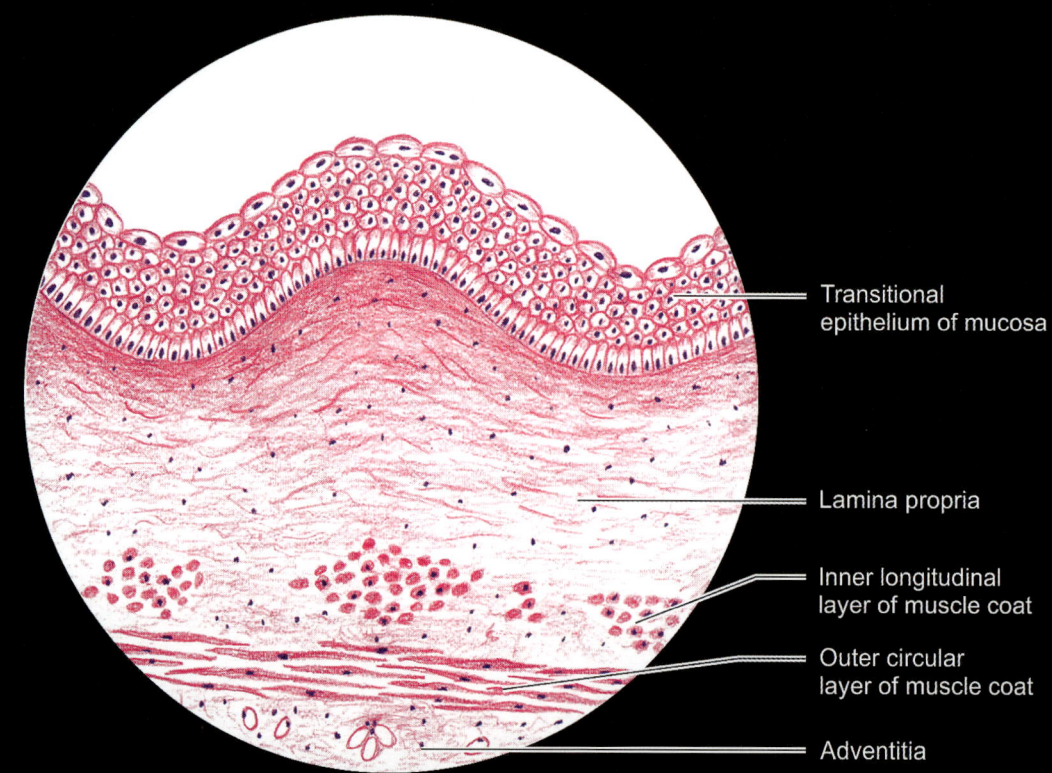

URETER

- Made of three layers:
  1. **Mucosa**
  2. **Muscle coat**
  3. **Adventitia**.
- **Mucosa** consisting of **transitional epithelium** and lamina propria.
- **Lamina propria** consists of supporting connective tissue rich in elastic fibers.
- **Mucosa** is thrown into folds giving **star-shaped** appearance.
- **Muscle coat**—consisting of smooth muscle fibers arranged in two layers.
  - **Inner longitudinal** layer.
  - **Outer circular** layer.
  - Additional **outer longitudinal** layer is present in lower 1/3rd of ureter located near the bladder.
- **Adventitia** is made up of loose connective tissue with blood vessels, lymphatics, nerves and adipose tissue.

Applied Anatomy

- A descending ureteric calculus produces loin to groin pain and is colicky type of pain.
- A ureteric calculus is often associated with hematuria.
- When the stone is imapcted, the colic goes off and causes a dull ache.
- Stone in the ureter is visualized using intravenous pyelography or cystoscopy.
- Transitional cell carcinoma is a common cause of ureteric cancer and other urinary tract cancers.

Viva voce

Q. What is the functional importance of thick muscular coat?
Ans. Urine is squeezed into the urinary bladder by means of peristalsis.
Q. What is functional importance of folded mucosa?
Ans. The folded mucosa protects against the reflux of urine when the bladder is full.

URINARY BLADDER

- Consists of three layers:
  1. **Mucosal** layer
  2. **Muscle coat**
  3. **Adventitia**
- **Mucosa**—made of **transitional epithelium** and lamina propria.
- **Transitional epithelium** or **urothelium** is binucleate and when the bladder is empty it exhibits five to six layers and folds.
- But when the bladder is distended, the epithelium is thin, consists of 3-4 layers and the superficial cells are flattened.
- **Muscle coat** is made up of three loosely arranged indistinctive layers of smooth muscle fibers:
  1. **Inner longitudinally** arranged layer
  2. **Middle circularly** arranged layer
  3. **Outer longitudinally** arranged layer
- Adventitia is made of fibroelastic connective tissue with blood vessels, nerves and lymphatics.

Applied Anatomy

- Transitional epithelium has the following function here:
  - Protects mucosa from being corroded by acidic pH of urine.
  - Acts as an osmotic barrier.
  - They are nonabsorptive in function.
- Detrusor muscle is layer of urinary bladder wall and problems with this muscle layer can lead to incontinence.

Viva voce

Q. Which part of the urinary bladder can undergo malignant changes?
Ans. Urothelium.
Q. What is the typical feature of transitional epithelium?
Ans. Transitional epithelium is binucleate and when the bladder is empty it exhibits five to six layers and folds and when the bladder is distended, the epithelium is thin, consists of 3-4 layers and the superficial cells are flattened.

URINARY BLADDER

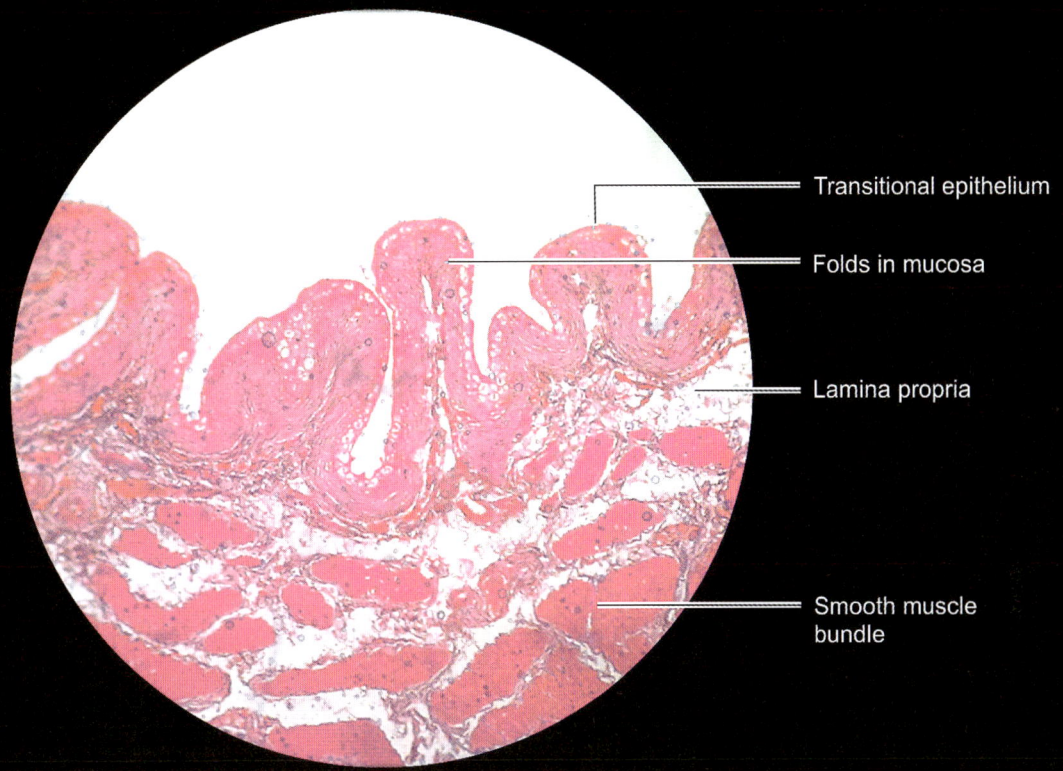

SP:
- Presence of transitional epithelial lining.
- Presence of ill-defined muscle coat.

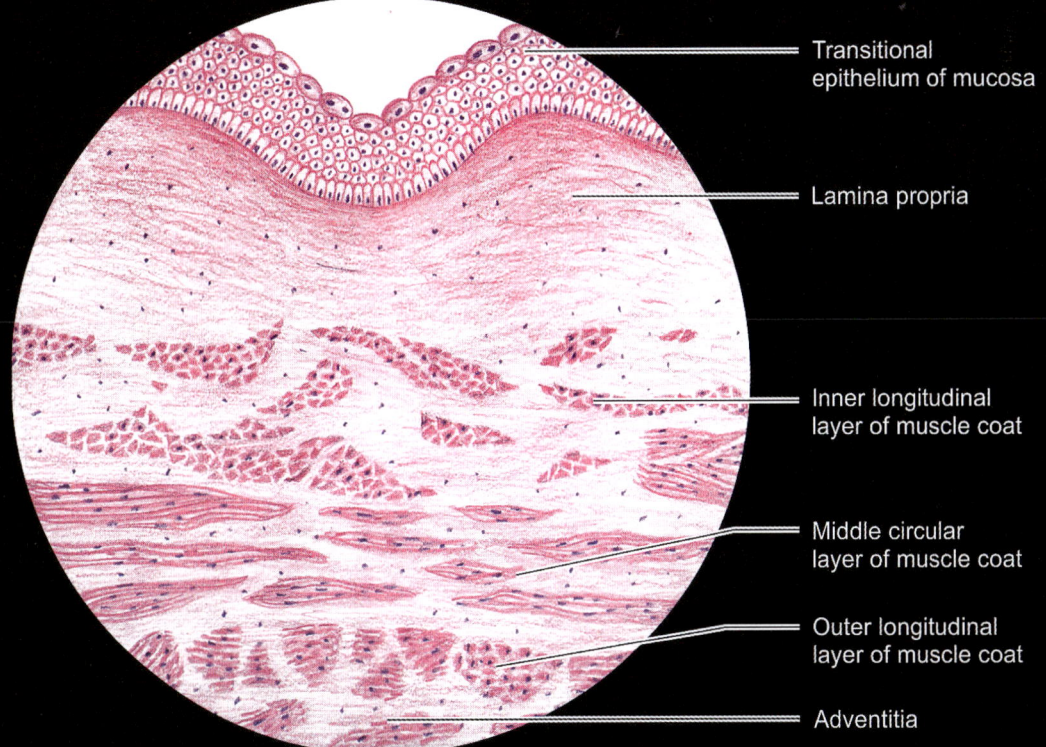

THICK SKIN

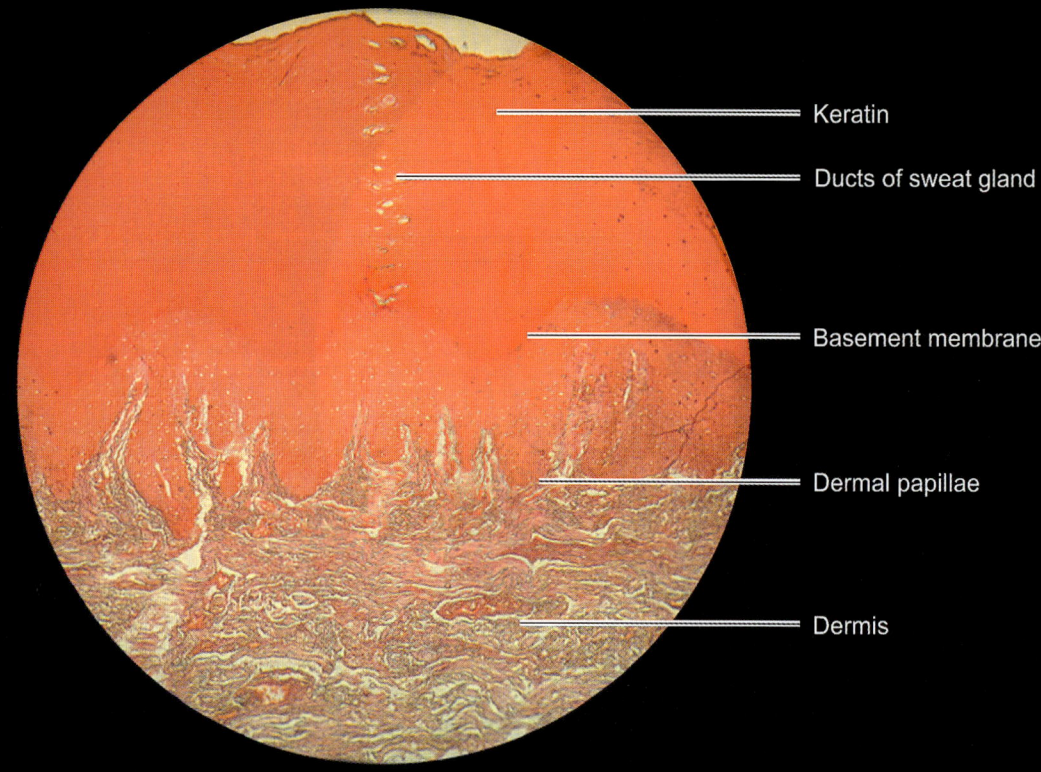

SP:
- Presence of dermis and thick epidermis.
- Presence of dermis with sweat glands.

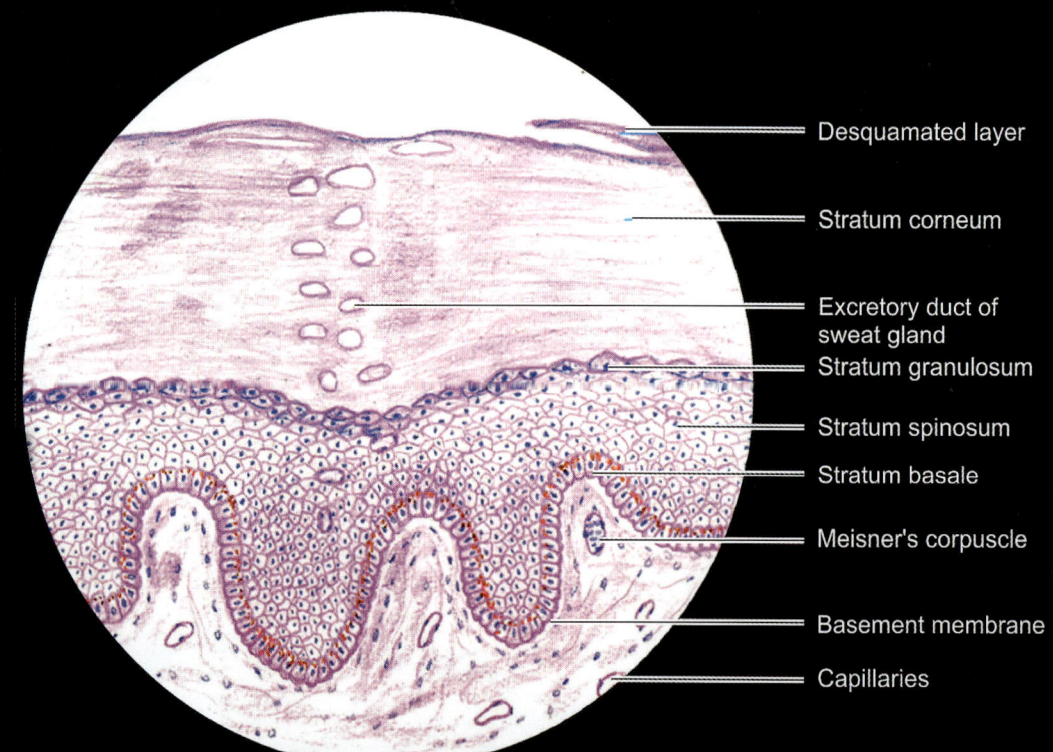

SKIN

GENERAL ASPECT

- Skin, its derivatives and appendages constitute the integumentary system.
- It is the largest organ in the body.
- Skin consists of two distinct regions viz. **epidermis and dermis**.
- These two layers are separated by a basement membrane.

Epidermis
- Superficial region.
- Lined by **keratinized stratified squamous epithelium**.
- Nonvascular.
- Five layers are seen in this region (from deep to superficial).
    I. **Stratum basale:**
        - Deepest layer of epidermis.
        - Consists of simple columnar cells.
        - Contains specialized sensory cells called **cells of Merkel**.
    II. **Stratum spinosum:**
        - Consists of several layers of polyhedral cells.
        - Cells are held together by **desmosomes**.
    III. **Stratum granulosum:**
        - Made up of 3–5 layers of flattened fusiform shaped cells.
        - Cells contain keratohyalin granules (basophilic) and membrane coating granules.
    VI. **Stratum lucidum:**
        - Homogenous glassy layer of flattened dead cells (eosinophilic).
        - Cytoplasm contains keratin.
        - Nuclei and organelles not evident.
    V. **Stratum corneum:**
        - Superficial layer of epidermis.
        - Made up of flattened, non nucleated, dead, scaly keratinized cells.
        - Cytoplasm filled with keratin.

Dermis
- This region is present inferior to epidermis.
- It is homologous to the lamina propria of the mucous membrane.
- Vascular in nature.
- Contains dense irregular connective tissue fibers.
- Dermis can be subdivided into two layers:
    1. **Superficial papillary layer:**
        - Contains sweat glands, loose connective tissue, fibroblasts, mast cells, etc.
        - Meisner's corpuscle (sensory receptor) present in this layer.
    2. **Deep reticular layer:**
        - Contains irregular collagenous connective tissue (type I).
        - **Pacinian corpuscle (sensory receptor)** present in this layer.

THICK SKIN

- **Epidermis** is very thick due to the thick stratum corneum layer.
- Hair follicles and sebaceous glands are **absent**.
- **Sweat glands** are present in dermis.

THIN SKIN
- **Epidermis** is very thin due to the thin stratum corneum.
- **Contains** hair follicles and sebaceous glands.
- Sweat glands present in dermis.

Applied Anatomy
- In squamous cell carcinoma cells of the stratum spinosum layer are affected.
- In psoriasis cells of the stratum basale layer proliferate very rapidly and undergo keratinization very early, it leads to increased thickness of skin and raised red patches under white scale.
- Membrane coating granules present in the cells discharge their contents into granular layer providing the epidermis a sealing effect against foreign materials.

Viva voce
Q. What are the cell junctions in the stratum spinosum?
Ans. Desmosomes
Q. Where are the melanocytes located?
Ans. Stratum basale
Q. Where are cells of Merkel present?
Ans. Stratum basale
Q. Where are Meisner's corpuscles present?
Ans. Superficial papillary layer of dermis
Q. Where are Pacinian corpuscles present?
Ans. Deep reticular layer of dermis.
Q. What are the characteristic features of the stratum lucidum layer?
Ans. Homogenous glassy layer of flattened dead cells, cytoplasm contains keratin, and nucleus and organelles are not evident.

THIN SKIN

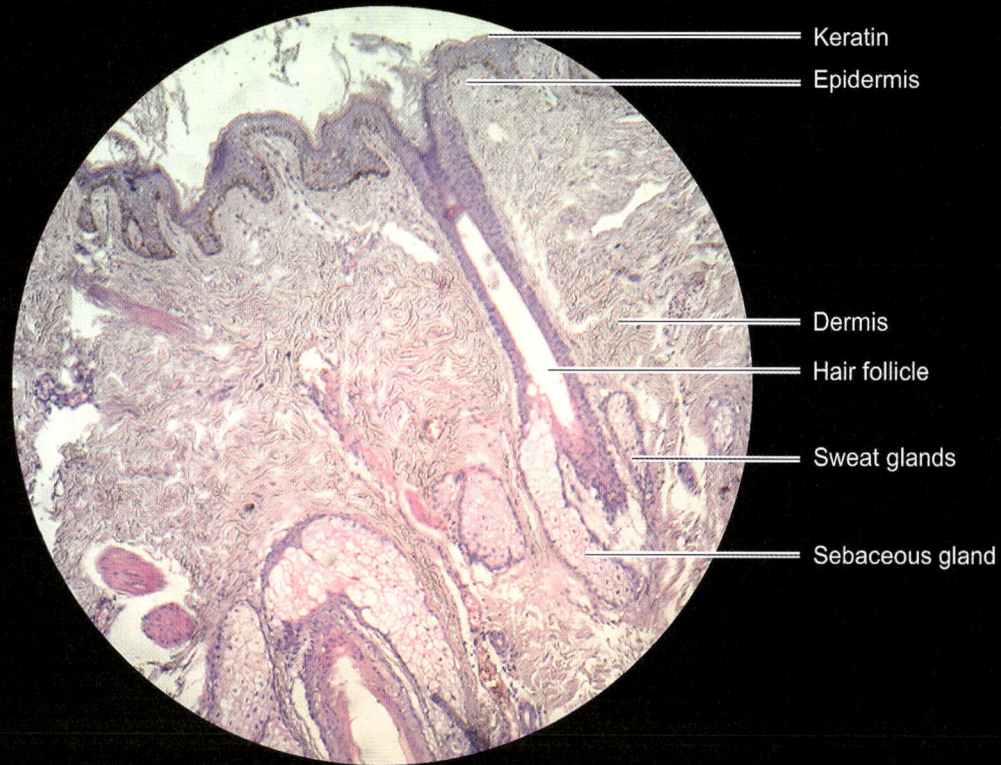

SP:
- Presence of dermis and epidermis.
- Presence of dermis with hair follicles and sebaceous glands.

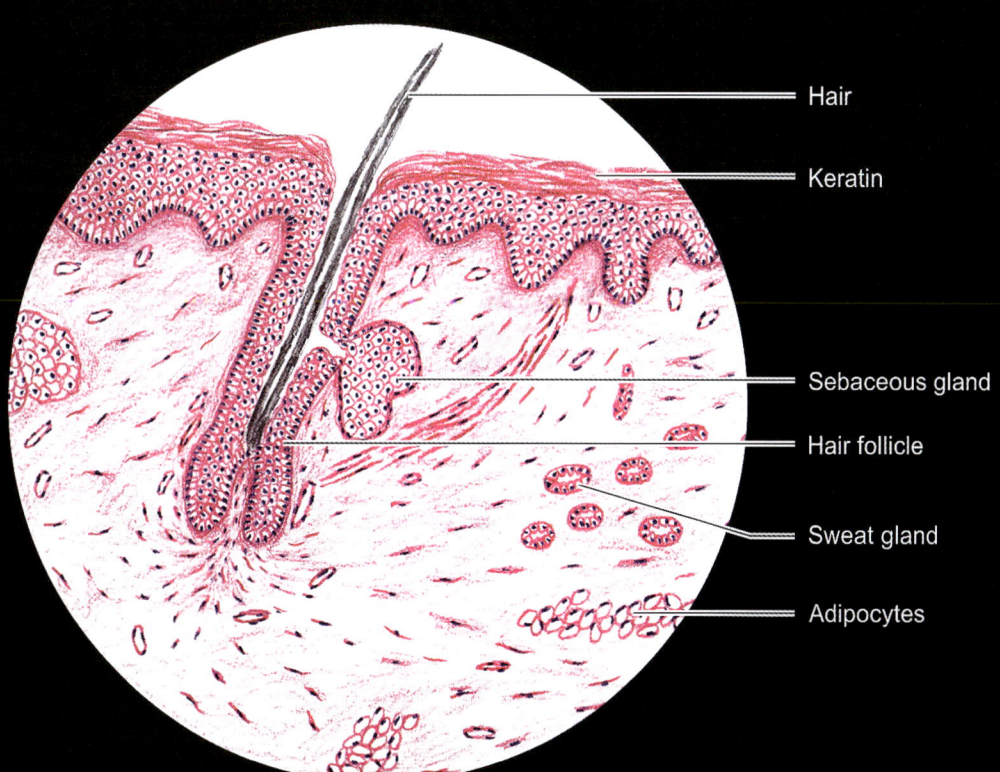

CORNEA

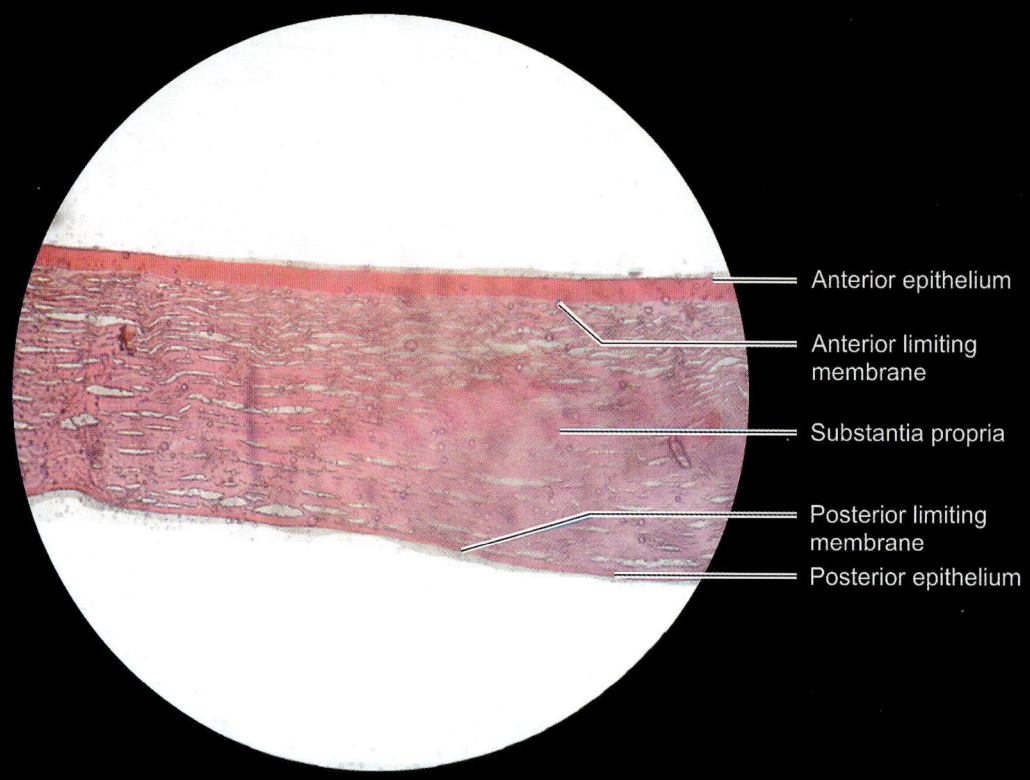

SP:
- Presence of anterior limiting lamina.
- Presence of thick substantia propria with keratocytes.

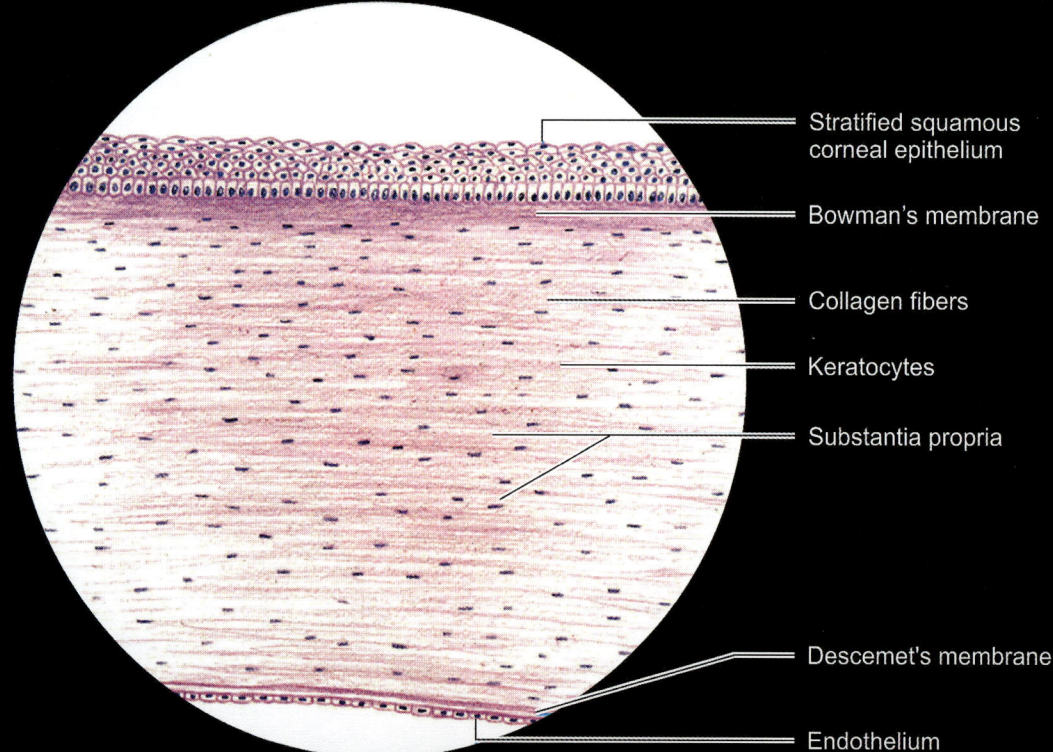

SPECIAL SENSES

CORNEA

- It is a **thick, transparent, and nonvascular** structure.
- It is composed of five layers.
    1. **Anterior (corneal) epithelium** made up of **nonkeratinized stratified squamous epithelium.**
    2. **Bowman's membrane (anterior limiting membrane)**: Acellular layer made up of compactly packed collagen fibers.
    3. **Corneal stroma (substantia propria)** consists of bundles of collagen fibers arranged in layers, parallel to the surface of the cornea.
    4. **Descemet's membrane (posterior limiting membrane)**: Made up of collagen fibers, separates substantia propria from endothelium.
    5. **Corneal endothelium** is lined by a single layer of squamous epithelium; it forms the posterior surface of cornea.

Applied Anatomy

- Due to its avascular nature:
    1. Transparency of cornea is maintained.
    2. Chances of endogenous infections are rare.
    3. Corneal transplants are not immunologically rejected.
- Corneal abrasion involves loss of surface epithelial layer due to trauma.
- In corneal dystrophy one or more parts loses its normal clarity.
- Corneal neovascularization is due to excessive ingrowth of blood vessels from limbal vascular plexus into the cornea caused by lack of oxygen from air.

Viva voce

Q. What is Descemet's membrane madeup of?
Ans. It is made up of collagen fibers and it separates substantia propria from endothelium.
Q. What is the other name of anterior limiting membrane?
Ans. Bowman's membrane.
Q. What kind of epithelium lines the corneal endothelium?
Ans. Corneal endothelium is lined by a single layer of squamous epithelium.

RETINA

- **Innermost coat** of the eyeball.
- In total, the retina is made up of **ten layers**.
- **Pigment layer** made of pigmented cuboidal cells.
- **Nervous layer** is a layer made by **outer and inner segments of rods and cones** whose tips are surrounded by processes of pigment cells.
- **External limiting membrane** separates rods and cones from the dense outer nuclear layer.
- **Outer nuclear layer** contains the nuclei of rods and cones and outer processes of **Müller's cells**.
- **Outer plexiform layer**, where the axons of rods and cones synapse with dendrites of horizontal cells.
- **Inner nuclear layer** is a dense layer of cell bodies of bipolar neurons.
- **Inner plexiform layer** where the axons of bipolar cells synapse with dendrites of ganglion and amacrine cells.
- **Ganglion cell layer** contains cell bodies of ganglion cells and neuroglial cells.
- **Optic nerve fiber layer** is made up of bundles of unmyelinated axons of ganglion cells and inner fibers of Müller's cells.
- **Internal limiting membrane**—formed by expanded basal ends of Müller's cells with basement membrane.

Applied Anatomy

- In nonproliferative type of diabetic retinopathy, there will be thickening of capillary basement membrane. Whereas in case of proliferative type of diabetic retinopathy there will be neovascularization of retina.
- **Retinoblastoma:** One of the common tumors of childhood. It arises from retinal neurons.
- Since the pigment cell layer is more firmly attached to the choroid than to the nervous layer, in myopies retinal detachment usually occurs, leading to blindness.
- Posterior (¾)th part of the retina is called the optic part since it is photosensitive and derived from the walls of the optic cup.

Viva voce

Q. What are Müller's cells?
Ans. These are supportive cells for the neurons of the retina and have the ability of dedifferentiation to form particular cells when there is injury.

RETINA

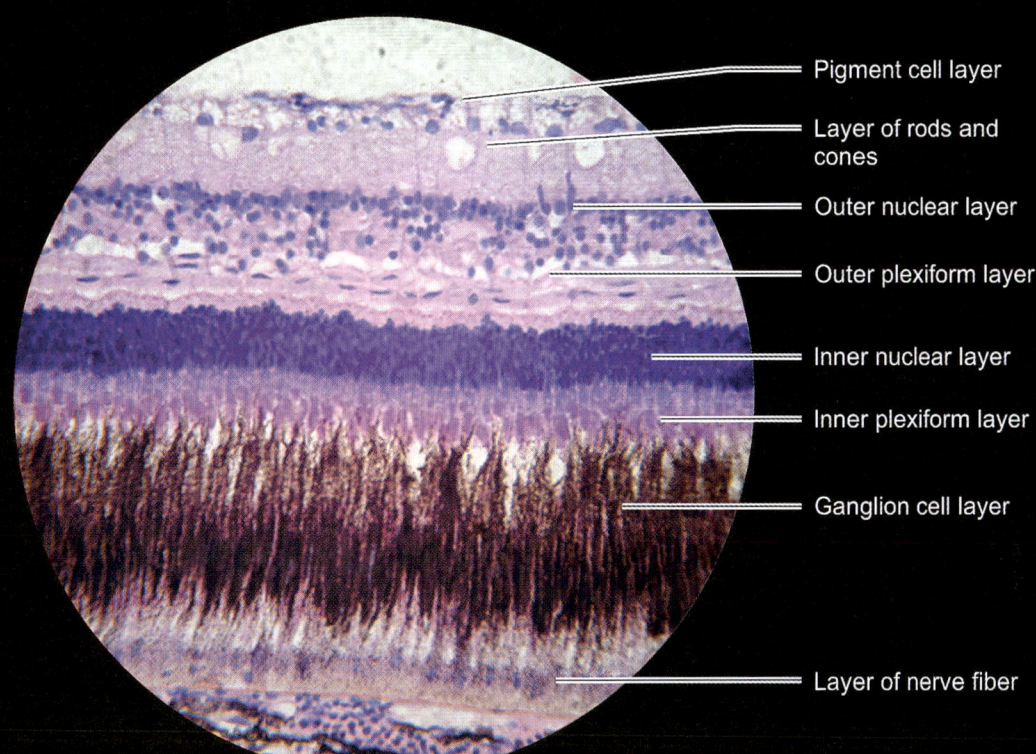

SP:
- Presence of ten layers.
- Presence of external and internal limiting lamina.

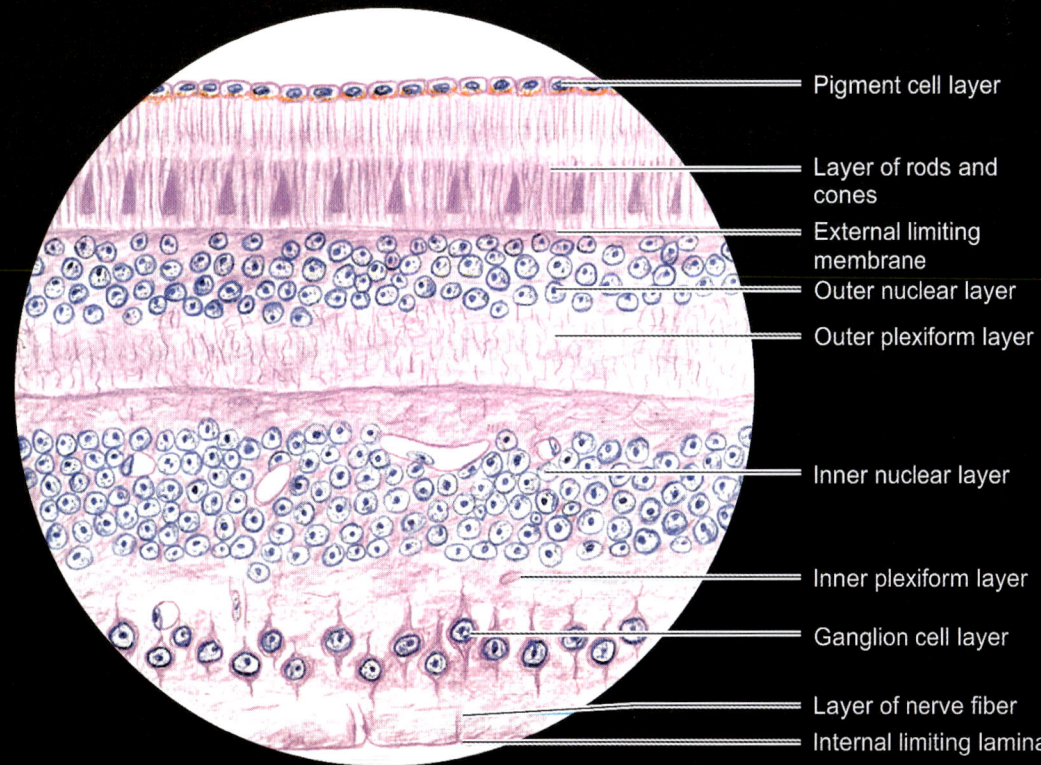

OPTIC NERVE

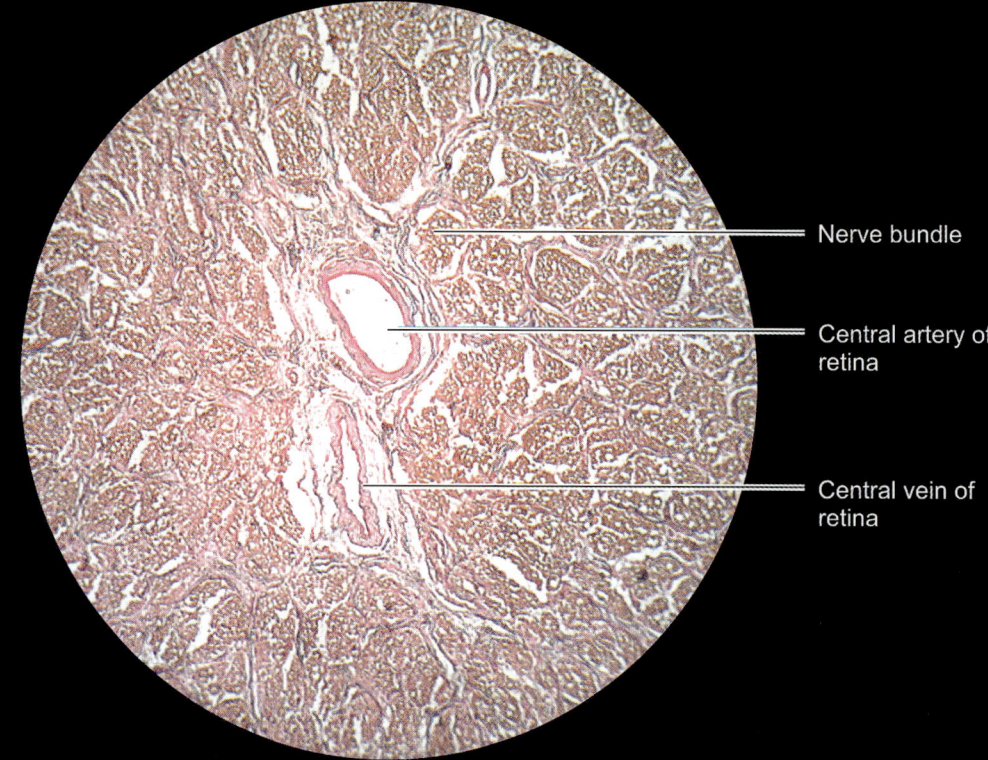

SP:
- Presence of three layers of meninges.
- Presence of central artery and vein along with nerve fiber bundles.

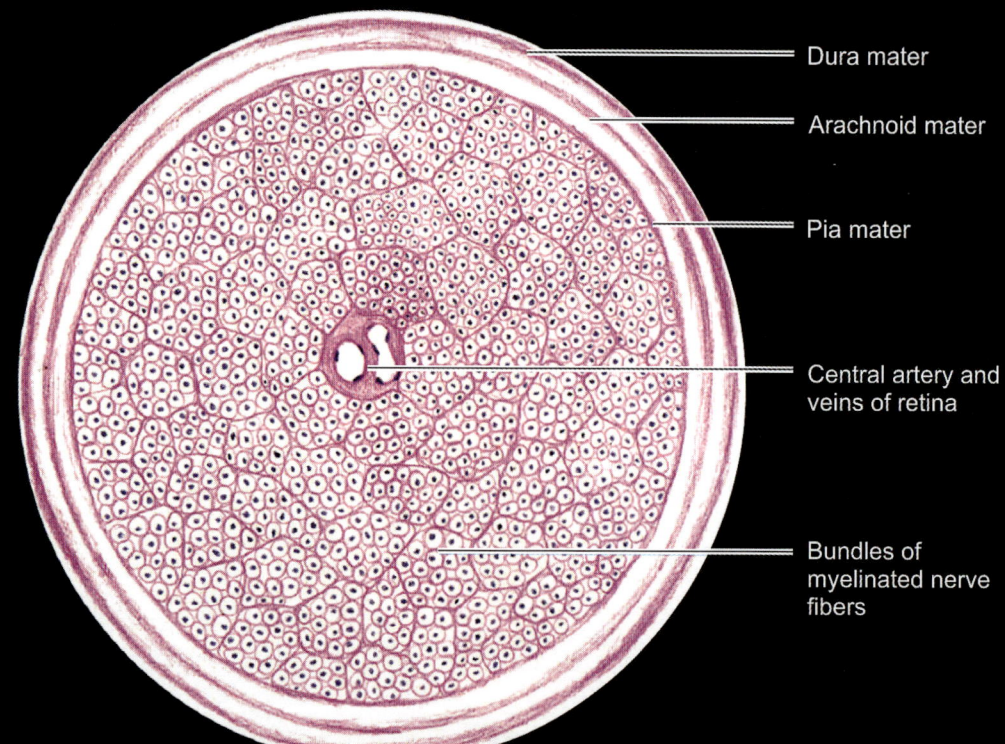

OPTIC NERVE

- It is covered by **dura mater, arachnoid mater and pia mater**.
- Within the covering bundles of nerve fibers surrounded by **astrocytes** are seen.
- Each bundle contains many **myelinated nerve fiber axons** of varying caliber.
- **Nerve fibers** are derived from the ganglion cells of the retina.
- These bundles also contain a small number of **pupillomotor fibers** and some **centrifugal fibers**.
- **A central artery and vein** are present at the center.

Applied Anatomy

- Optic nerve is not covered by neurilemma, which is present in other peripheral nerves. As a result, the optic nerve can not regenerate when it is cut.
- The optic nerve fibers develop from the nerve fiber layer of the retina which grow into optic stalks by passing through choroidal fissure and pass posteriorly into the brain.
- Lesions of the optic nerve are characterized by marked loss of vision or complete blindness on the affected side and associated with loss of direct light reflex in the ipsilateral side.
- Common lesions of optic nerve include optic atrophy, trauma, avulsion, indirect optic neuropathy, acute optic neuritis, etc.
- Congenital anomalies of optic nerve include medullated or opaque nerve fibers and result in enlargement of blind spot.

Viva voce

Q. What are the supportive cells present in the optic nerve?
Ans. Astrocytes
Q. From which structure do nerve fibers of the optic nerve develop from?
Ans. Nerve fibers are derived from the ganglion cells of the retina.

FEMALE REPRODUCTIVE SYSTEM

MAMMARY GLAND

- Consists of mainly parenchyma and stroma.
- Both of these components differ in case of lactating gland as well as a nonlactating one.

In nonlactating gland:
- **Parenchyma** consists of **less glandular tissue, poorly developed alveoli** having a solid cord of cells, extensive branching of the duct system, duct lumen poorly visible, tubules and ducts are lined by **cuboidal epithelium**.
- **Stroma** contains more connective tissue and adipose tissue, interlobular connective tissue septum is **thick**, abundant intralobular loose connective tissue with numerous **fibroblasts**.

In lactating gland:
- **Parenchyma** having **more glandular tissue** with **proliferated tubules** enlarged to alveoli which is highly developed, external branching of alveolar ducts and large ducts being lined by **stratified epithelium**.
- **Lumen is filled** with milk and contains fat droplets.
- **Stroma: Less connective tissue** and adipose tissue, interlobular connective tissue septum is **thin**, intralobular connective tissue is less and contains **lymphocytes and plasma cells**.

Applied Anatomy

- In normal mammary gland alveoli are small and few in number whereas in lactating one alveoli are enlarged and distended and number of ducts also increase.
- The cancers arising from the ductal portion of breast are called ductal carcinomas and cancers arising from the lobules are called lobular carcinomas.
- Metastasis from one breast to another or to other sites can occur.

Viva voce

Q. What are the major hormones responsible for the cyclic changes in the mammary gland?
Ans. Estrogen and progesterone.

MAMMARY GLAND

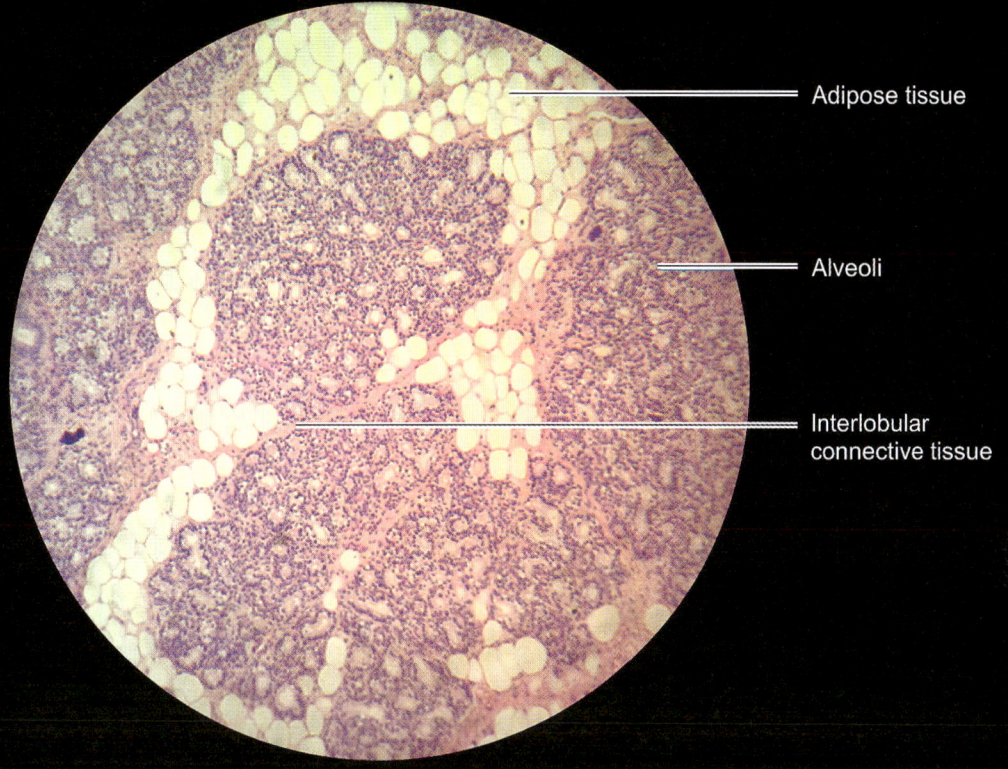

SP:
- Presence of secretory acinar tissue.
- Presence of intralobular CT, interlobular CT and their ducts.

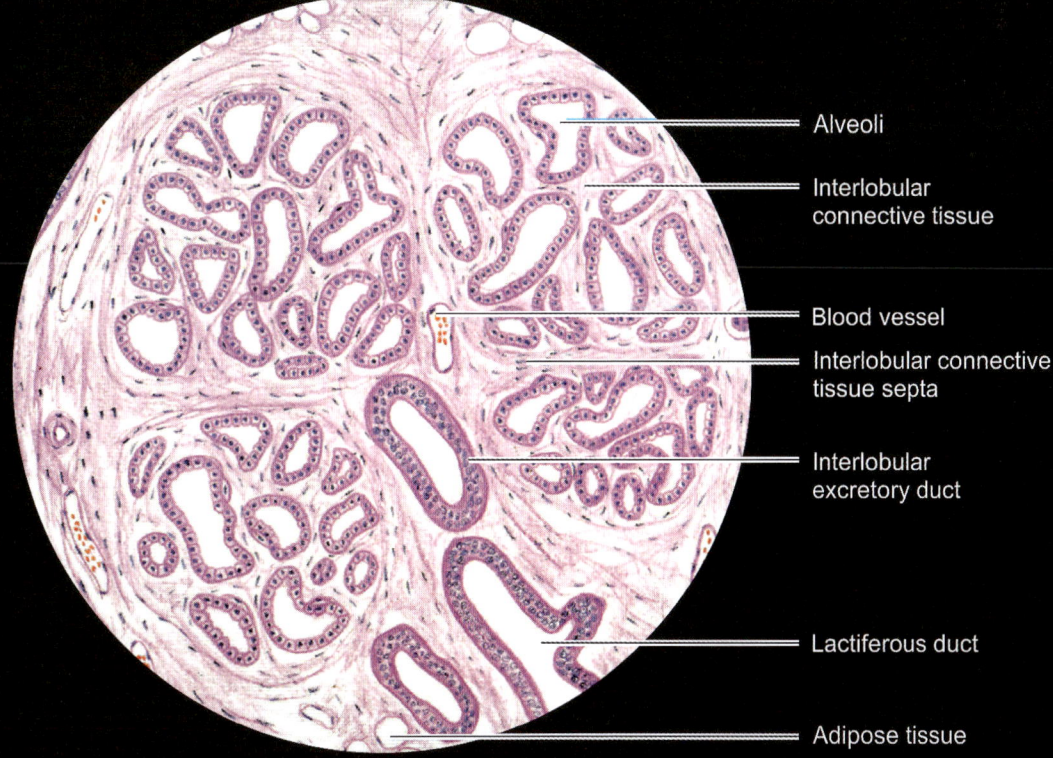

OVARY

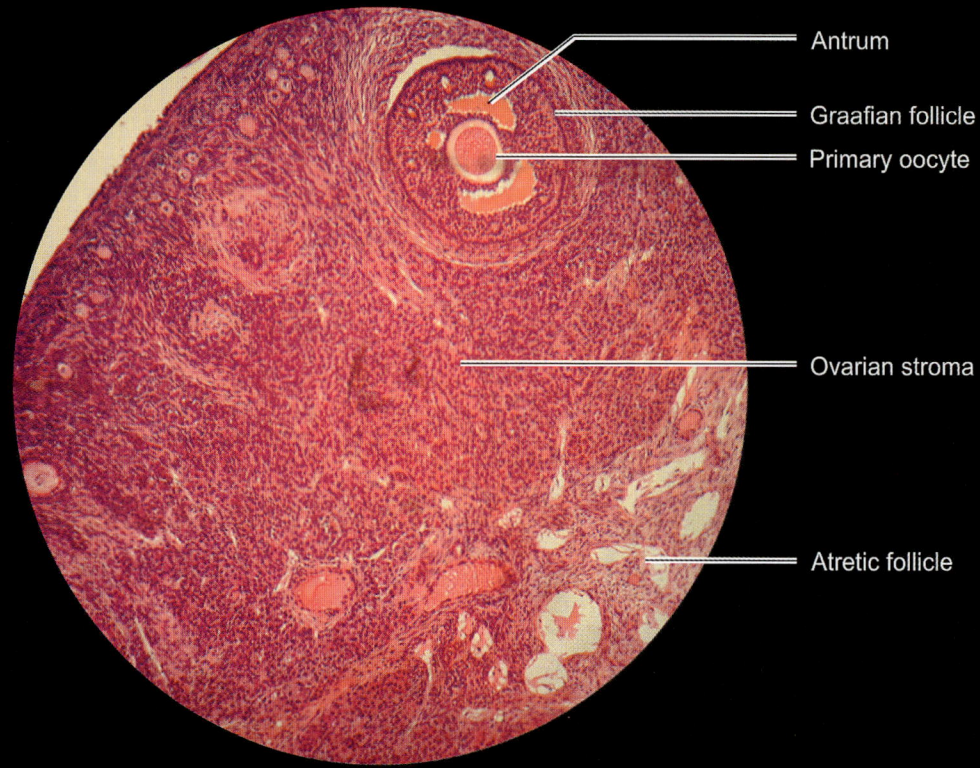

SP:
- Presence of follicles with oocytes in different stages of maturity.
- Presence of germinal epithelium.

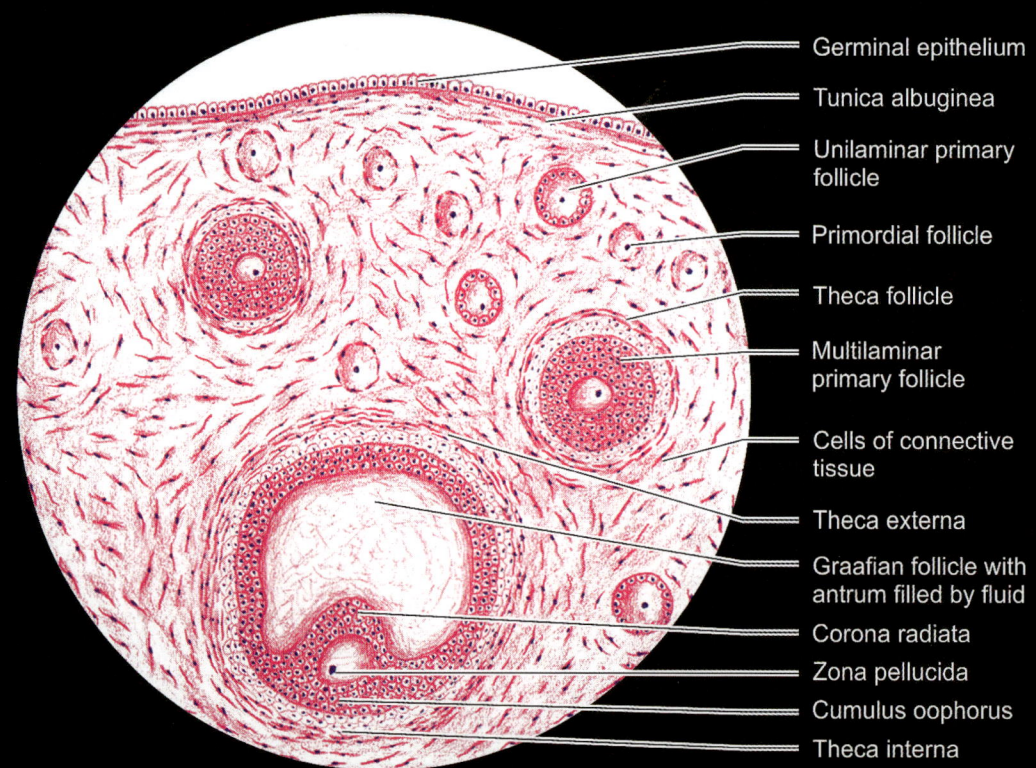

OVARY

- Lined by **simple cuboidal epithelium called as germinal epithelium** which is continuous with mesothelium of peritoneum.
- Beneath the epithelium a layer of dense connective tissue is present called **tunica albuginea**.
- Exhibits cortex and medulla arrangement.
- **Cortex** occupies the most part and contains **stroma** (dense reticular fibers and spindle shaped cells with no fibrils) and **ovarian follicles** of different stages (also **atretic follicles, corpus luteum, corpus albicans**).
- **Medulla** is made of loose fibroelastic connective tissue and contains blood vessels, lymphatics and nerves and is continuous with the mesovarium of the peritoneum.
- **The primary ovarian follicles** and corpus luteum follicles possess a large central cell and a surrounding flattened cell layer whereas the secondary follicle is multilayered.
- And the largest of all the **Graafian follicle** is seen with varying sizes and lines near surface and consists of:
    - **Oocytes** surrounded by **ooplasm** or yolk.
    - **Ovum** covered by **zona pellucida**.
    - Surrounded by **membrana granulosa** having **cumulus oophorus** and **discus proligerus** and a follicular cavity embedded in it called **antrum folliculi**.
    - **Theca folliculi** comprising of theca externa and theca interna.

Applied Anatomy

- **Polycystic ovary:** It is a condition characterized by the presence of numerous cysts in the ovary. The cysts are lined by granulosa cells.
- **Mucinous tumor of ovary:** Also cystic tumors, it consists of hundreds of cysts which are filled with mucin.

Viva voce

Q. What is the lining epithelium of the ovary?
Ans. Lined by simple cuboidal epithelium called as germinal epithelium.
Q. What is the primary ovarian source of estrogenic hormones?
Ans. Granulosa cells.

FALLOPIAN TUBE

- Also known as uterine tubes.
- Made up of three layers:
  1. **Mucosa**
  2. **Muscle coat**
  3. **Serosa**
- **Mucosa** includes lining epithelium and lamina propria.
- Lined by **simple ciliated columnar epithelium**.
- Apart from **ciliated columnar cells**, it also contains some **nonciliated secretory peg cells**.
- **Ciliated columnar cells** are short and are more prominent in the proliferative phase.
- **Nonciliated peg cells** are longer than ciliated columnar cells.
- **Mucosa** consists of extensive folds, as a result the lumen becomes highly irregular which helps in providing nutrition to fertilized ovum from all sides.
- **Muscle coat** is made of two layers smooth muscles:
  1. **Inner circularly** arranged layer.
  2. **Outer longitudinally** arranged layer.
- **Serosa** consists of mesothelium (peritoneum of broad ligament) and supported by connective tissue.

Applied Anatomy

- Tubal obstruction forms one of the major causes of infertility in females.
- Tubal patency is assessed by using procedures like hysterosalpingography, laparoscopy.
- Surgical removal of fallopian tubes is called a salpingectomy.
- Propulsion of gametes and embryos is achieved by complex interaction between muscle contractions, ciliary activity and the flow of tubal secretions.

Viva voce

Q. What is the lining epithelium of mucosa of the fallopian tube?
Ans. Lined by simple ciliated columnar epithelium and nonciliated secretory peg cells.
Q. What are the characteristics of columnar cells in the proliferative phase?
Ans. The columnar cells are prominent and short in the proliferative phase.

FALLOPIAN TUBE

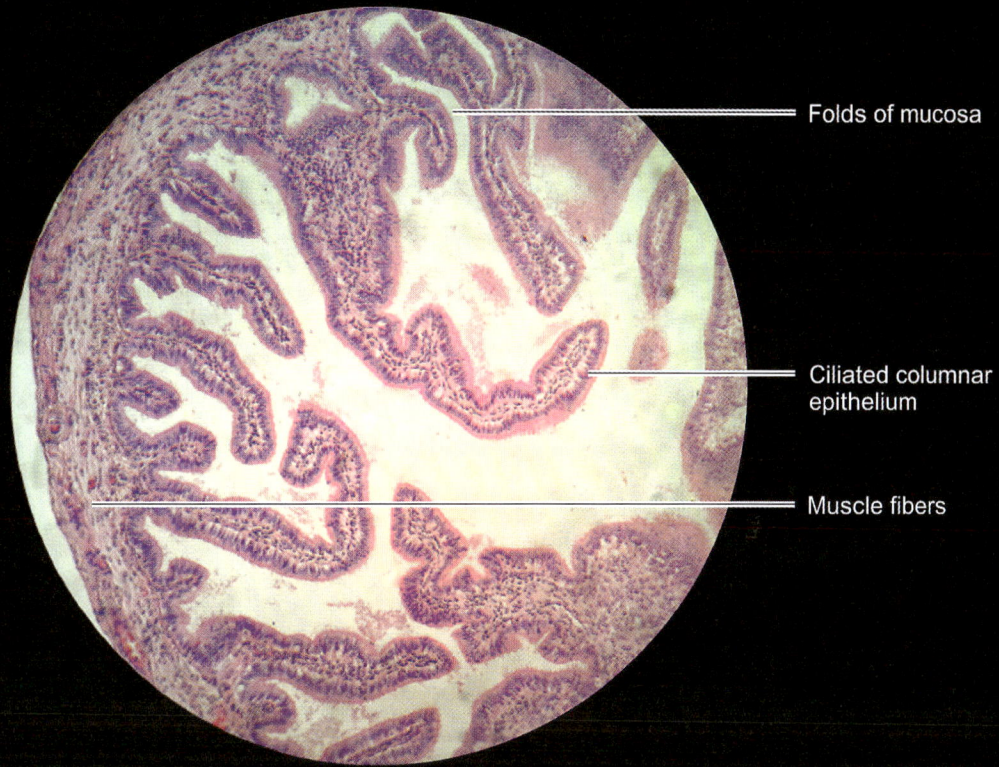

- Folds of mucosa
- Ciliated columnar epithelium
- Muscle fibers

SP:
- Presence of 1°, 2°, 3° mucosal folds and its lumen.
- Presence of circular muscle coat.

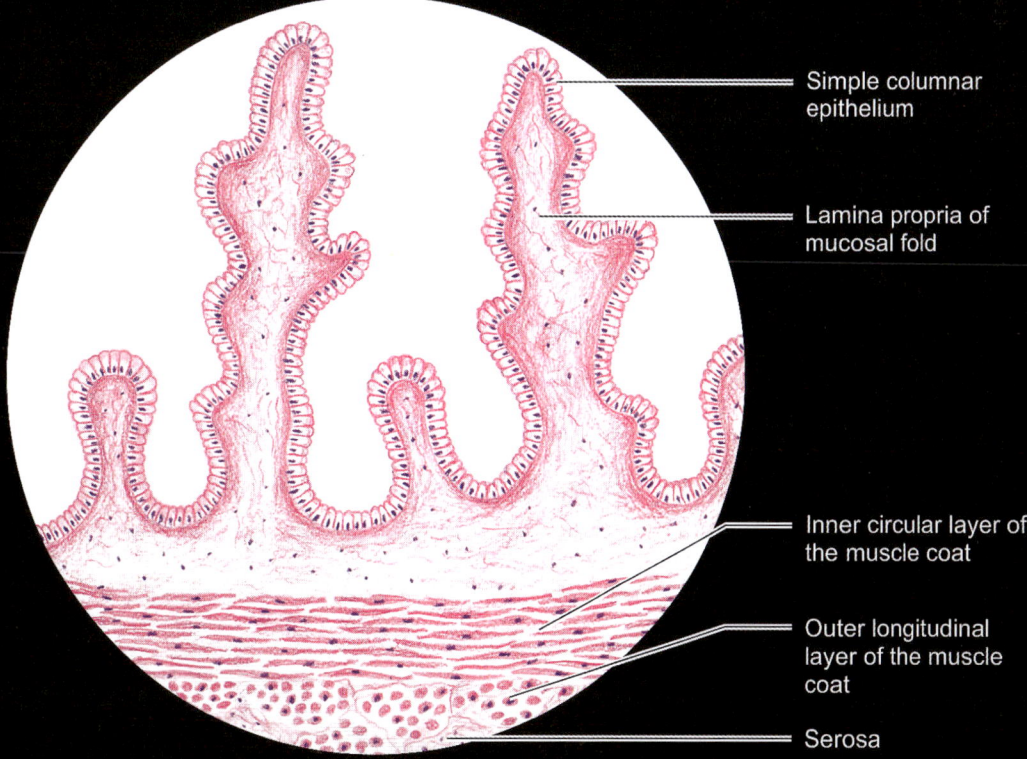

- Simple columnar epithelium
- Lamina propria of mucosal fold
- Inner circular layer of the muscle coat
- Outer longitudinal layer of the muscle coat
- Serosa

UTERUS

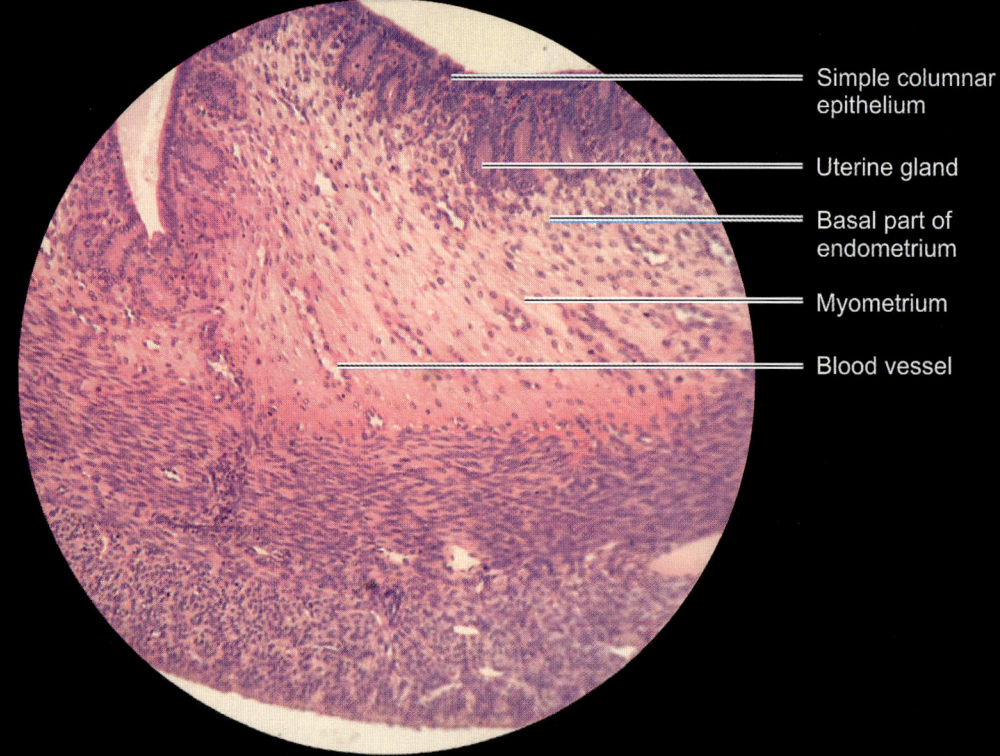

SP:
- Presence of thick myometrium with smooth muscle.
- Presence of uterine glands in endometrium.

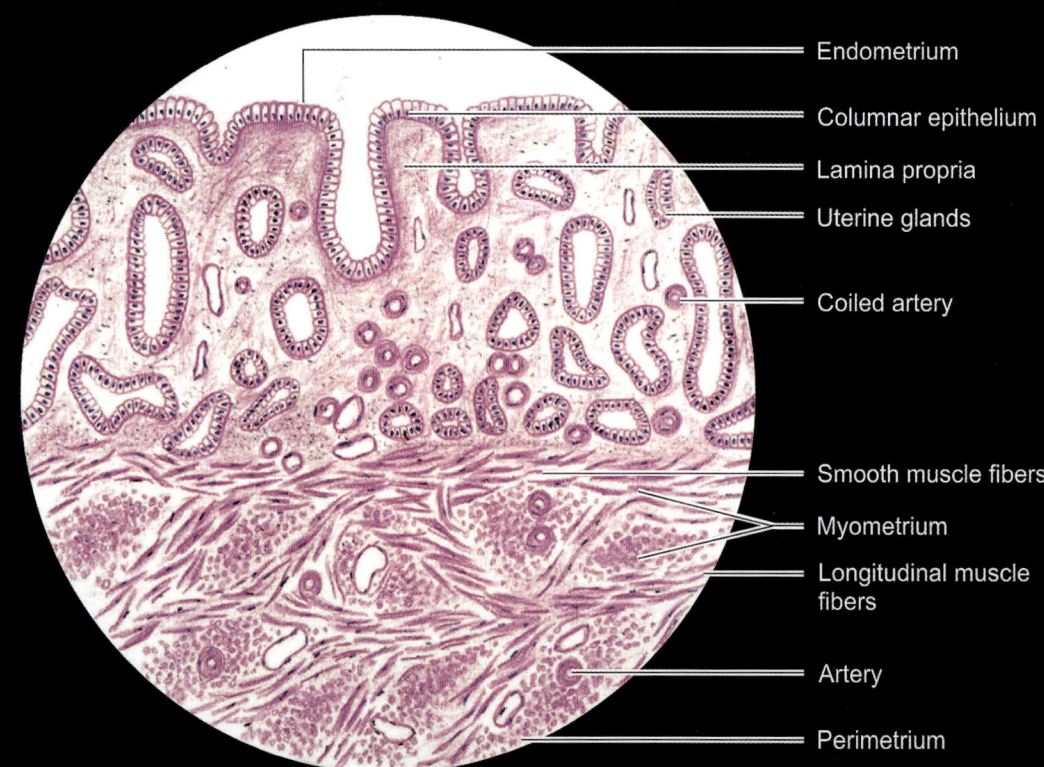

UTERUS

Proliferative Phase
- Made up of three layers (outer to inner):
  1. **Perimetrium (serosa)**
  2. **Myometrium (muscle coat)**
  3. **Endometrium (mucosa)**
- **Perimetrium** is lined by simple squamous epithelium, supported by connective tissue and contains numerous blood vessels and elastic fibers.
- **Myometrium** is a thick muscular layer, composed of smooth muscle fibers arranged in three indistinctive layers:
  1. **Outer longitudinal layer.**
  2. **Middle circular layer (thickest of the three).**
  3. **Inner longitudinal layer.**
- **Myometrium** is highly vascular having areolar tissue, blood vessels and lymphatics.
- **Endometrium** lined by simple columnar epithelium. Beneath it, a layer called **lamina propria** is present which is highly cellular.
- Lining epithelium extends down into the lamina propria and forms long tubular uterine glands.
- Uterine endometrium is divided into **superficial stratum functionalis** and **deep stratum basalis**.

Applied Anatomy
- **Leiomyoma:** Benign tumor of smooth muscle affecting the uterus.
- **It is seen in the uterus mainly at three sites:** Submucosa, intramural and subserosa.
- **Adenomyosis:** Islands of endometrial tissue found deep in the myometrium.
- It is mainly the stratum functionalis where the changes occur in response to hormones and is usually shed when fertilization does not occur.

Viva voce
Q. What are the layers of uterine endometrium?
Ans. Uterine endometrium is divided into superficial stratum functionalis and deep stratum basalis.

PLACENTA

- Consists of the fetal portion and as well as maternal portion.
- **Fetal portion** is formed by the **chorionic plate** and its villi.
- **Maternal portion** is formed by the **decidua basalis of endometrium**.
- **The chorionic plate** is formed by:
  - **Trophoblast cells** are present just below the connective tissue layer, which is located below the lining of the amniotic surface.
  - Section shows cross sections of **chorionic villi** of different sizes and shapes scattered in intervillous spaces filled with maternal blood.
- In early stages of pregnancy:
  - The **chorionic villi form chorionic plate** which contain
    1. Connective tissue core.
    2. Fetal blood vessels (including branches of umbilical arteries and vein).
    3. Mesenchyme cells.
    4. Macrophages.
  - The villi are separated by **intervillous space**.
  - Maternal blood reaches the intervillous space through spiral arteries of the decidua and bathes the villi containing fetal blood cells.
- In full term of pregnancy:
  - The **chorionic villi** shows:
    - Chorionic epithelium reduced to **syncytiotrophoblast**.
    - Connective tissue having more fibers and fibroblasts.
    - Fetal blood vessels of increased complexity.
    - The intervillous space surrounded by maternal blood cells.

Applied Anatomy

- **Placental site trophoblastic tumor:** It is a trophoblastic tumor mainly composed of monomorphic population of intermediate trophoblasts. The tumor cells are irregular, large polyhedral cells with hyperchromatic nuclei.
- **Choriocarcinoma:** This is also a carcinoma affecting placenta arising from the trophoblast.

Viva voce

Q. What are the parts of the placenta?
Ans. Fetal part formed by chorionic plate and villi and maternal portion by decidua basalis.

PLACENTA

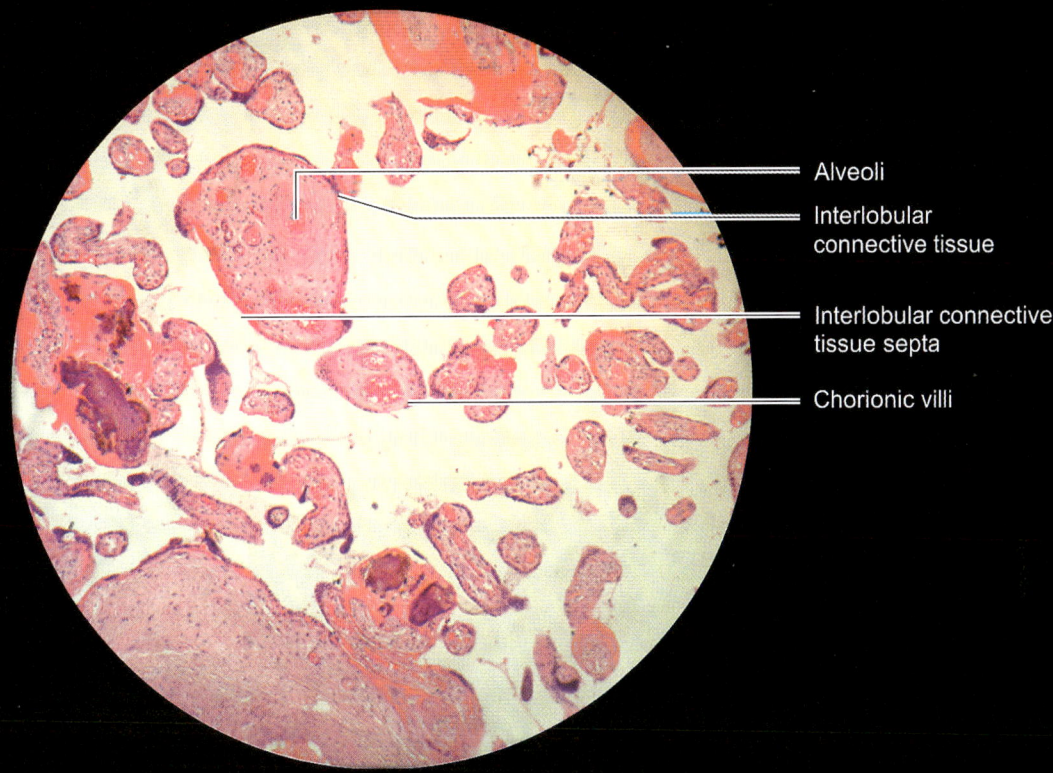

SP:
- Chorionic villi of different stages seen.
- Intervillous space filled with maternal blood and RBCs.

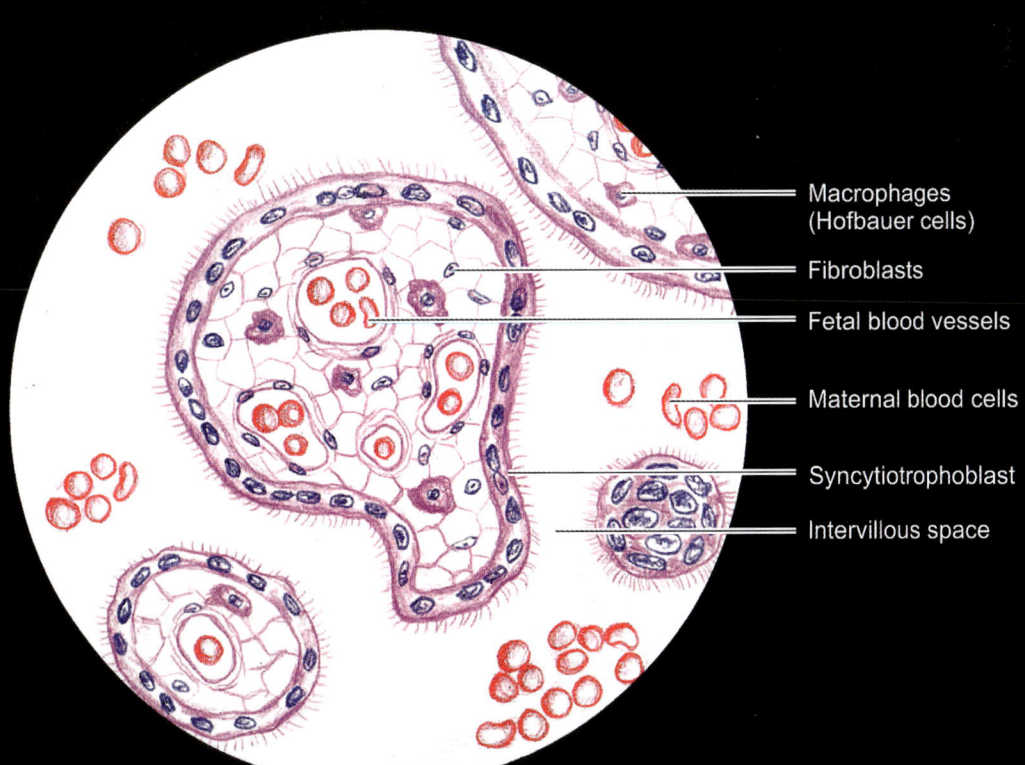

UMBILICAL CORD

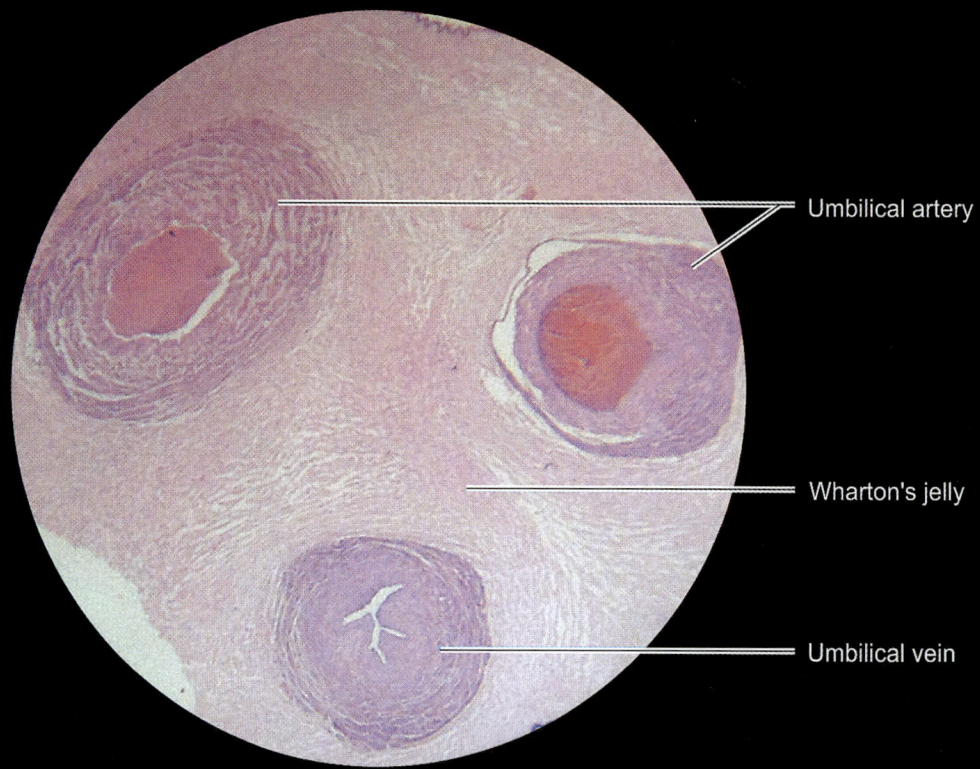

SP:
- Presence of two umbilical arteries and one umbilical vein.
- Presence of Wharton's jelly.

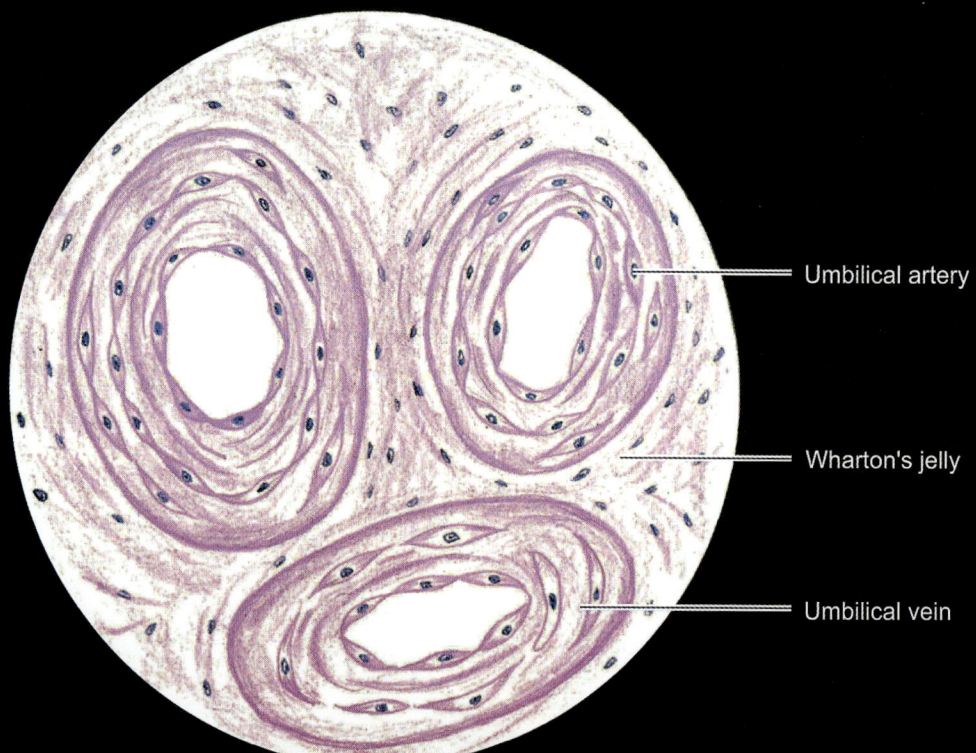

UMBILICAL CORD

- Consists of a single umbilical vein, two umbilical arteries, Wharton's jelly, and a layer of amnion.
- **Umbilical vein** is a thin-walled structure with wider lumen and brings oxygenated blood from placenta to fetus.
- **Umbilical artery** is thick walled in nature and has a narrow lumen and takes deoxygenated blood from fetus to placenta.
- **Wharton's jelly** is a mass of gelatinous mucoid connective tissue which holds together the umbilical vessels.
- A thin single layered amnion covers all the above structures.
- **Amnion** is made up of a single layer of cuboidal epithelium.

Applied Anatomy

- The nonpatent obliterated part of the umbilical artery is the medial umbilical ligament.
- The umbilical vein of the newborn baby is used as a site for regular transfusion in case of hemolytic disease of the newborn since the umbilical vein remains patent for at least a week after birth.
- After a week since birth the umbilical vein is completely obliterated and is replaced by a fibrous cord called ligamentum teres of the liver.

Viva voce

Q. What is Wharton's jelly?
Ans. Wharton's jelly is a mass of gelatinous mucoid connective tissue which holds together the umbilical vessels.
Q. What is the function of the umbilical artery?
Ans. Umbilical artery is thick walled in nature and has a narrow lumen and takes deoxygenated blood from fetus to placenta.
Q. What is the function of the umbilical vein?
Ans. Umbilical vein is a thin-walled structure with wider lumen and brings oxygenated blood from placenta to fetus.
Q. What is the lining epithelium of amnion?
Ans. Single layer of cuboidal epithelium.

MALE REPRODUCTIVE SYSTEM

TESTIS

- Each testis is enclosed within an outer thick connective tissue capsule called **tunica albuginea** and inner vascular layer of loose connective tissue called the **tunica vasculosa**.
- **Connective tissue** that extends inward into the testes and surrounds, binds, supports the seminiferous tubules is called **interstitial connective tissue**.
- Thin fibrous septa divides the testes into compartments called **lobules**.
- Within each lobule one to four seminiferous tubules are present.
- **Seminiferous tubules** are lined with stratified epithelium called germinal epithelium containing **spermatogenic cells** producing sperms.
- **Germinal epithelium** roots on basement membrane.
- Supportive **Sertoli cells** in the seminiferous tubules nourish the developing sperm and produce hormones like **inhibin, anti-Mullerian hormone, etc**.
- **Leydig cells (interstitial cells)** situated in the interstitial connective tissue produce testosterone.
- Alongwith the Leydig cells, clusters of epithelial cells, blood vessels, loose connective tissue cells are also present in the interstitial connective tissue.

Applied Anatomy

- Seminoma is the most common testicular tumor arising from germ cells.
- Cryptorchidism is undescent of testis which can predispose to testicular tumors.
- Leydig cell tumors are functional tumors (hormone producing) arising from the interstitial cells of Leydig.

Viva voce

Q. What is the difference between spermatogenesis and spermiogenesis?
Ans. Spermatogenesis is the entire process of formation of sperm from stem cell to spermatozoon. Spermiogenesis is the maturation process from spermatid to spermatozoon.
Q. What are the components of the blood-testis barrier and what is its significance?
Ans. Tight junctions between Sertoli cells isolate developing sperm from the vasculature (prevent their immunological rejection).
Q. What is the primary source of testosterone?
Ans. The Leydig cells.

TESTIS

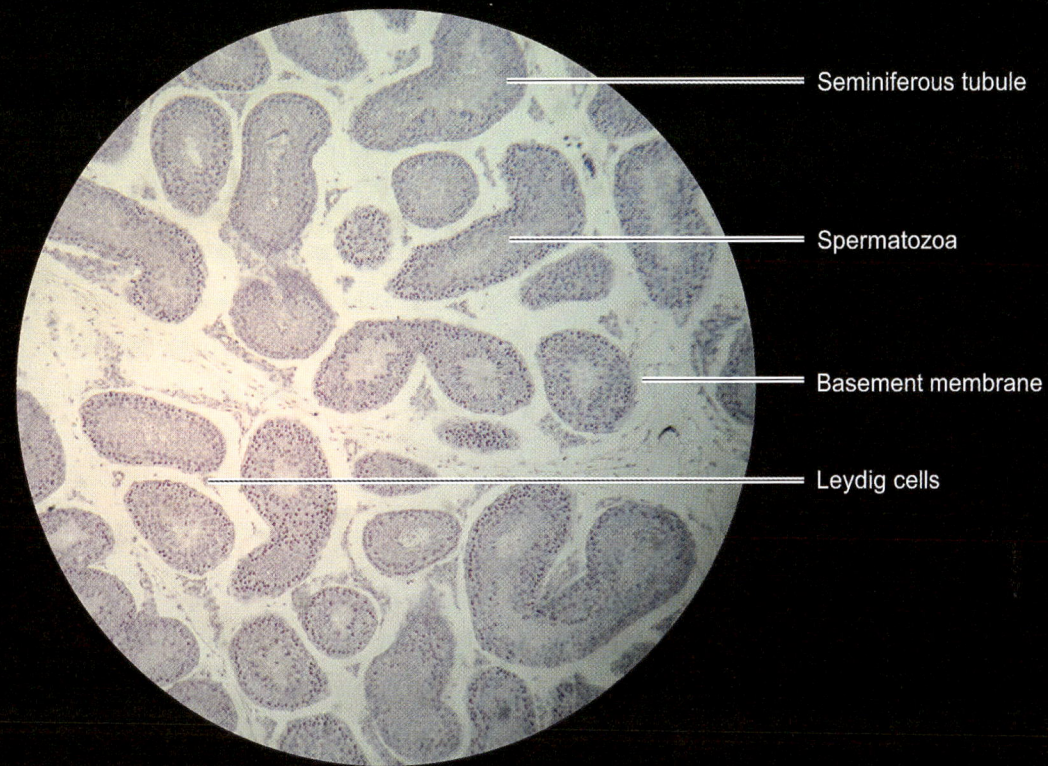

SP:
- Presence of seminiferous tubules with spermatozoa.
- Presence of interstitial cells between the tubules.

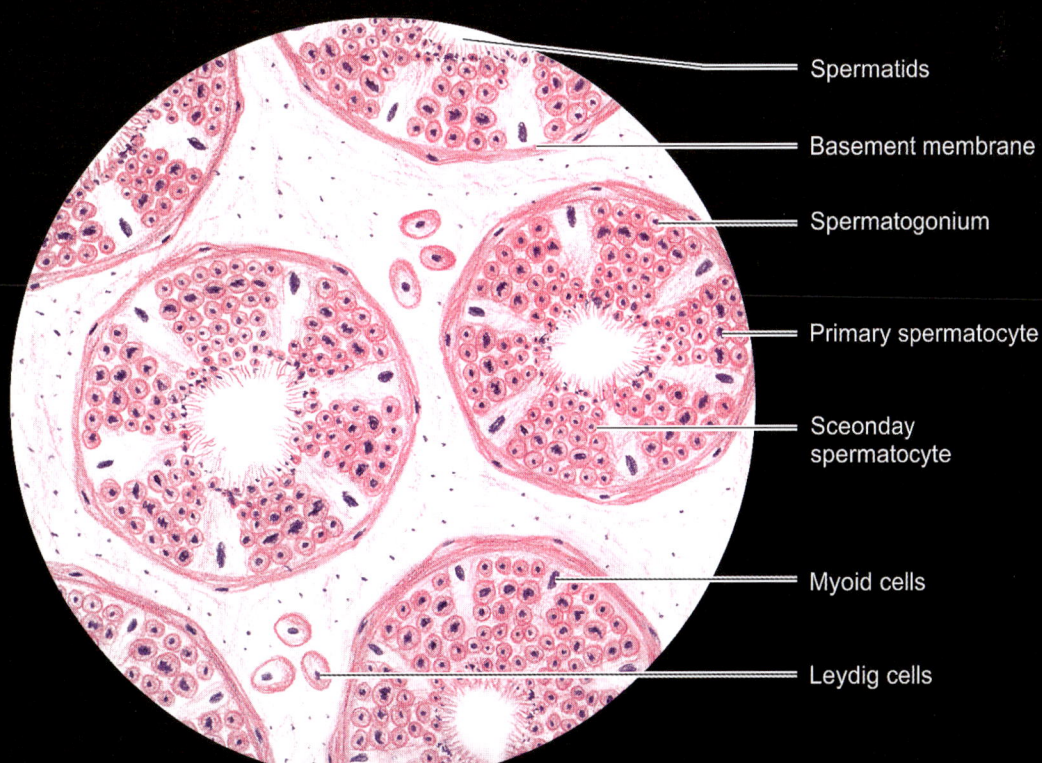

EPIDIDYMIS

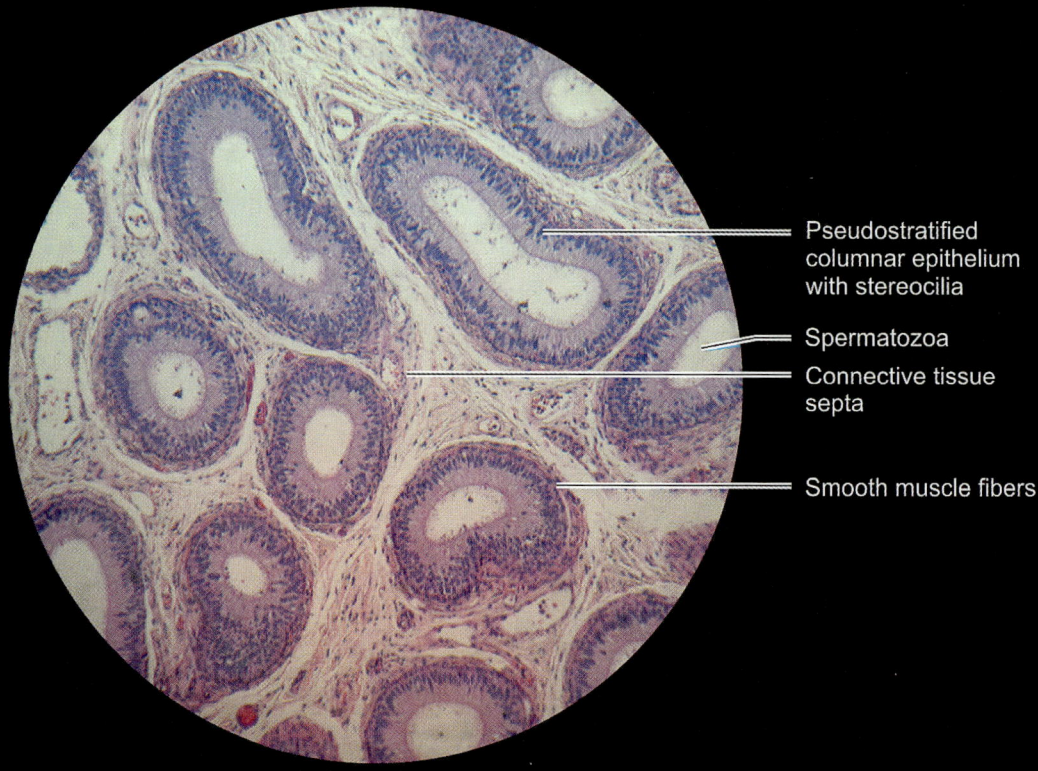

SP:
- Presence of highly convoluted efferent ductules with stereocilia.
- Presence of smooth muscle around the ductules.

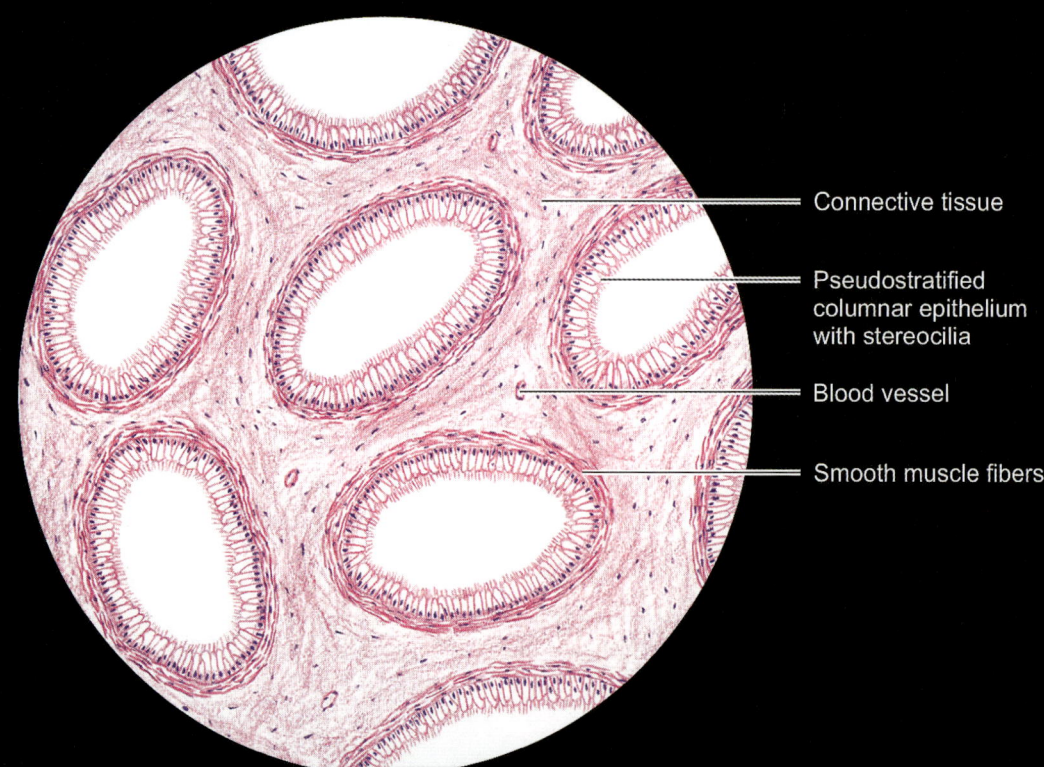

EPIDIMYMIS

- Contains highly convoluted efferent ductules called **ductus epididymis.**
- These are surrounded by connective tissue and thin smooth muscle layer.
- Lumen of ductus epididymis is lined by **pseudostratified columnar epithelium** with two types of cells:
  1. **Tall columnar principal cells.**
  2. **Small basal cells.**
- The **tall columnar cells** bear microvilli called stereocilia.
- Some parts of the ductus contain mature sperm.

Applied Anatomy

- The stereocilia present in the epididymis are responsible for the absorption and removal of the sperm which fails to leave the epididymis.
- The name stereocilia is a misnomer as it does not move like the other cilia, and it is moreover like the villi of gut.

Viva voce

Q. Where is the principal site of storage and mobility acquisition of spermatozoa in the male reproductive system?
Ans. Epididymis.
Q. What are the two types of cells present in the lining of lumen of epididymis?
Ans. Tall columnar cells and small basal cells.

VAS DEFERENS

- Consists of mainly three layers.
- **Mucosa** is lined by **pseudostratified columnar epithelium** and provided with stereocilia in the extra-abdominal part of the duct.
- The mucosa is thrown into longitudinal folds which permit expansion of the duct during ejaculation.
- Underlying **lamina propria** consists of compact collagen fibers and a fine network of elastic fibers.
- **Muscular layer** consists of three smooth muscle layers.
    1. **Thin inner longitudinal** layer
    2. **Thick middle circular** layer, and
    3. **Thinner outer longitudinal** layer.
- **Adventitia** is made up of fibroelastic connective tissue having abundant blood vessels, venules, arterioles and nerves.
- The lumen may carry sperms.

Applied Anatomy

- The unexpelled sperms produced daily are mainly absorbed by the pseudostratified columnar epithelium of vas deferens. And the absorbed sperms are engulfed and lysed by the macrophages.
- The same thing happens in men who have undergone vasectomy procedure.

Viva voce

Q. What type of epithelium lines the mucosa of vas deferens?
Ans. Mucosa is lined by pseudostratified columnar epithelium and has stereocilia in extra-abdominal part of the duct.
Q. What does lamina propria of vas deferens contain?
Ans. Lamina propria consists of compact collagen fibers and a fine network of elastic fibers.

VAS DEFERENS

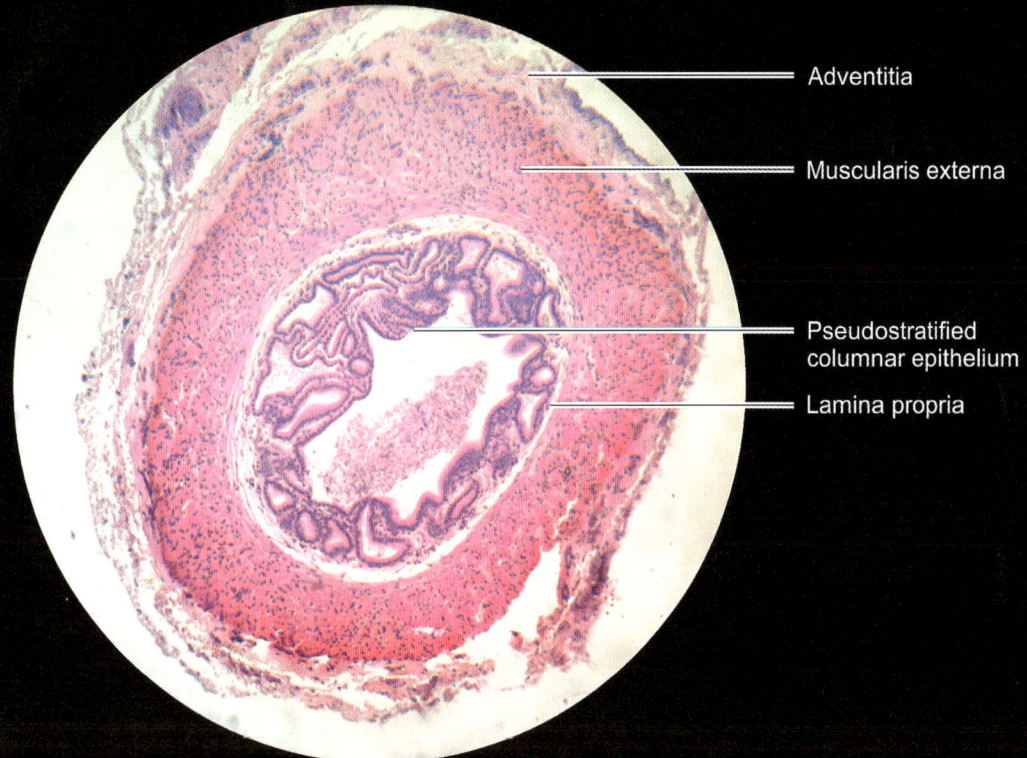

SP:
- Presence of narrow irregular lumen with mucosal folds.
- Presence of thick circularly arranged muscle coat.

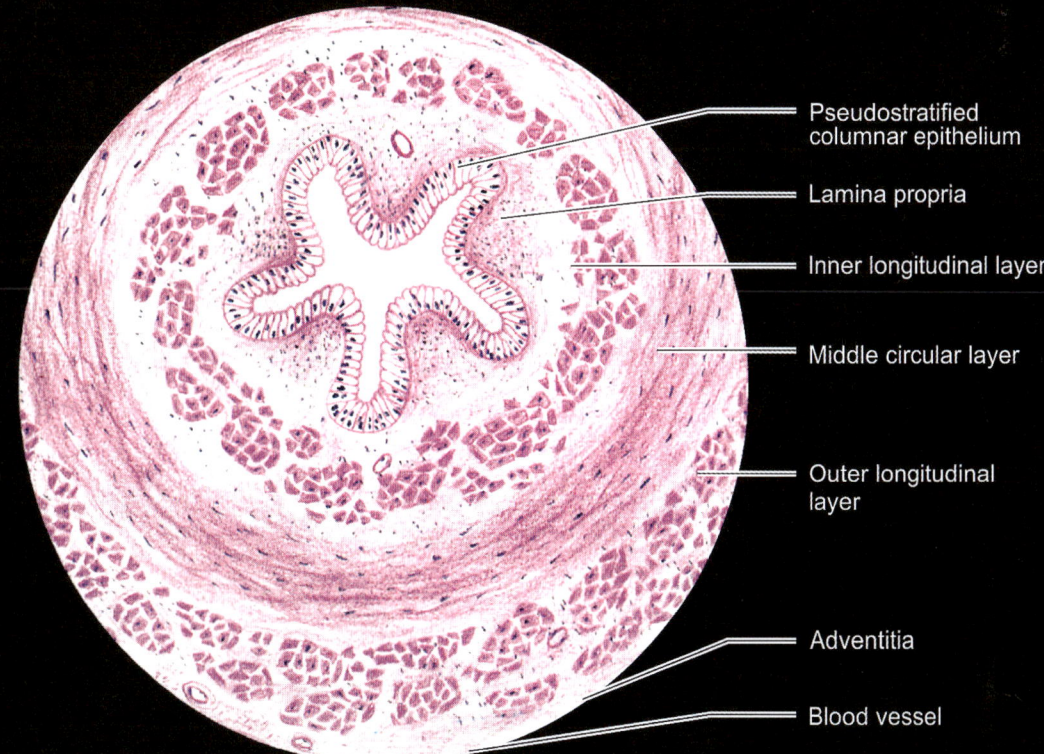

PROSTATE GLAND

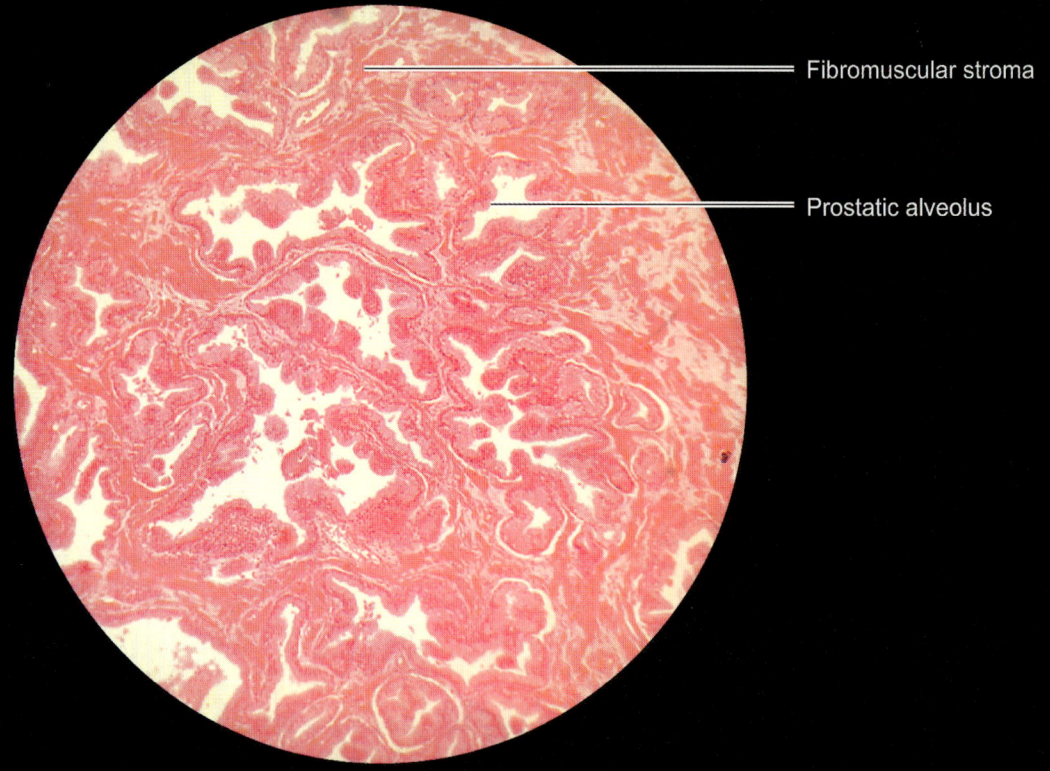

SP:
- Presence of prostatic acini separated by fibromuscular tissue.
- Presence of amyloid body.

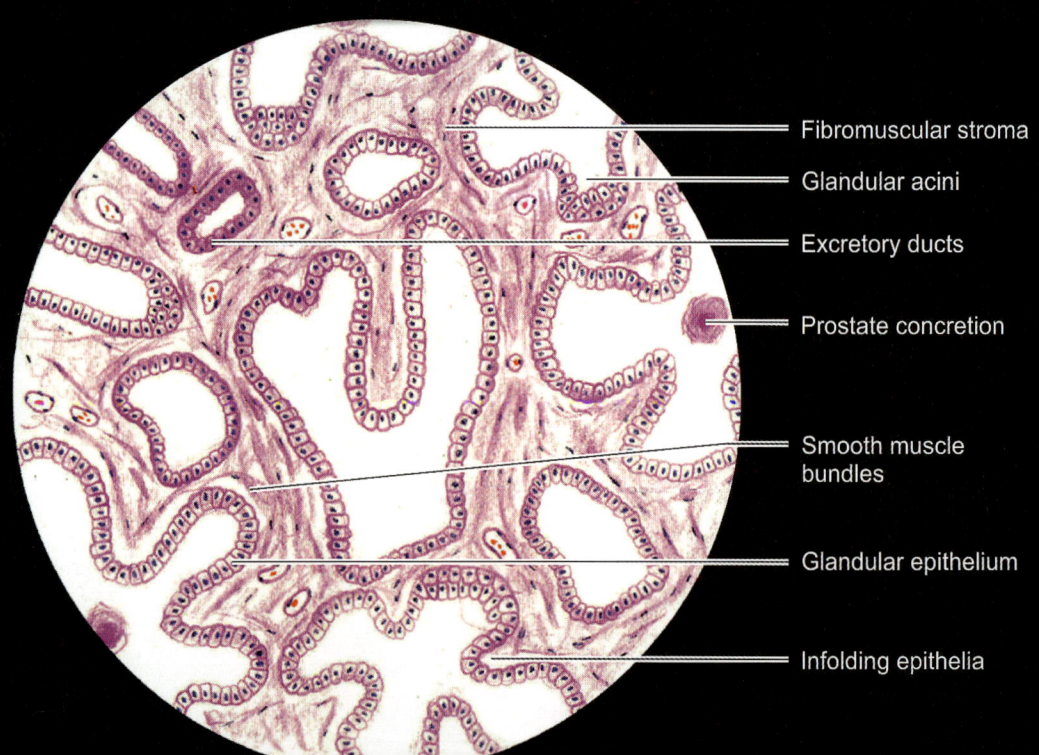

PROSTATE GLAND

- **Prostate** is covered by:
  - **Inner capsule**—formed by condensation of fibromuscular stroma.
  - **False capsule**—formed by pelvic fascia.
- It is composed of 30–50 branched tubuloalveolar glands embedded in **fibromuscular stroma**.
- The ducts of the gland open into prostatic urethra which is lined by **transitional epithelium**.
- The **parenchyma** is made up of large irregular prostatic alveoli with wide lumen which is lined by epithelium varying from **cuboidal to columnar** depending on its activity.
- The lumen of prostatic alveoli contains condensed prostatic secretions called **prostatic concretion or amyloid bodies**.
- The **fibromuscular stroma** supports the parenchyma and is made of smooth muscle fibers with connective tissue fibers.
- Stroma also contains blood vessels, lymphatics and nerves.

Applied Anatomy

- In nodular hyperplasia of the prostate, there will be hyperplasia of all three tissue elements— glandular, fibrous and muscular, in which glandular hyperplasia predominates.
- In adenocarcinoma of the prostate, malignant acini have little or no stroma between them.
- Prostatic secretions along with the secretions from seminal vesicles from the major part of semen.

Viva voce

Q. What are prostatic concretions?
Ans. The lumen of prostatic alveoli contains condensed prostatic secretions called prostatic concretion or amyloid bodies.
Q. What is the type of epithelium lining the prostatic alveoli?
Ans. The prostatic alveoli is lined by cuboidal to columnar type of epithelium depending on its activity.
Q. What is the fibromuscular stroma of the prostate made of?
Ans. The fibromuscular stroma is made of smooth muscle fibers and connective tissue fibers.

ENDOCRINE SYSTEM

ADRENAL GLAND

- Consist of capsule, cortex, medulla.
- **Cortex**—consists of the following layers from outer to inner.
  - **Zona glomerulosa**—cells arranged in clumps (inverted 'U' shape), cytoplasm stains pink. This layer produces **mineralocorticoids**.
  - **Zona fasciculata**—widest layer, cells arranged in vertical columns or radial plates, lightly stained due to the presence of numerous lipid droplets. This layer produces **glucocorticoids**.
  - **Zona reticularis**—close to medulla, cells form anastomosing cords. This layer produces **sexcorticoids**.
- **Medulla**—not sharply demarcated from cortex.
  - Consists of polyhedral cells which are modified sympathetic neurons and are seen singly or in groups.
  - The cell groups are separated by wide sinusoidal capillaries.
  - Adrenal medullary cells produce **adrenaline and noradrenaline**.
  - After tissue fixation fine brown granules become visible in cells called **chromaffin cells** indicating presence of medullary hormones.
- The hormones produced by cortex are:
  1. **Zona glomerulosa—mineralocorticoid**.
  2. **Zona fasciculata—glucocorticoid**.
  3. **Zona reticularis—sex corticoids**.
- The hormones synthesized by **medulla** include:
  1. **Epinephrine.**
  2. **Norepinephrine**.

Applied Anatomy

Pheochromocytoma: They are tumors arising from chromaffin cells of the adrenal medulla. The tumor cells are polygonal in shape and are arranged in groups surrounded by a fibrovascular septa.

Viva voce

Q. How is medullary function regulated?
Ans. Through presynaptic nerves and glucocorticoids.

ADRENAL GLAND

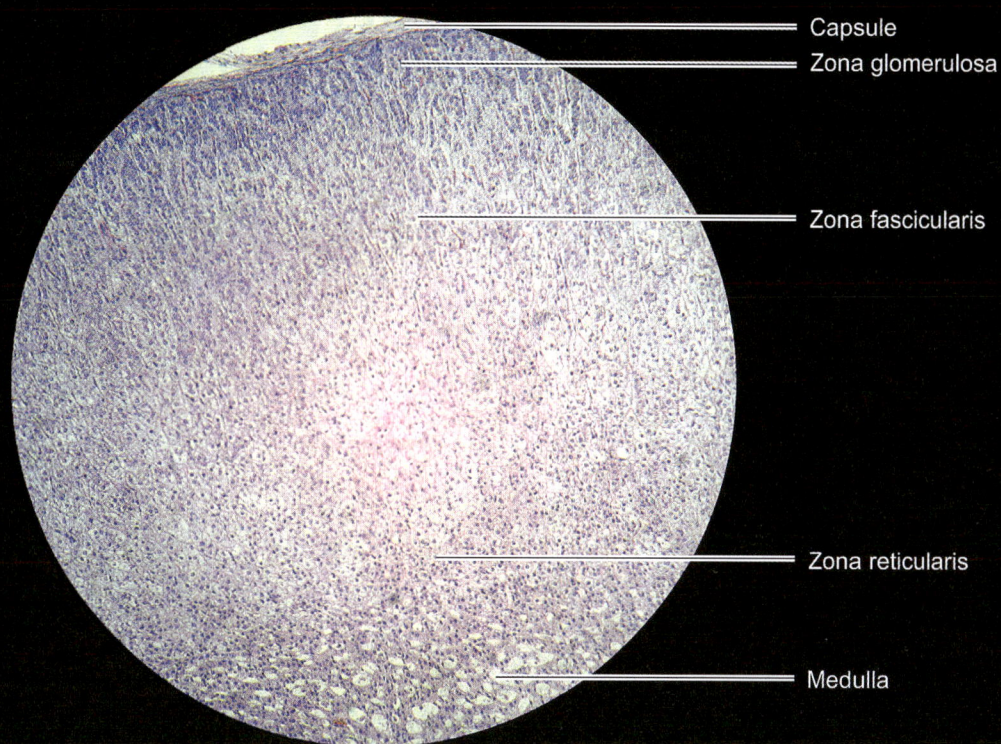

- Capsule
- Zona glomerulosa
- Zona fasciculars
- Zona reticularis
- Medulla

SP:
- Presence of cortex and medulla.
- Presence of secretory cells and sympathetic neurons.

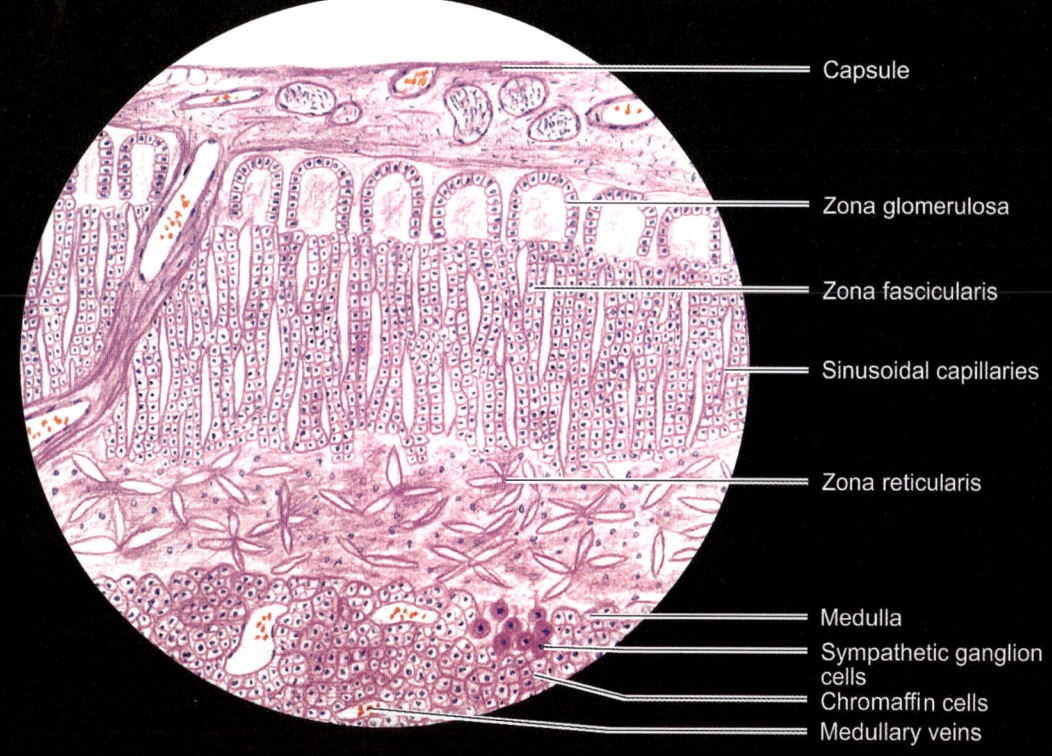

- Capsule
- Zona glomerulosa
- Zona fasciculars
- Sinusoidal capillaries
- Zona reticularis
- Medulla
- Sympathetic ganglion cells
- Chromaffin cells
- Medullary veins

THYROID GLAND

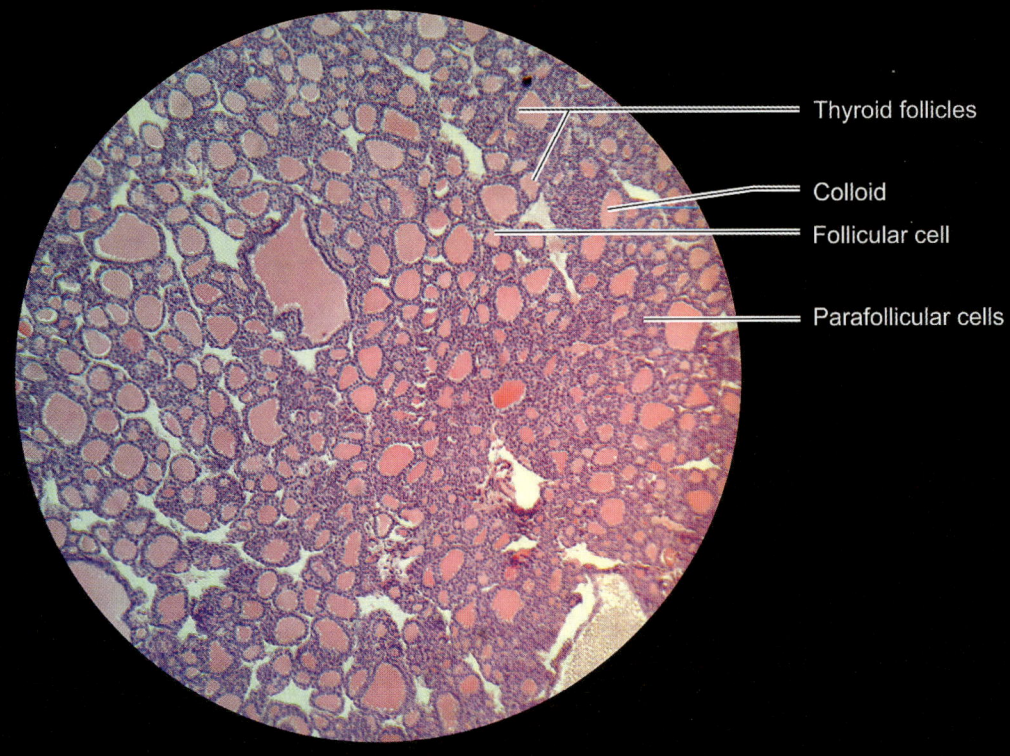

SP:
- Presence of thyroid follicles filled with colloid.
- Presence of parafollicular cells.

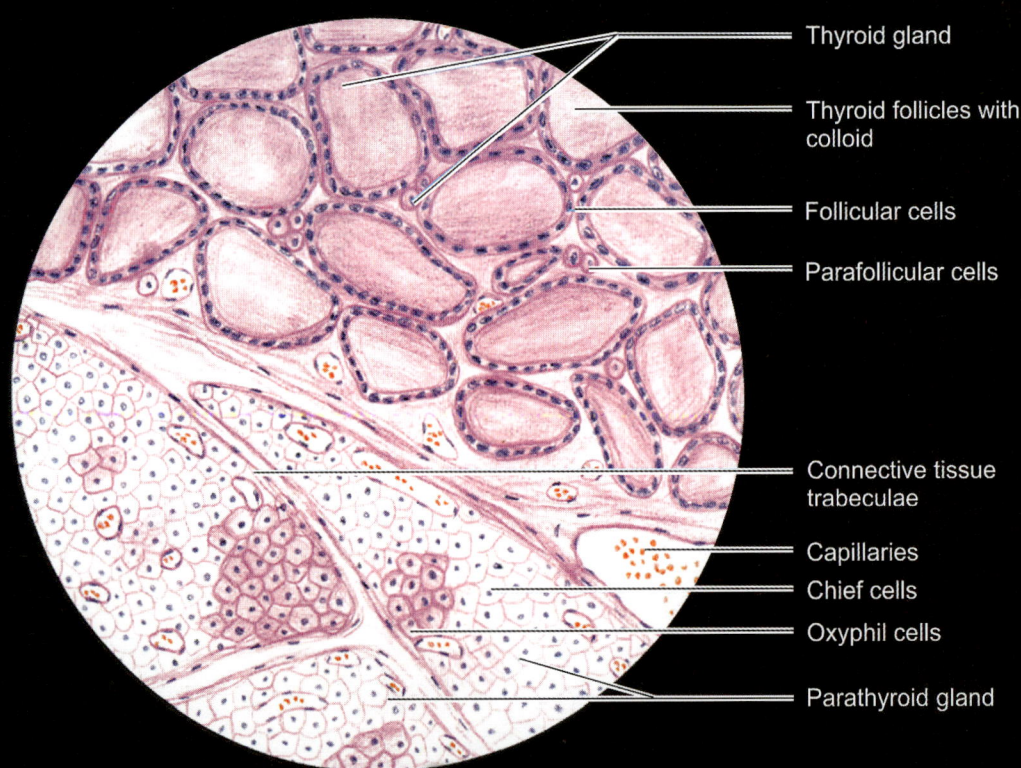

THYROID GLAND

- Consists of mainly follicular cells.
- **Follicular cells** are arranged spherically into follicles.
- These **follicles** are the structural and functional units of thyroid gland.
- In highly **active follicles**, epithelium is **cuboidal** whereas in **less active ones** the epithelium is **flat**.
- All follicles are filled with colloid but some of them may show retraction due to preparation.
- **Parafollicular cells** are seen within follicular epithelium or in between follicles.
- Surrounding the thyroid follicles and follicular cells, thin interfollicular connective tissue is present containing blood vessels and capillaries.
- The follicular cells are responsible for the production of thyroid hormones.
- Parafollicular cells secrete **calcitonin**.

PARATHYROID GLAND

- They lie in close relation to thyroid gland.
- **Glands** are covered by a connective tissue capsule from which septa extend into the substance of the gland.
- The **stroma** is formed by a network of reticular fibers and adipocytes.
- The **parenchyma** consist of mainly two types of cells viz. **chief cells and oxyphil cells** which are arranged in a cord-like manner.
- The **chief cells** are small round cells with vesicular nuclei.
- The **oxyphil cells** are larger cells with granules.
- The chief cells produce parathormone.
- The oxyphil cells have the ability to produce autocrine/paracrine factors (parathyroid hormone-related protein and calcitriol).

Applied Anatomy

- In Graves disease, the follicular epithelial cells are tall and thrown into small papillae. The papillae project into the lumen of the follicle.
- In Hashimoto thyroiditis, the thyroid tissue shows dense infiltration lymphocytes and plasma cells. The lymphocytes form lymphoid follicles with germinal centers.

PITUITARY GLAND

- Mainly divided into **adenohypophysis and neurohypophysis**.
- **Adenohypophysis** consists of pars distalis (anterior lobe), pars tuberalis, pars intermedia.
- **Neurohypophysis** consisting of **pars nervosa, infundibulum, and median eminence**.
- **Pars nervosa** forms the largest portion of neurohypophysis.
- **Pars distalis** consists of **chromophobe cells** (cells that do not take stain), and **chromophil cells** (cells that take stain—acidophils, basophils).
- **Pars intermedia** contains colloid filled cystic follicles.
- **Pars nervosa** consists of axons and supporting pituicytes with oval nuclei. It also contains accumulation of neurosecretory material called **herring bodies**.

Applied Anatomy

- **Pituitary adenomas:** In this condition there will be presence of tumor cells arranged in nests surrounded by thin connective tissue. Cells can also be arranged in a cord-like manner.
- Damage to hypothalamus which stores antidiuretic hormone produced by neurohypo-physis, causes deficiency of ADH and leads to diabetes insipidus.

Viva voce

Q. What kinds of cells are in the neurohypophysis?
Ans. Pituicytes (glia), endothelial cells.
Q. What do herring bodies represent?
Ans. Sites for storage or degradation of neurotransmitters.
Q. What hormones might you expect to find in herring bodies?
Ans. Vasopressin (antidiuretic hormone) and oxytocin.
Q. Where are the hormones of the neurohypophysis synthesized?
Ans. Hypothalamus.
Q. What are chromophil and chromophobe cells?
Ans. Chromophobe cells are cells that do not stain, and chromophil cells are cells that take stain and include acidophils, basophils.
Q. What is the functional significance of the hypothalamo-hypophyseal system?
Ans. It allows for rapid and direct delivery of hypothalamic products with releasing and inhibiting effects on anterior pituitary cells.

PITUITARY GLAND

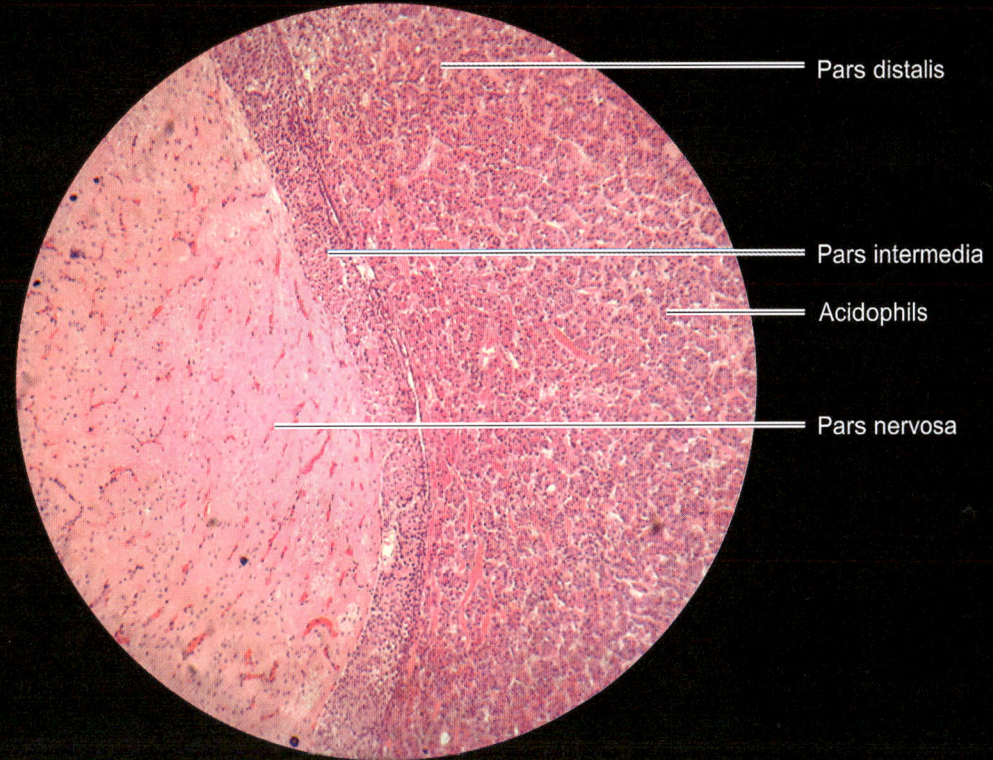

SP:
- Presence of pars anterior with acidophils and basophils.
- Presence of pars nervosa with pituicytes and pars intermedius with colloid.

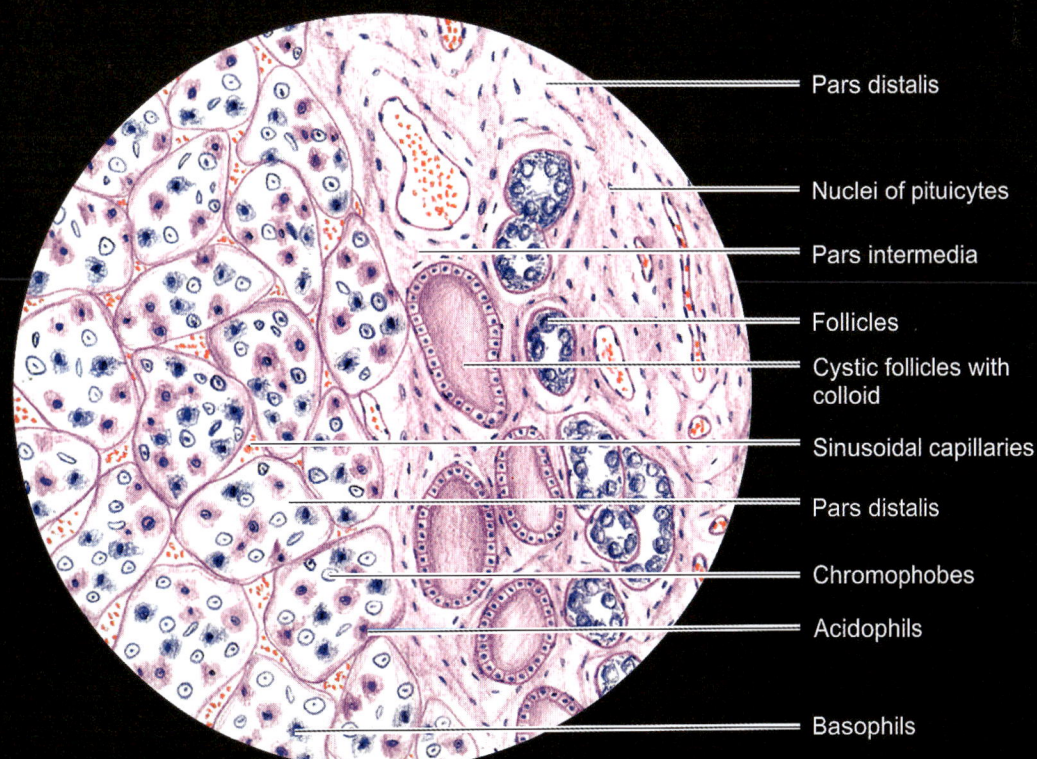

SPINAL CORD

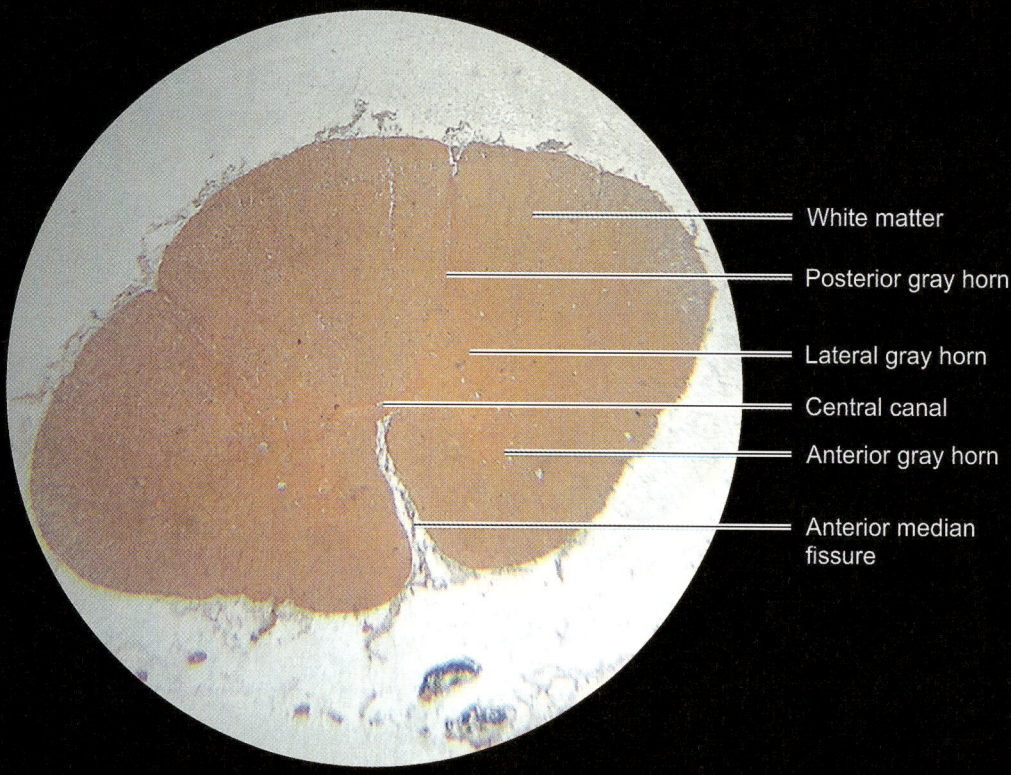

SP:
- Presence of H-shaped gray mater.
- Presence of central canal.

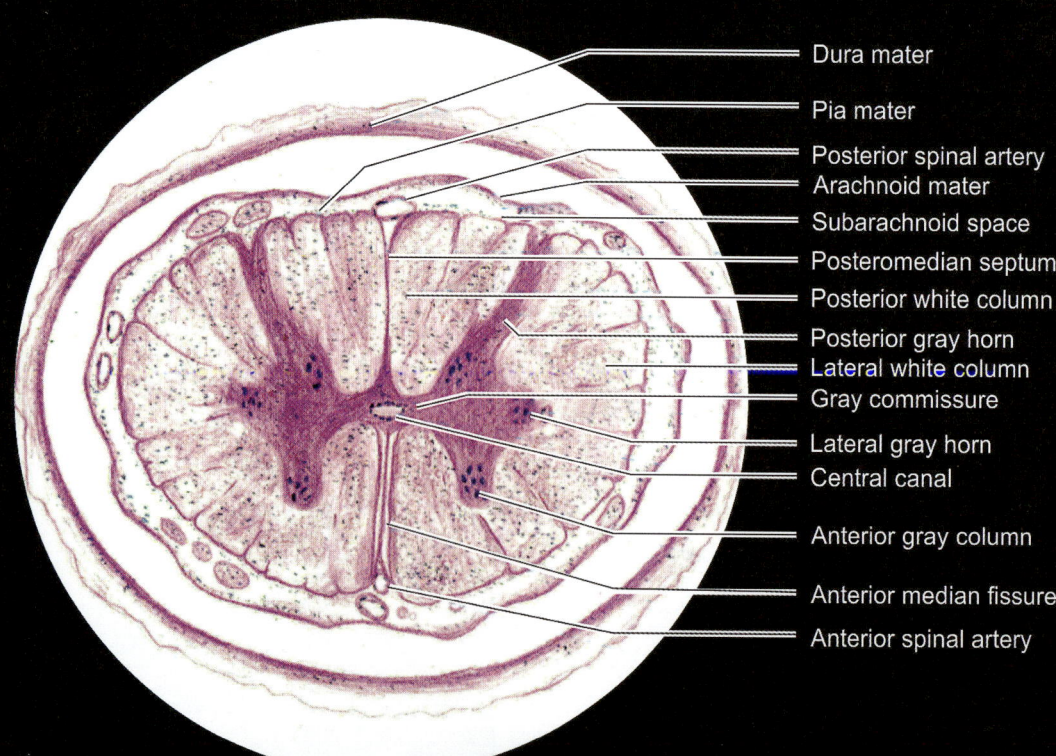

CENTRAL NERVOUS SYSTEM

SPINAL CORD

- In the transverse section (TS) of the thoracic segment of the spinal cord, we can see gray matter inside and white matter on the periphery.
- **Gray matter** is almost an H-shaped or butterfly-shaped structure.
- Each half of the gray matter can be divided into three portions namely:
  1. **Anterior gray horn:** Large anterior mass, this region consists of multipolar motor neurons.
  2. **Posterior gray horn:** Narrow and elongated part, which is located posteriorly, **Clark's column or dorsal nucleus** is present in the medial part of the base of the posterior horn.
  3. **Lateral gray horn:** It is a wedge-shaped lateral projection of gray matter between anterior and posterior gray horns. This region consists of sympathetic preganglionic visceral motor neurons.
- **Lateral gray horn** is limited to the thoracic and upper two lumbar segments of the spinal cord.
- Two halves of gray matter are connected by the gray commissure at the midline.
- **A central canal** is present at the midpoint of the horizontal limb of H.
- Central canal is lined by **ependymal cells** and it represents the lumen of the neural tube.
- **White matter** which lies in the periphery is divided into two halves: Right and left
  1. **Anteriorly by anterior median fissure.**
  2. **Posteriorly by posterior median septum.**
- **Anterior spinal artery** is present in the anterior median fissure.
- Similar to gray matter, the white matter of each half can be divided into three portions:
  1. **Anterior white column:** White matter anterior and medial to anterior gray horn.
  2. **Posterior white column:** White matter medial to posterior gray horn.
  3. **Lateral white column:** White matter lateral to anterior and posterior gray horns.
- White matter of each half is connected to each other anteriorly by the **anterior white commissure**.
- A sulcus is present just behind the posterior most end of posterior median septum called as posterior median sulcus.

Applied Anatomy

- Damage to the lateral horn can lead to Horner's syndrome.
- **Poliomyelitis:** Inflammation of gray matter of spinal cord.

CEREBELLUM

- **Cortex** is highly folded.
- These folds are called **cerebellar folia**.
- Folds are separated by transverse fissures called **sulci**.
- **Folium** contains an inner core of white matter and an outer cortex of gray matter covered by the thin connective tissue called **pia mater**.
- **Cortex** consists of three layers:
  1. **External molecular layer:** Superficial layer, thick, and made of nerve fibers and cells: **stellate cells** above and basket cells below.
  2. **Purkinje cell layer:** Made up of **Purkinje cells** (large sized, flask-shaped neurons arranged between molecular and granular layer in single row). Dendrite of Purkinje cells synapses with axons of granular cells.
  3. **Granular layer:** Densely packed with very small granule neurons (smallest cells in the body), they exhibit intensely stained nuclei, few Golgi cells are also present. Dendrite of granule cells and axons of Golgi cells synapses with mossy fibers to form glomeruli (lightly stained).
     - **Mossy fibers** are afferent fibers ending in a granular layer.
     - **White matter** consists of myelinated nerve fibers.

Applied Anatomy

- Rett syndrome is a cerebellar pathology characterized by loss of Purkinje cells, atrophy, astrocytic gliosis of the molecular and granular layers.
- Cerebellar diseases result in lack of coordination and disturbances of accuracy movements causing a constellation of symptoms and motor signs.

Viva voce

Q.   What are Purkinje cells?
Ans. These are large sized, flask-shaped neurons arranged between molecular and granular layers in a single row.
Q.   What are the characteristics of granular layers?
Ans. The layer is densely packed with very small granule neurons (smallest cells in the body), they exhibit intensely stained nuclei, and few Golgi cells are also present.
Q.   What are mossy fibers?
Ans. These are afferent fibers ending in a granular layer.

CEREBELLUM

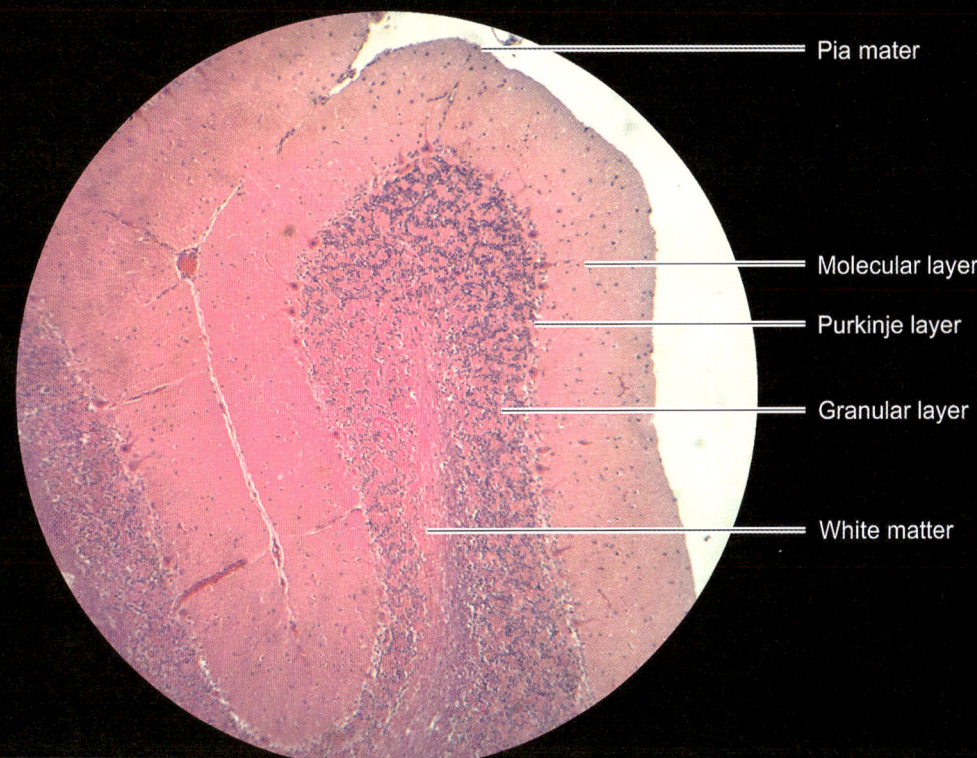

SP:
- Presence of molecular layer and granular layer and white matter.
- Presence of Purkinje cells in Purkinje cell layer.

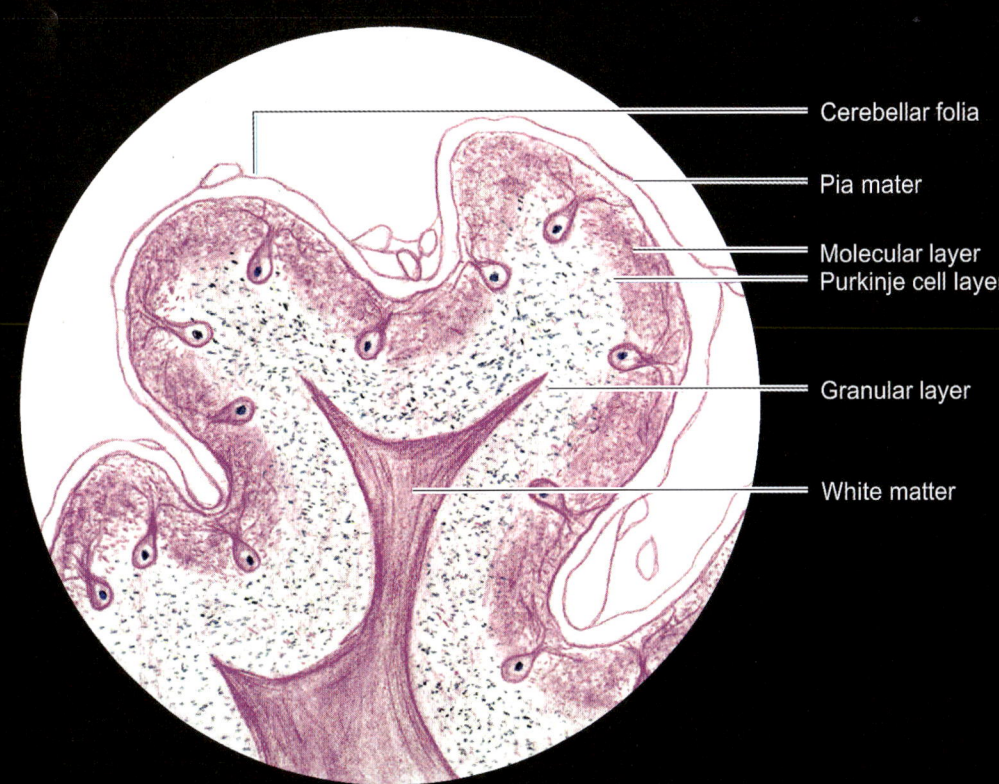

CEREBRUM

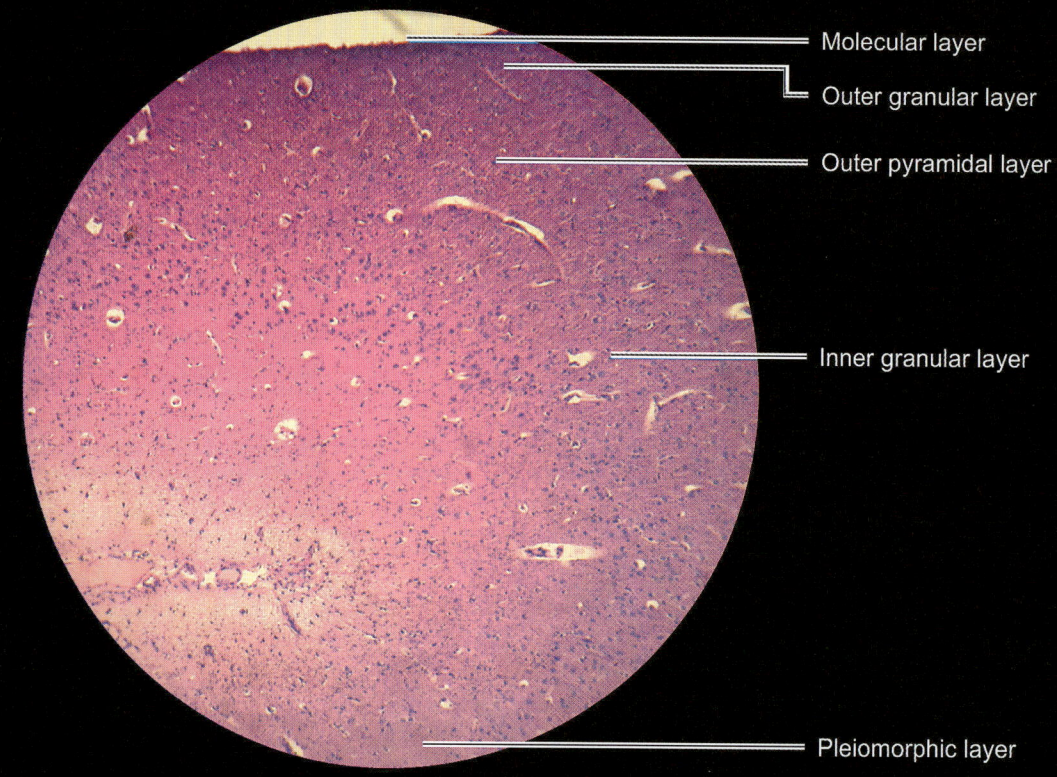

SP:
- Presence of superficial pia mater and inner white matter.
- Presence of stellate cells and giant pyramidal cells.

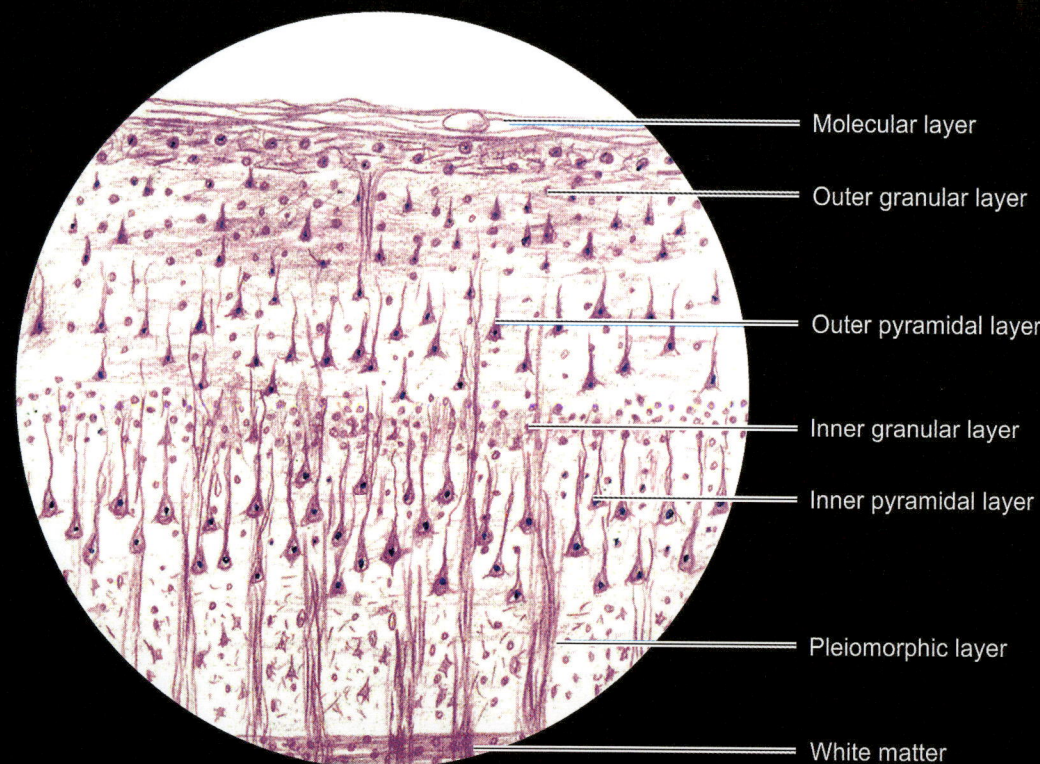

CEREBRUM

- Cortex is made up of gray matter.
- Cortex consists of nerve fibers, nerve cells, neuroglia and blood vessels.
- **Neuroglia** are highly branched cells that support neurons.
- Made up of six layers of nerve cells and associated fibers.
- A layer called **superficial pia mater** is also present, it is a layer of pia mater overlying and covering the molecular layer.
- Layers from above to below.
    - **Molecular layer/plexiform layer**—superficial layer, well defined, mainly consists of neuroglial cells and horizontal cells of Cajal.
    - **External granular layer**—it consists of **stellate cells** and **small pyramidal cells**.
    - **External pyramidal layer**—made up of mainly medium sized pyramidal cells, few stellate cells and **cells of Martinotti** (small multipolar cells).
    - Internal granular layer is a thin layer containing stellate cells which are closely packed and nerve fibers which are arranged horizontally called the outer band of Baillarger.
    - **Internal pyramidal layer/ganglionic layer**—consists of numerous **large pyramidal cells (Betz cells)** located mainly on the motor area, also containing few stellate cells and cells of Martinotti. The nerve fibers are arranged horizontally, called the **inner band of Baillarger**.
    - **Multiform layer**—polymorphic cell layer, deepest layer, contains mainly **fusiform cells**, few **stellate cells** and also **cells of Martinotti** are present. They are mixed with nerve fiber which runs from and to the white matter beneath.

Applied Anatomy

- In Huntington disease (autosomal dominant), striatal neurons are lost from the cerebral cortex and putamen.
- **Ganglioglioma:** Tumor affecting temporal lobe. There will be presence of a mixed population of neoplastic astrocytes and abnormal ganglion cells.

Viva voce

Q. What is the inner band of Baillarger?
Ans. The nerve fibers of the pyramidal layer are arranged horizontally. And this is known as the inner band of Baillarger.
Q. Where are horizontal cells of Cajal present?
Ans. They are present in the molecular or plexiform layer.

CHAPTER 2: Embryology

OUTLINE

- General Embryology
- Systemic Embryology
- Genetics

Embryology

GENERAL EMBRYOLOGY

■ EMBRYOGENESIS (FIG. 1)

- Sperm + Oocyte → Zygote → Cleavage → Morula → Differentiate → Inner cell mass (embryoblast) + Trophoblast → Blastocyst → Embryonic Disc
- Inner cell mass (embryoblast) has two parts:
  1. Epiblast (ectoderm) → Embryo, amnion
  2. Hypoblast (endoderm) → Yolk sac
- Trophoblast → Syncytiotrophoblast + Cytotrophoblast → Placenta (fetal part).

■ IMPLANTATION (FIG. 2)

- Post shedding of the ovum, it reaches uterus via uterine tubes and undergoes fertilization.
- A fertilized ovum as it reaches uterus, it would have become a morula.
- Trophoblast cells of embryo have a property to stick to any tissue which it comes in contact with.
- Morula covered by zona pellucida prevent morula from sticking to the walls of uterine tube.
- After zona pellucida disappears the trophoblast cells become exposed and gets sticked to uterine endometrium. This is known as implantation.

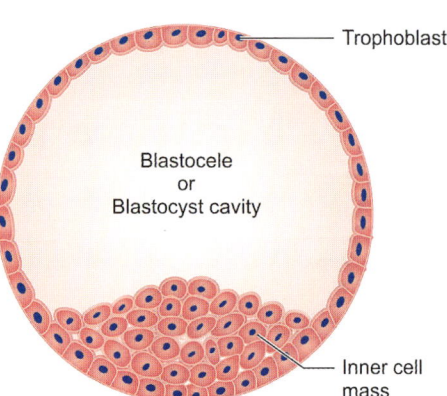

Fig. 1: Blastocyst.

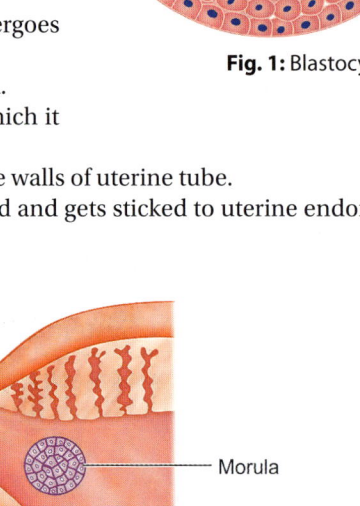

Fig. 2: Implantation.

Interstitial Implantation

In humans, the trophoblast of blastocyst after sticking to the uterine endometrium burrow and grow deep into it and finally whole of embryo comes under the substance of endometrium.

Applied Anatomy

Abnormal Implantation

- *Extrauterine implantation/ectopic pregnancy:* Sites include ovary, uterine tubes, abdominal cavity (common), very rarely in cesarean scar.
- *Abnormal intrauterine implantation:* Placenta previa, it occurs in the lower part of uterine cavity.

Embryology

DECIDUA (FIG. 3)

- Uterine endometrium after implantation is known as decidua.
- Stromal cells become enlarged and vacuolated and stores glycogen and lipids, also nuclei become rounded, volume of cell increases, etc., this change in stromal cells is termed as **decidual reaction**.
- Decidua consists of three parts:
  1. *Decidua basalis:* Maternal source of placenta, firmly attached to chorion, present at embryonic pole and also called decidual plate and contain large cells with high lipid content.
  2. *Decidua capsularis:* Separates embryo from uterine lumen.
  3. *Decidua parietalis:* It lines the uterine cavity.

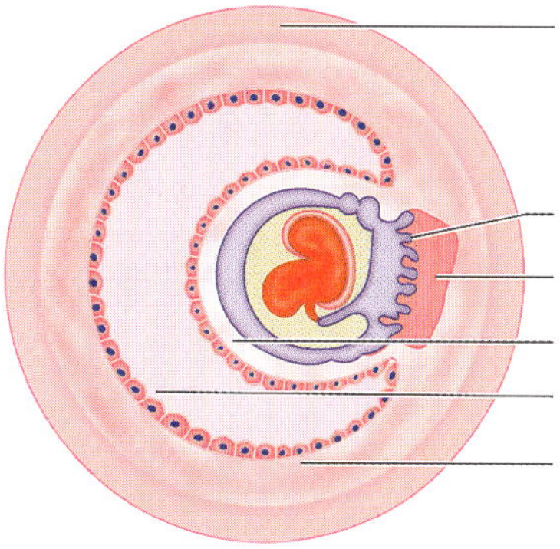

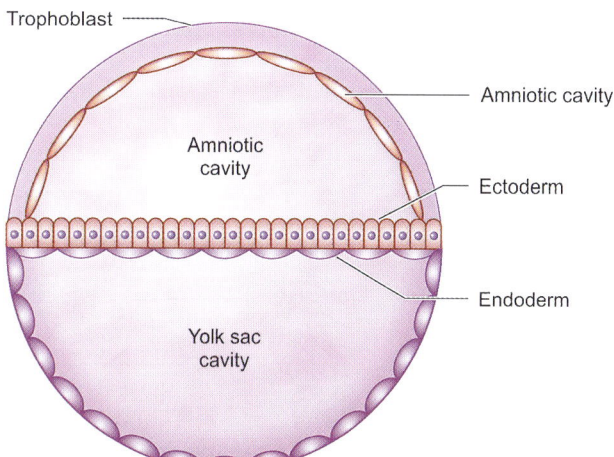

Fig. 3: Decidua.

EMBRYONIC DISC AND GERM LAYERS (FIG. 4)

- Some cells of the inner cell mass differentiate into flat cells and come to lower end and form endoderm, remaining cells become columnar and form ectoderm.
- A space arises between trophoblast and ectoderm called amniotic cavity.
- Some cells of trophoblast gets seperated and forms the roof of amniotic cavity. These cells are called amniogenic cells.
- Flat cells from endoderm cover blastocystic cavity and the newly formed cavity is called primary yolk sac.
- The cells of trophoblast form a mass called extraembryonic mesoderm. Gradually small spaces form inside these mass of cells and form a cavity called extraembryonic celom.
- As a result extraembryonic mesoderm is split into two layers—the outermost part called somatopleuric or parietal extraembryonic mesoderm and innermost, i.e., just outside the yolk sac called the splanchnopleuric or visceral extraembryonic mesoderm.
- But the extraembryonic celom is not continuous where extraembryonic mesoderm attaches the amniotic cavity to trophoblast. And this unsplit part of extraembryonic mesoderm forms the **connecting stalk**.
- **Chorion** is formed by parietal extraembryonic mesoderm and overlying trophoblast.
- Amnion is formed by amniogenic cells derived from trophoblast.
- The primary yolk sac undergoes reduction in size and cells become cubical forming secondary yolk sac.
- In the disc formed, in an area near the margin, the cubical cells of endoderm becomes columnar and this area is called **prochordal plate**.
- Soon some of the cells lying along the central axis of prochordal plate proliferate and bulge and form elevation called **primitive streak**.

Fig. 4: Embryonic germ layers.

INTRAEMBRYONIC MESODERM

Cells present on both sides of primitive streak proliferates, these cells migrate craniolateraly between endoderm and ectoderm layers and forms the intraembryonic mesoderm. It get's divided into four parts:
1. **Paraxial mesoderm** → somites, neuromers.
2. **Intermediate cell mass** → nephrons, smooth muscles and connective tissue of respiratory system.
3. **Lateral plate mesoderm** → somatopleuric mesoderm, splanchnopleuric mesoderm and septum transversum.
4. **Endothelium** of vessels and endocardium of heart.

SOMITES

- Paraxial mesoderm on either side of notochord differentiates, which gives rise to cuboidal paired bodies, known as somitomeres which further differentiates into somites.
- It extends from cranial end of notochord to coccygeal end, somites contains a slit like cavity called **myocele**.
- Each somite is subdivided into three parts, each part give rise to specialized structure they are:
    1. **Sclerotome** (ventromedial part)—gives rise to vertebral column and ribs.
    2. **Dermatome** (lateral part)—gives rise to dermis of skin and subcutaneous tissue.
    3. **Myotome** (intermediate part)—gives rise to striated muscles.

NOTOCHORD (FIG. 5)

- The cranial end of primitive streak gets thickened and this part is known as **primitive knot**.
- A depression appears in the center of primitive knot called as **blastopore**. Cells in the primitive knot multiply and pass cranially in between ectoderm and endoderm and reaches the caudal margin of prochordal plate resulting in formation of a solid cord known as **notochordal process**.
- The cells of notochordal process undergoes various degree of rearrangements and finally forms a solid rod called **notochord**.
- Notochord mostly disappears after development but small portion of it persist as **nucleus pulposes** in intervertebral discs.

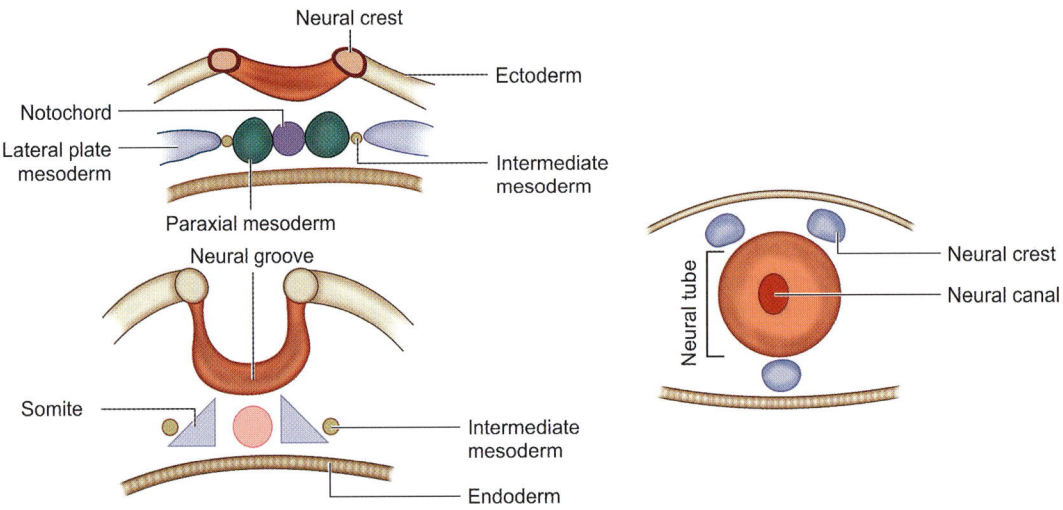

Fig. 5: Notochord and neural tube formation.

NEURULATION

- It is the process of formation of neural tube from the precursor neural plate and neural folds. Ectoderm overlying the notochord undergoes thickening.
- This thickened plate is known as **neural plate**.
- Notochord induces the formation of neural plate.
- Neural plate gets depressed in the midline to form **neural groove**.
- Neural groove has raised lateral edges known as the **neural folds**.
- Neural folds begins fusing at the middle and the fusion extends cranially and caudally.
- Since initially the middle part is becoming tubular, the neural tube opens cranially and caudally, forming the **anterior neuropore** and **posterior neuropore** respectively.
- Anterior neuropore closes 2–3 days before the closure of posterior neuropore.
- Neurulation is completed by the complete closure of the neuropores, resulting in formation of **neural tube**.
- Neural tube can be divided into:
    1. Enlarged cranial part → Brain ← Prosencephalon / Mesencephalon / Rhombencephalon
    2. Tubular caudal part → Spinal cord.

NEURAL CREST

- During the formation of neural plate few cells located between neural plate and rest of ectoderm undergo differentiation and become specialized.
- These specialized neuroectodermal cells are called **neural crest** cells.
- At the point of separation of neural tube from ectoderm surface, the neural crest cells lies on the dorsolateral aspect of neural tube.
- Later, the neural crest cells becomes free and migrate to distant sites, they mainly forms the peripheral nervous system.
- Structures derived from neural crest include arachnoid and piamater, neurons of dorsal root ganglion, Schwann cells, melanoblasts, chromaffin tissue, cardiac semilunar valves, tooth enamel, thyroid parafollicular cells, derivatives of pharyngeal arches, etc.

LAMINA TERMINALIS

- Derived from wall of neural tube.
- Closes cranial end of **prosencephalon**.

PLACENTA (FIG. 6)

- Formed from two sources:
  1. Fetal source—**chorion frondosum**
  2. Maternal source—**decidua basalis**
- The essential part of placenta is chorionic villi surrounded by maternal blood and fetal blood circulates through capillaries in villi.
- Syncytiotrophoblast part of trophoblast proliferates and grow towards the decidua basalis and capsularis.
- Trophoblast proper with primary mesoderm forms chorion.
- Lacunar spaces appear within the syncytiotrophoblast and decidua basalis.
- Trabeculae containing cords of syncytial cells are present between these lacunar spaces.
- Lacunae enlarge and contain uterine vessels.
- Then the cytotrophoblast extends into the core of trabeculae, converts them into **primary chorionic villi**.
- Now lacunar spaces are called **intervillous** spaces.
- In the development of chorionic villi it undergoes three stages:
  1. **Primary villi** consisting of a central core of cytotrophoblast covered by syncytiotrophoblast.
  2. **Secondary villi** having layers extraembryonic mesoderm, cytotrophoblast and syncytiotrophoblast.
  3. **Tertiary villi** having blood capillaries in extraembryonic mesoderm.
- Cytotrophoblast spreads outwards at tips of primary villi, resulting in outer cytotrophoblastic shell.
- Primary mesodermal cells invade central core of primary villi to form secondary villi.
- Fetal vessels derived from umbilical vessels appear within primary mesoderm, forming the tertiary villi.
- Tertiary chorionic villi attached to decidua basalis forms the chorion frondosum. Rest of the villi attached to the embryonic pole degenerates. This results in the formation of placenta from chorion frondosum and decidua basalis.

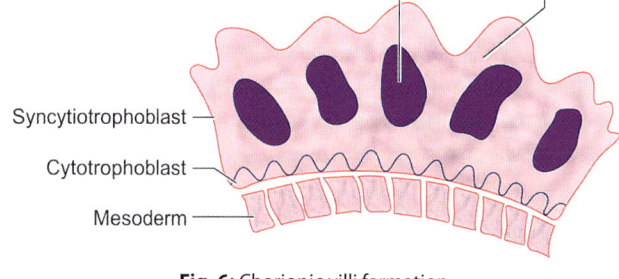

Fig. 6: Chorionic villi formation.

Anomalies

Chorion epithelioma: It is a malignant tumor, results when endometrium is too resistant to blastocyst.

SYSTEMIC EMBRYOLOGY

PHARYNGEAL ARCHES (FIG. 7)

- Series of mesodermal thickenings appear in the wall of cranial part of primitive foregut, known as **pharyngeal arches**.
- Each arch contains an outer lining of **ectoderm**, inner core of **mesoderm**, and an inner lining of **endoderm**.
- At first there will be **six arches**, later the **fifth arch disappears**.
- Each arch extends into the floor of primitive pharynx and meet's its corresponding arch at the midline.
- At this stage the cranial end of pharynx is separated from stomatodeum by **buccopharyngeal membrane**.
- Buccopharyngeal membrane ruptures soon.
- In the gap between successive arches the endoderm is pushed outside and ectoderm is pushed inside, giving rise to endodermal pouches and ectodermal clefts respectively.
- Each pharyngeal arch consists of three elements:
  1. **Skeletal element:** It is cartilaginous in beginning, it remains as such or form bone or disappears.
  2. **Striated muscle:** Supplied by special nerve of the arch, first attached with skeletal elements, may retain or not retain these attachments in future. May subdivide to give distinct muscles. Sometimes these muscles moves away from arch but takes it's nerve with it.
  3. **Arterial arch (aortic arch):** Arteries develop ventral and dorsal to foregut, known as ventral and dorsal aortae respectively. Two arteries of a pharyngeal arch are connected by an aortic arch of its own. Artery gets modified during the course of time.
- Important derivatives of pharyngeal arches:
  1. **First arch (mandibular arch):** Meckel's cartilage, maleus, incus, muscles of mastication, etc.
  2. **Second arch (hyoid arch):** Superior part of hyoid, stapes, styloid process, muscles of face, etc.
  3. **Third arch:** Greater part of hyoid, stylopharyngeus, etc.
  4. **Fourth arch and sixth arch:** Larynx (cartilaginous part), muscles of larynx and pharynx, etc.

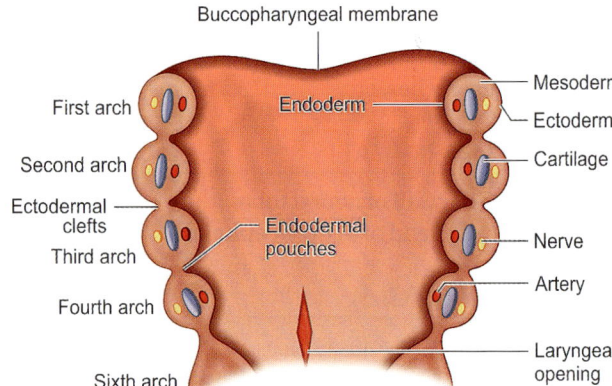

Fig. 7: Pharyngeal arches.

PALATE (FIG. 8)

Palate is developed from:
- **Maxillary process**, which is two in number.
- **Frontonasal process**

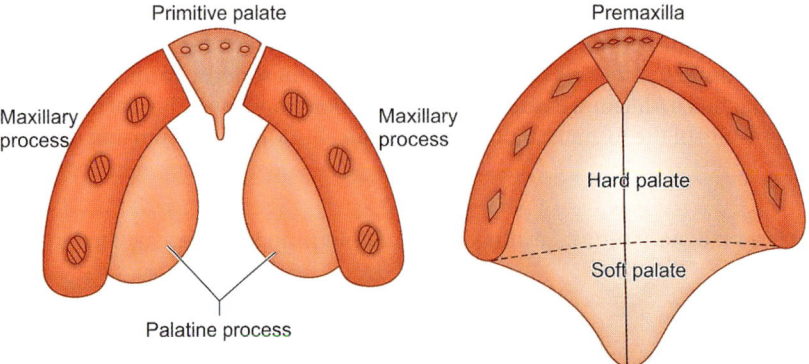

Fig. 8: Development of palate.

Steps of Fusion
- From each maxillary process, a plate like shelf grows medially known as **palatal process**.
- Primitive palate is formed by the fusion of medial nasal folds.
- Medial nasal folds are folds of frontonasal process.
- Now palate proper is formed by the fusion of these three components, i.e., two palatal processes and one primitive palate.
- Each palatal process fuses with posterior margin of primitive palate.
- Each palatal processes fuses with each other at midline.
- Also palatal process fuses with lower free edge of nasal septum separating nasal cavity into two.
- Most of palate gets ossified to form **hard palate** and unossified posterior part forms **soft palate**.

Cleft Palate
It is a developmental anomaly **(Fig. 9)** due to defective fusion of various components of palate.
1. Bilateral complete cleft palate:
    - Occurs due to complete non-fusion.
    - Give rise to Y-shaped cleft.
    - Associated with bilateral cleft lip.
2. Unilateral complete cleft palate:
    - Due to complete arrest of fusion of palatine process of one side with primitive palate and nasal septum.
    - Associated with unilateral hair lip.

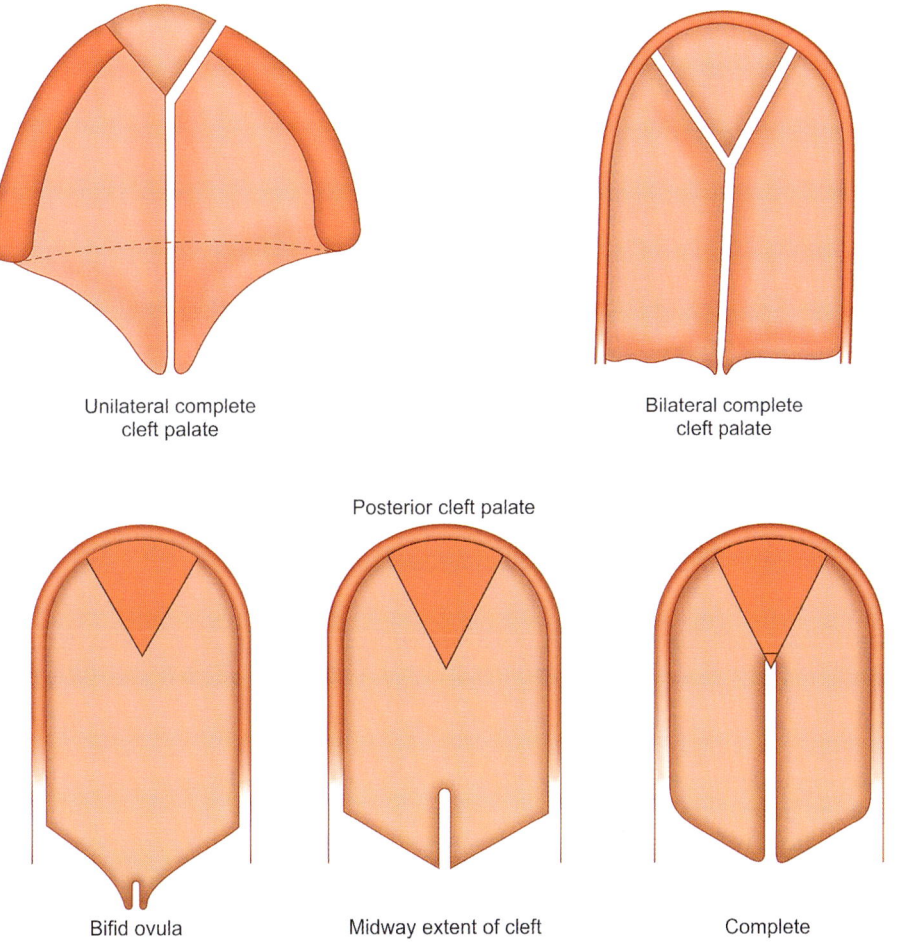

Fig. 9: Anomalies of palate.

3. Partial midline cleft:
    - Due to complete failure of fusion of palatine process with each other.
    - Cleft of soft palate
4. Due to complete failure of fusion of palatine process with each other in the dorsal 1/4th part.

FACE (FIG. 10)

- Face develops from various processes (eminences), that develop around the stomatodeum, due to proliferation of underlying mesoderm.
- The neural crest cells that migrate into the head and neck region are responsible for the differentiation of mesoderm.
- The various processes are:
  1. Frontonasal process
  2. A pair of mandibular and maxillary processes
  3. A pair of lateral and medial nasal processes
- Mesoderm infront of the prosencephalon proliferates and forms the frontonasal process.
- **Mandibular process** (formed from mandibular arch) develops dorsolaterally to stomatodeum and it is directed medially.
- **Maxillary process** is formed as a branch from the dorsolateral part of mandibular process.
- On each side of frontonasal process, an ectodermal elevation occurs called as **nasal placodes or olfactory placodes**.
- Mesoderm surrounding the margins of nasal placodes starts to proliferate and gets raised.
- As a result the nasal placodes sinks and this give rise to **nasal pits or olfactory pits**.
- The raised margins are divided into two:
  1. **Medial nasal process**, present medially
  2. **Lateral nasal process**, present laterally
- Frontonasal process gives rise to forearm, dorsum of nose and nasal septum.
- Mandibular process grows medially and fuses with each other, resulting in formation of lower jaw, lower lip, etc.
- Mandibular and maxillary processes combinedly gives rise to cheeks, in addition maxillary process forms the lateral part of upper lip.
- Medial nasal process fuses with each other and forms the **philtrum**.
- Lateral nasal process gives rise to lateral wall of nose.

Anomalies

Macrostomia: Due to incomplete fusion of mandibular and maxillary processes leading to large mouth.

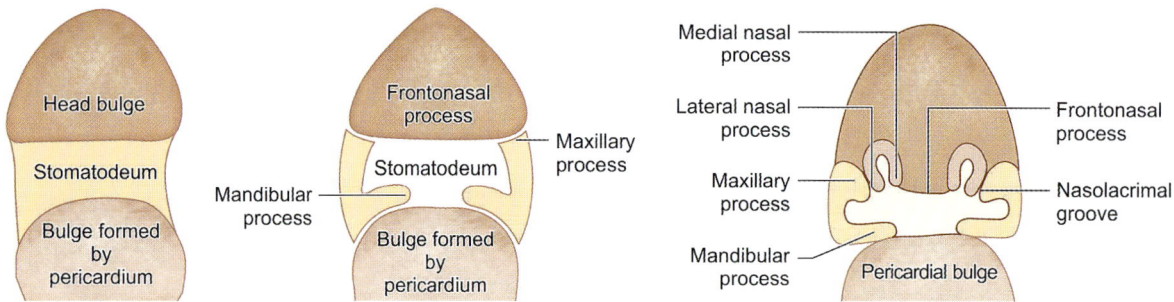

Fig. 10: Development of face.

UPPER LIP

Developed principally from fusion **lateral and medial nasal process** with **right and left maxillary process**.

Steps of Fusion

- **Maxillary and lateral nasal process** are initially separated by a **nasolacrimal groove**.
- Both maxillary process grows medially.
- Maxillary process first fuses with lateral nasal process.
- Secondly fuses with medial nasal process.
- Medial and lateral nasal process also then fuses with each other.
- Median part of upper lip or philtrum is derived from **frontonasal process**.
- By the formation of upper lip, nasal pits are cut off from the stomatodeum.

TONGUE (FIG. 11)

- Medial most part of first pharyngeal arches proliferates and forms two **lingual swellings**.
- Lingual swellings are partially separated by a median swelling called **tuberculum impar**.
- Another midline swelling called **hypobranchial eminence** is also formed from mesoderm of 2nd, 3rd, and 4th arches.
- Anterior 2/3rd of tongue is formed by the fusion of two lingual swellings with tuberculum impar.
- The cranial part of hypobranchial eminence (3rd arch) give rise to posterior one-third of tongue.
- Posterior most part is formed from fourth arch.
- Connective tissue is derived from mesenchyme.
- Tongue muscles are derived from occipital myotomes.

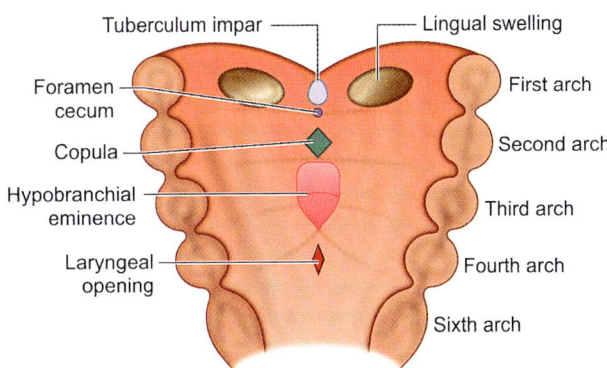

Fig. 11: Tongue.

Anomalies

Ankyloglossia (tongue tie): Here frenulum extends to tip of tongue as a result tongue become anchored to floor of mouth.

THYROID GLAND (FIG. 12)

- Thyroid gland develops from an endodermal **thyroid diverticulum** arising from the floor of pharynx.
- At the floor of pharynx, medial ends of two mandibular arches are separated by a midline swelling called **tuberculum impar**.
- Endodermal cells dorsal to tuberculum impar proliferate to cause a surface elevation at the midline (at the junction of anterior one-third and posterior two-thirds of tongue).
- Later, this elevation get depressed and cells get evaginated caudally, and forms a narrow thyroid diverticulum.
- It grows downwards into the neck. As the lower end of diverticulum reaches ventral to the proximal part of trachea, it bifurcates and forms a bilobed mass. This bilobed mass develops into thyroid gland.
- Rest of diverticulum remains narrow and is known as thyroglossal duct (usually disappears).
- The cranial end of disappeared thyroglossal duct persist as foramen cecum.
- Lower end of thyroglossal duct may persist as pyramidal lobe.
- Parafollicular cells are derived from caudal pharyngeal complex called ultimobranchial body.
- Remnants of thyroglossal ducts may sometimes results in thyroglossal fistula.

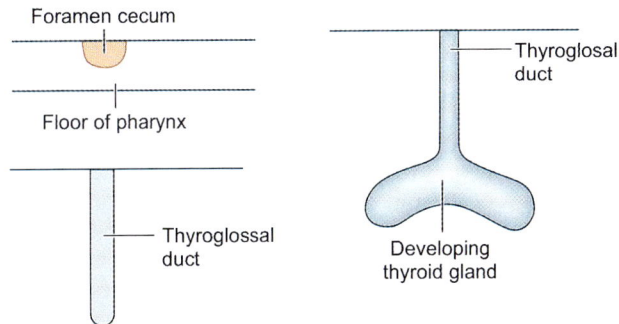

Fig. 12: Thyroid gland.

LUNGS

- Lungs developed from lung buds which develops at the caudal end of laryngotracheal tube.
- It divides into two knob like bronchial buds, which grows into celomic ducts, the primordia of pleural cavities.
- They are surrounded by splanchnic mesenchyme.
- Each bronchial bud enlarges to form primary bronchus.
- Primary bronchus on right side forms superior and inferior secondary bronchi, on the left side forms two secondary bronchus for superior and inferior lobes.
- Secondary bronchus forms tertiary bronchus. Ten on right and nine on left side each.
- Surrounding mesenchyme gives rise to a bronchopulmonary segment.
- Cartilage, smooth muscles, connective tissue, and capillaries are derived from surrounding splanchnic mesenchyme.
- Visceral pleura from splanchnic mesoderm and parietal pleura from somatopleuric mesoderm.

HEART TUBE (FIG. 13)

- Mesodermal in origin.
- During 3rd week angioblastic cords are formed from intraembryonic mesoderm.
- Angioblastic cords are paired endothelial strands formed in cardiogenic area.
- Cords undergo canalization and forms heart tubes.
- Firstly heart is right and left endothelial tubes which fuse together to form single tube.
- Single tube undergo dilatation separated by constrictions from top to bottom.
- These dilatations from above to below are later identified as:
  1. Bulbus cordis has three parts:
     i. *Truncus arteriosus*: Distal 1/3rd part, forms ascending aorta and pulmonary trunk, truncus arteriosus continuous distally with aortic sac.
     ii. *Conus*: Middle 1/3rd, forms outflow tracts of ventricles.
     iii. *Proximal*: 1/3rd part, forms primitive right ventricle.
  2. Primitive ventricle, form trabeculated part of left ventricle.
  3. Primitive atrium
  4. Sinus venosus
- Sinus venosus has prolongations at caudal end called right and left horns.
- Each horn is joined by a vitelline vein, umbilical vein and common cardinal vein.

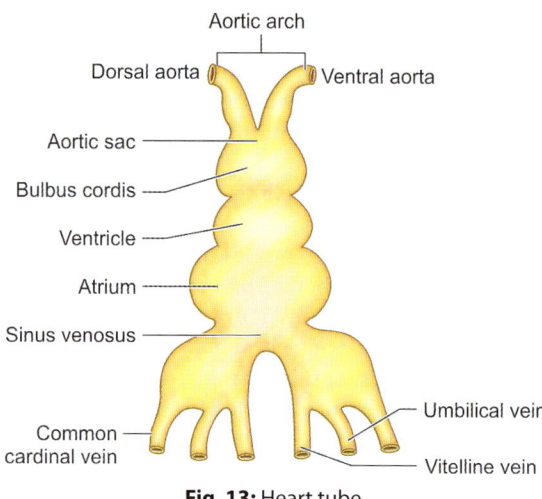

Fig. 13: Heart tube.

RIGHT ATRIUM

- Mainly formed from the right half of primitive atrium.
- Rough anterior part develops from right horn of sinus venosus.
- Sinus venosus and right half of atrioventricular canal get absorbed into right atrium.
- Smooth posterior part along with right auricle develops from primitive atrium.

INTERATRIAL SEPTUM (FIGS. 14A TO D)

- It develops from two septa (septum primum and septum secondum) arising from the roof of atrial chamber.
- Septum primum arise from roof of atrial chamber and grows downwards towards septum intermedium.
- Initially there will be a gap between septum primum and septum intermedium known as **foramen primum**.
- Finally septum primum fuses with septum intermedium.
- Before the fusion, the upper part of septum primum breaks down leaving a free upper edge.
- And a new foramen is created known as **foramen secondum.**
- Another septum called as septum secondum start to grow from the right of the septum primum, towards septum intermedium.
- Another septum called as septum secondum start to grow from the right of the septum primum, towards septum intermedium.
- Septum secondum overlaps the upper margin of septum primum, creating an oblique passage between septum primum and secondum called as **foramen ovale.**

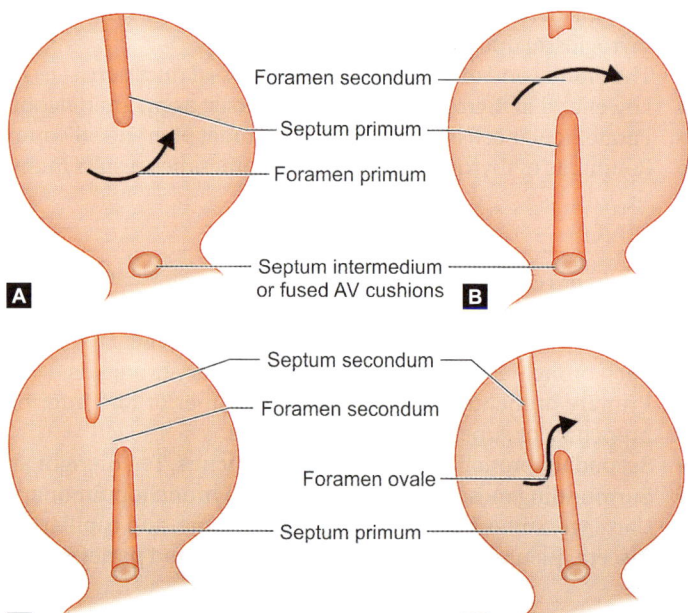

Figs. 14A to D: Development of interatrial septum.

- In fetal life, foramen ovale allows the blood to flow from right to left atrium.
- Finally by the fusion of septum secondum and septum primum, the foramen ovale is obliterated.
- Thus upper and lower half of interatrial septum is formed by septum secondum and primum respectively.

FALLOT'S TETRALOGY

Congenital condition characterized by:
- Stenosis of pulmonary trunk.
- Large ventricular septal defect (VSD).
- Overriding of aortic orifice above VSD
- Right ventricular hypertrophy due to high BP in RV.
- Results in severe cyanosis.

DIAPHRAGM

- Central tendon from septum transversum.
- Dorsal paired portion of diaphragm from pleuroperitoneal membrane. Circumferential portion from lateral thoracic wall.
- Dorsal unpaired portion from dorsal mesentery of esophagus.

GUT

Endoderm differentiates into foregut, midgut and hindgut.

Foregut Derivatives

Epithelium of pharynx, esophagus, stomach, duodenum till ampulla of Vater, respiratory system auditory tube and mucous membrane of tongue, parenchyma of liver, pancreas, thyroid, parathyroid, etc.

Midgut Derivatives

Epithelium of duodenum from ampulla of Vater to junction of right 2/3rd and left 1/3rd of transverse colon.

Hindgut Derivatives

Mucous membrane of large intestine from left 1/3rd of transverse colon to mucocutaneous junction of anal canal, parenchyma of prostate, epithelium of urinary bladder, urethra, etc.

ESOPHAGUS

- Developed from posterior most part of foregut.
- It is short in the beginning but it lengthens quickly due to descend of heart and lungs.
- Musculature is derived from the splanchnic mesenchyme surrounding the foregut.

STOMACH (FIG. 15)

- Distal part of foregut shows a fusiform dilatation.
- This dilatation represents the primitive stomach.
- Primitive stomach has anterior and posterior borders, right and left surfaces. The posterior border grows faster than anterior border.
- It undergoes 90° clockwise rotation along vertical axis.
- As a result left and right surfaces becomes anterior and posterior surfaces, posterior and anterior borders give rise to greater (left border) and lesser (right border) curvatures respectively.

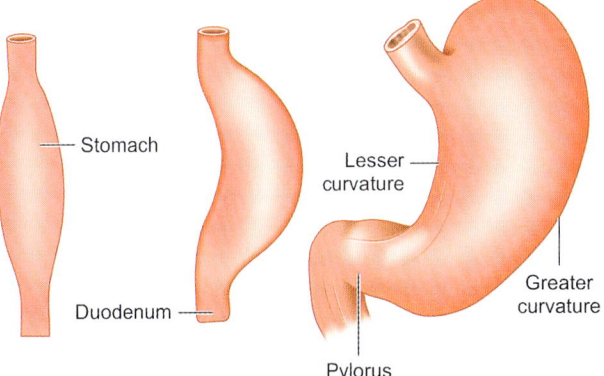

Fig. 15: Development of stomach.

MECKEL'S DIVERTICULUM (FIG. 16)

- Midgut communicate with yolk sac at embryological stage through vitellointestinal duct
- Normally vitellointestinal duct involutes and disappears, occasionally the duct closes at umbilical end but remain patent at intestinal end.
- Patent vitellointestinal duct gives rise to Meckel's diverticulum.
- This patent part appears as out pocketing of ileum.
- Occurs in 2% subjects, 2 inches long and situated 2 ft proximal to ileocecal valve, occurs most commonly in children under 2, and is symptomatic in 2% of patients.

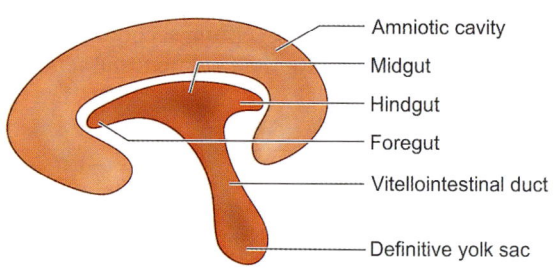

Fig. 16: Meckel's diverticulum.

PANCREAS (FIG. 17)

- Pancreas is developed from two endodermal buds (ventral and dorsal buds), formed at the junction of foregut and midgut.
- Dorsal bud lies at dorsal aspect of gut. Ventral bud lies below hepatic bud.
- Large part of pancreas develops from dorsal bud.
- Ventral bud gives rise to inferior part of head of pancreas and uncinate process.
- Dorsal bud gives rise to upper part of head of pancreas, body and tail of pancreas.
- Dorsal and ventral buds give rise to primitive ducts.
- Proximal part of the duct of dorsal bud form accessory pancreatic duct.
- Distal part of duct of dorsal bud and duct of ventral bud, together forms main pancreatic duct.

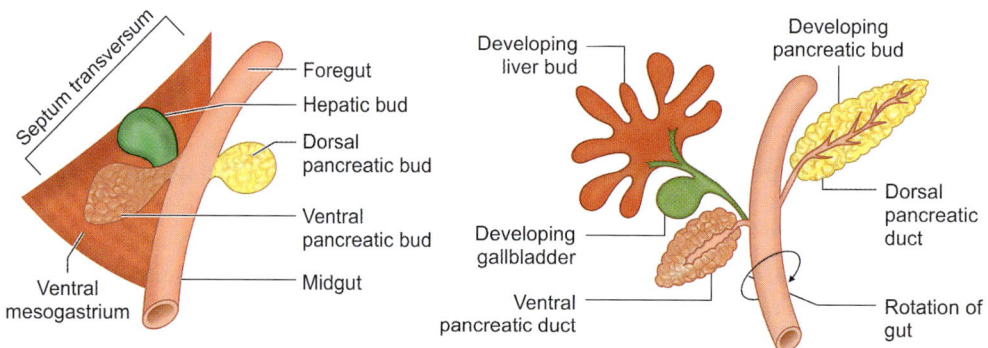

Fig. 17: Development of liver and pancreas.

Anomalies

Annular pancreas: Pancreatic tissue surrounds the duodenum and obstructs it.

LIVER AND GALLBLADDER (FIG. 17)

- Liver is derived from an endodermal bud known as hepatic bud.
- Hepatic bud is formed at the junction between foregut and midgut.
- It grows into the septum transversum via ventral mesogastrium.
- The bud enlarges and divides into:
  - Large cranial part called **pars hepatica**.
  - Small caudal part called **pars cystica**.
- Pars hepatica divides into two parts, that later forms the parenchyma of right and left lobes, Kupffer's cells and blood cells are formed from mesoderm of septum transversum.
- Pars cystica forms the gallbladder and cystic duct.

KIDNEY (FIG. 18)

- Kidney develops from the intermediate cell mass.
- Intermediate cell mass lies between paraxial mesoderm and lateral plate mesoderm.
- Paraxial mesoderm gives rise to somites.

- Intermediate cell masses extends craniocaudally on both sides of primitive dorsal aorta.
- In cervical and upper thoracic region it shows segmentation called nephrotomes.
- Remaining unsegmented portion below give rise to nephrogenic cord.
- Nephrogenic cord later divides into three parts, from above to below pronephros, mesonephros, metanephros.
- Excretory tubules of kidney are formed from metanephros.
- Collecting part of kidney is formed from a diverticulum called **ureteric bud**.
- Ureteric bud is derived from lower part of mesonephric duct.
- Horse-shoe kidney—lower pole of two kidneys fuse together to form an isthmus.

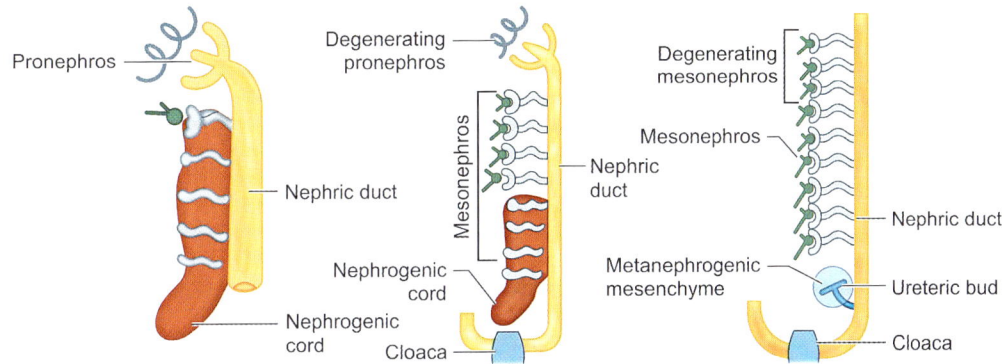

Fig. 18: Development of kidney.

URINARY BLADDER

- Cloaca is subdivided by urorectal septum into:
  - Anterior primitive urogenital sinus
  - Posterior anorectal canal
- Cranial and largest part of urogenital sinus is called **vesicourethral canal**.
- Vesicourethral canal forms most of the urinary bladder.
- Trigone of bladder is formed by absorption of mesonephric duct.
- Apex of bladder is derived from urachus.
- Splanchnopleuric mesoderm gives rise to muscular and serous walls of the bladder.
- *Ectopia vesicae*: Congenital anomaly in which posterior wall of bladder is exposed to outside, anterior wall of bladder is missing.
- *Hour glass bladder*: Urinary bladder become divided into upper and lower part by a middle constriction, thus giving an appearance of an hour glass.

UTERUS (FIG. 19)

- Paramesonephric ducts (Müllerian ducts) gets fused to form uterovaginal canal.
- Epithelium of uterus is developed from uterovaginal canal.
- Myometrium is formed from surrounding mesoderm.
- Unfused horizontal parts of two paramesonephric ducts partially get embedded in substance of myometrium to form the fundus of uterus.
- Soon after, cervix is also recognized as a separate region.
- *Didelphys uterus*: Complete duplication of uterus.
- *Unicornuate uterus*: One-half of uterus absent.

UTERINE TUBE (FIG. 19)

Derived from unfused parts of paramesonephric ducts.

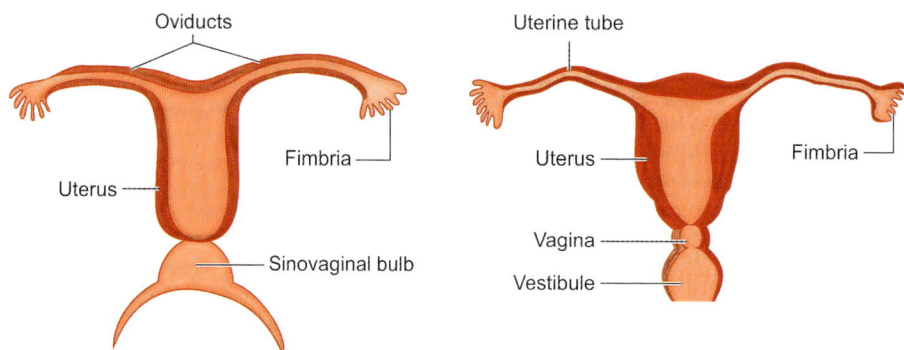

Fig. 19: Development of uterus and uterine tubes.

DEVELOPMENT OF GONADS (TESTIS AND OVARIES) (FIG. 20)

- The development of testis and ovaries begins in a similar manner but parts way at a particular point.
- Gonads develop from three sources:
  1. **Intermediate mesoderm**—which is present medial to middle part of mesonephros.
  2. **Coelomic epithelium**—which covers the intermediate mesoderm.
  3. **Primordial germ cells** from the wall of yolk sac near the allantois.
- Coelomic epithelium begins to proliferate and it gets thickened.
- Mesoderm below the coelomic epithelium condenses due to thickening of coelomic epithelium.
- Both these process lead to formation of genital ridge.
- Coelomic epithelial cells continue to proliferate and they invade the condensed mesoderm in the form of solid cords, known as the **"sex cords"**.
- Primordial germ cells from the wall of yolk sac migrate along the dorsal mesentery of hindgut towards the developing gonad.
- Sex cords and primordial germ cells get intermixed.
- Till this point the development of testis and ovaries are the same.

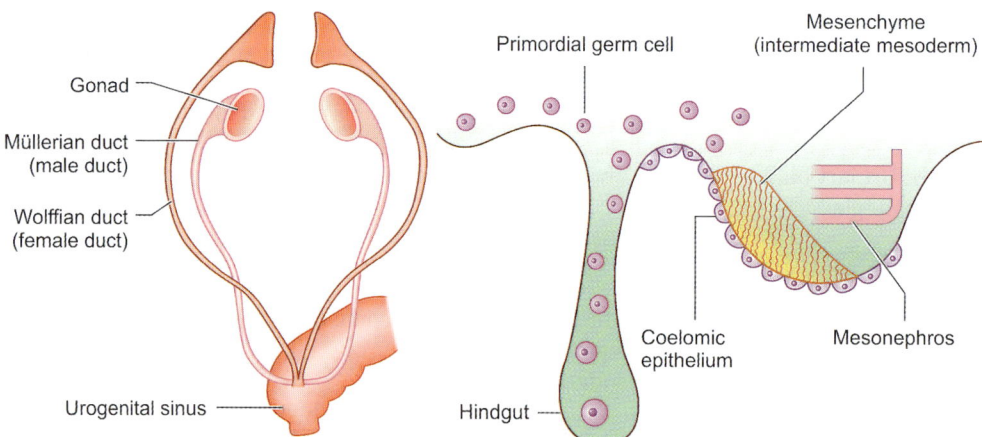

Fig. 20: Development of gonads.

Testis

- Sex cords increase in length and extend into the medulla of developing gonad. Sex cords are now called as **medullary cords**.
- The sex cords anastomoses with each other and canalize resulting in formation of seminiferous tubules.
- The ends of seminiferous tubules anastomoses with one another giving rise to rete testis.
- Two types of cells lines the seminiferous tubules:
  1. *Spermatogenic cells:* Formed from primordial germ cells.
  2. *Sertoli cells:* Formed from coelomic epithelium.

- A dense fibrous layer is formed by mesoderm which separates the sex cords from coelomic epithelium, known as **tunica albuginea**. Mesoderm also gives rise to:
  1. Leydig cells.
  2. Connective tissue around seminiferous tubules.
  3. Mediastinum testis.
- The canal of epididymis and vas deferens develop from mesonephric duct.

Descend of Testis
- Testis which develops in relation to lumbar region of the posterior abdominal wall starts to descend.
- It gradually descend to the scrotum through iliac fossa (3rd month) and inguinal canal (7th month), finally reaching scrotum by the end of 8th month. It is a mandatory developmental process to ensure that the mature testis promotes normal spermatogenesis.
- Some factors responsible for descend of testis are:
  - Increased intra-abdominal pressure.
  - *Gubernaculum:* Guiding force for descent.
  - Differential growth of body wall.

Anomalies
- *Cryptorchidism:* Descend of one or both testis may fail to occur or is arrested somewhere in the pathway.
- *Ectopic testis:* Testis may lie in abnormal positions like in the femoral canal, under the skin of penis or on the front of thigh, behind the scrotum in perineum.

Ovary
- Unlike the development of testis where the sex cords increase in length and extend into the medulla, the sex cords of female do not extend into medulla.
- Instead they get fragmented into small mass of cells.
- Each mass of cells surround a primordial germ cell, forming a primordial follicle.

RECTUM AND ANAL CANAL
- Upper part of rectum develops from endoderm of hind gut. Lower part of rectum and upper part of anal canal are developed from the anorectal canal.
- Lower part of anal canal developed from proctodeum.

PROSTATE
- Prostate develops from a large number of buds arising from the prostatic urethra.
- Buds arising from the endodermal part of prostatic urethra forms the glandular part of prostate.
- Buds arising from mesodermal part of prostatic urethra forms the stroma of prostate.

AMNIOCENTESIS
- Amniocentesis is a medical procedure used to obtain a sample of the amniotic fluid.
- Amniotic fluid contains cells shed by the fetus along with various enzymes, proteins, hormones, and other substances.
- These cells possess genetic information of the fetus and can be used to diagnose genetic abnormalities like chromosomal disorders and open neural tube defects (ONTDs).
- Amniocentesis can be performed in late pregnancy to check fetal well-being, such as lung maturity, infections, etc.
- Amniocentesis is generally done in women who are at high risk for chromosome abnormalities. Commonly between 15th to 20th weeks of pregnancy.
- Sex of fetus can also be determined by this procedure.

The steps of embryonic development is shown in **Figure 21**.

Embryology

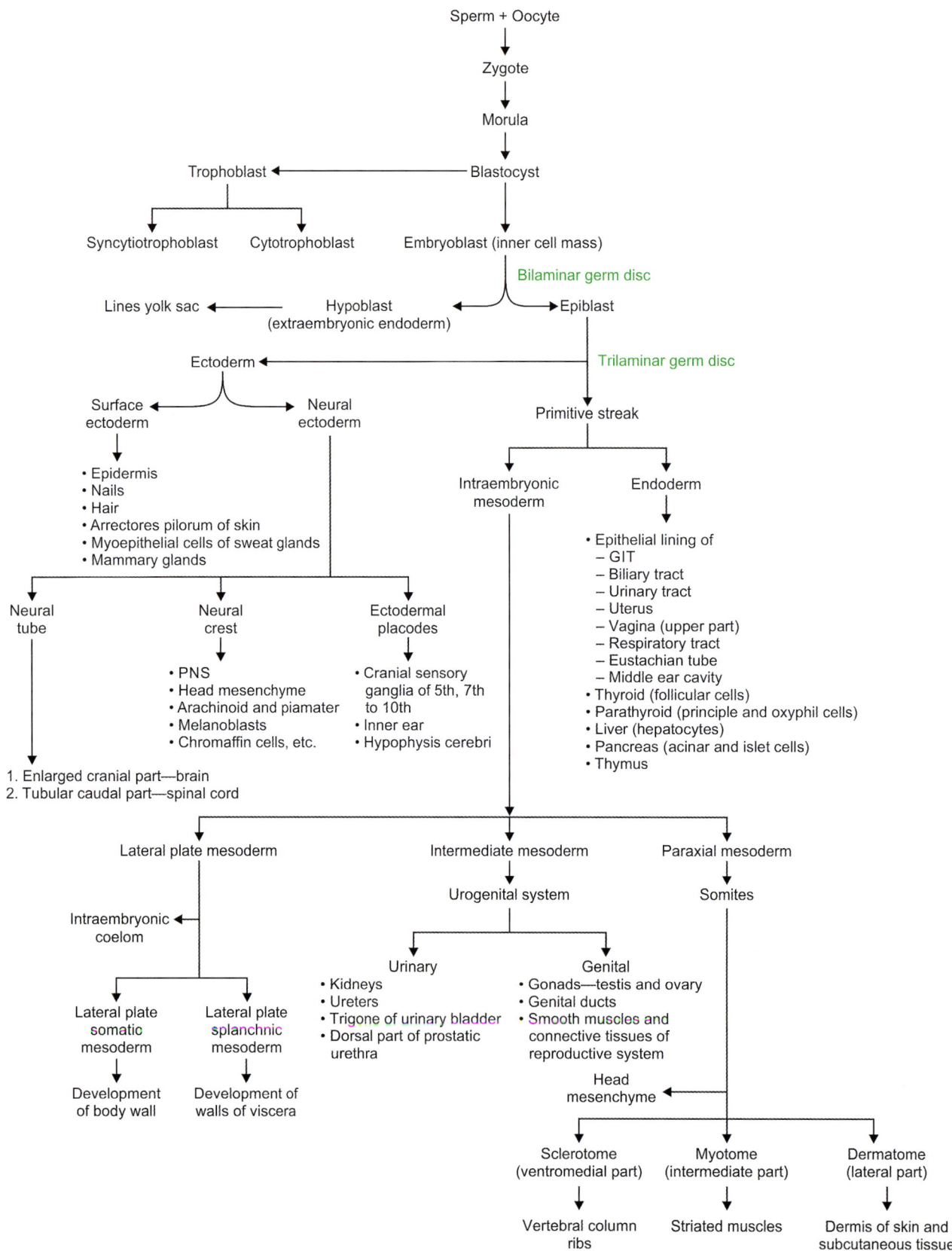

Fig. 21: Embryonic development: It is a complex process and in many places there will be contradictions. A chart can never illustrate the complete processs, so thorough reading is necessary for proper understanding of the concept. This chart is given to simplify the process by giving the student a basic idea of how the process goes. (PNS: peripheral nervous system; GIT: gastrointestinal tract)

GENETICS

BARR BODY (SEX CHROMATIN)

- Found by Barr and Bertram.
- This is seen in those species whose sex is determined by the presence of Y-chromosome.
- It is a densely stained, inactivated and condensed X-chromosome in a female somatic cell.
- It is found attached to the nuclear membrane.
- They are inactivated by a process known as lyonization. In lyonization the chromosome is inactivated by packing it in a way such that it has a transcriptionally inactive structure.
- Lyon's hypothesis (N-1 Rule)
- N = Number of X chromosomes
- It states that in cells with multiple X chromosomes, all the X chromosomes except one are inactivated.
- So in human female, XX, no. of Barr body: 2 – 1 = 1
  Male, XY, no. of Barr body : 1 – 1 = 0

CHROMOSOME BANDING

- It is also known as G-banding or Giemsa banding. Since Giemsa staining is most commonly used.
- It is a technique used in cytogenetics for precise identification of individual chromosomes or its parts.
- Methods:
  1. Cells are treated with tubulin inhibitors (colchicine's) which depolymerize the spindle and arrest the cells in metaphase.
  2. Cells are spread on glass slide.
  3. Chromosomes are then treated with trypsin and stained with Giemsa stain.
  4. This will give rise to dark regions (bands) and light regions (bands) in all the chromosomes.
  5. Each chromosome has a unique alternating dark and light staining pattern.
- Banding techniques used are:
  1. G-Banding (Giemsa stain)
  2. Q-Banding (quinacrine fluorescence stain)
  3. R-Banding (reverse Giemsa staining)
  4. C-Banding (constitutive heterochromatin demonstration)
- *Applications:* Chromosome mapping, to check for chromosomal rearrangements in malignancies, look for deletion and inversion in case of mutations.

KARYOTYPING

- Karyotype is the photographic representation of the stained preparation of chromosomes.
- Karyotyping is the classification of chromosomes based on their:
  1. Banding pattern.
  2. Length.
  3. Position of centromere.
- Chromosomes are arranged in the descending order of their length
- Identical chromosome sarepaired and numbered from 1 to 22 (1 is the longest chromosome).
- These chromosomes are divided into seven groups **(Fig. 22)**:
  1. Group A (CHR 1-3)
  2. Group B (CHR 4-5)
  3. Group C (CHR 6-12)
  4. Group D (CHR 13-15)
  5. Group E (CHR 16-18)
  6. Group F (CHR 19-20)
  7. Group G (CHR 21-22)
- *Applications:* To study chromosomal aberrations, to identify abnormal chromosome, to gather information about past evolutionary events, etc.

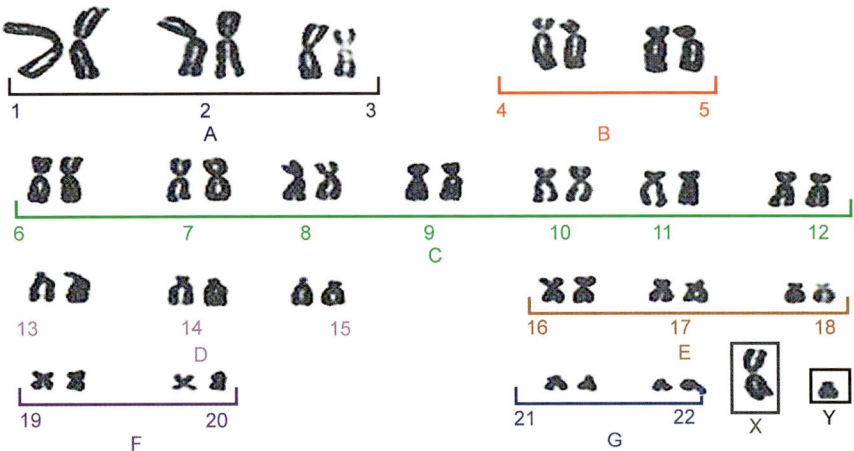

Fig. 22: Groups of chromosome.

NONDISJUNCTION

- It is the failure of chromosomes to separate from each other during anaphase of meiosis one.
- It occurs due to faulty spindle formation, slow chromatid movement, viruses, etc.

KLINEFELTER SYNDROME

- Male hypogonadism or testicular dysgenesis due to two or more X and one or more Y chromosomes respectively (trisomy).
- Incidence is 1 in 100 males.
- Occurs due to nondisjunction of sex chromosomes during meiosis.
- Extra X chromosome could be of maternal or paternal origin.
- Risk of recurrence increases with maternal age.
- Clinical features:
    - Testicular dysgenesis—small testis and penis.
    - Increased length between soles and pubic bones.
    - Poorly developed secondary sexual characters.
    - High pitched voice.
    - Gynecomastia.
    - Osteoporosis, due to deficient testosterone production.
    - Mild mental retardation.

TURNER'S SYNDROME

- Hypogonadism.
- Due to complete or partial loss of one X chromosome (monosomy).
- Incidence is 1 in 500 females.
- Monosomy occurs due to nondisjunction.
- Clinical features:
    - Short stature.
    - Webbing of neck.
    - Broad chest.
    - Low hairline.
    - Cubitus valgus (increased carrying angle).
    - Atrial septal defect.
    - Low hair line.

DOWN SYNDROME

- Trisomy in chromosome 21.
- Incidence 1/700 live birth.
- Risk of incidence more in elderly gravida (pregnancy at age 45 years or more).
- Causes are nondisjunction, translocation, and mosaicism.
- Clinical features:
    - Mental retardation.
    - Flat face.
    - Small, low bridged nose.
    - Mongoloid appearance due to epicanthal folds of eye.
    - Hypotonia.
    - Atrial and ventricular septal defect and cataract.

CHAPTER 3: Radiology

OUTLINE

- Basics
- Plane Radiography
- Contrast Radiography
- Computed Tomography (CT)
- Positron Emission Tomography (PET) Scan
- Ultrasonography (USG)
- Doppler
- Magnetic Resonance Imaging (MRI)
- Atlas of Radiological Imaging

BASICS

IMAGING MODALITIES

The principal imaging modalities used today are:
- **Using ionizing radiations like X-rays, gamma rays**
   a. Plane radiography
   b. Contrast radiography
   c. Computed tomography (CT)
   d. Positron emission tomography (PET) scan
- **Using nonionizing radiations**
   a. Ultrasonography
   b. Doppler
   c. Magnetic resonance imaging (MRI).

IMAGING MODALITIES WITH IONIZING RADIATIONS

CONCEPT OF RADIO-OPACITY

The fundamental principle of all radiographic tests using X-rays is that different body tissues have a different capacity to block or absorb X-rays. The tissue densities (in order of increasing radio-opacity, i.e., whiteness on conventional radiographic film or computerized tomograms) which are usually seen on a radiograph are:
1. **Air**, as found, for example, in the trachea and lungs, the stomach and intestine, and the paranasal sinuses.
2. **Fat**.
3. **Soft tissues**, e.g., heart, kidney, muscles (these are all approximately the density of water).
4. **Calcific** (due to the presence of calcium and phosphorus), for example, in the skeleton.
5. **Enamel** of the teeth.
6. **Dense foreign bodies**, for example, metallic fillings in the teeth. Also radio-opaque contrast media, such as a barium meal in the stomach or intravascular contrast.

PLANE RADIOGRAPHY

- Here no contrast media is used.
- Produced by passage of X-rays through subject and then exposing on a radiographic film.
- Bone absorbs most radiation causing least film exposure, thus developed film appears white in such regions.
- On the other hand air absorbs least radiation causing maximum exposure, so film appears black on the corresponding areas.
- Between these extremes, large differential tissues absorb radiation producing gray scale image.

Commonly Used Views in X-ray

- **Posteroanterior (PA) view:**
  - The beam of rays enters from back to front of the subject.
  - Here the structures visible are mostly the anterior most structures.
- **Anteroposterior (AP) view:**
  - The beam enters from front to the back of the subject.
  - Here the structures visible are mostly the posterior most structures.
- **Lateral view:**
  - The beam passes through the lateral part of the body or it passes through sideways of the body.

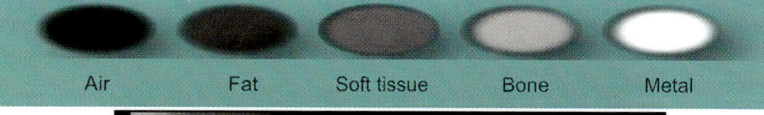
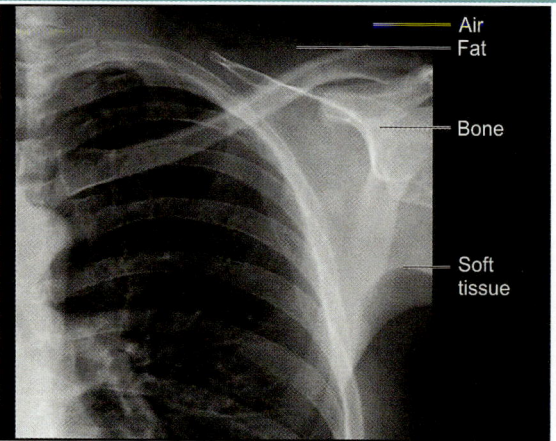

- **Oblique view:**
  - The beam enters any part at a particular angle so that the structures which are not seen in all other three views can be visualized.

HOW TO READ A CHEST RADIOGRAPH (PA VIEW)?

- **Check the patient's name and age.** First make sure that you are looking at the correct chest X-ray.
- **Read the date of the chest radiograph.** The date of the radiograph provides important context for interpreting any findings. For example, a mass that has become bigger over 3 months is more significant than one that has become bigger over 3 years.
- **Identify the type of film and view.** The standard view of the chest is the posteroanterior radiograph, or "PA chest." Posteroanterior refers to the direction of the X-ray passing the patient from posterior to anterior. This film is taken with the patient upright, in full inspiration. Other types of chest radiographs include:
  - The **anteroposterior (AP) chest radiograph** is obtained with the X-ray passing the patient from anterior to posterior, usually obtained with a portable X-ray machine from very sick patients, those unable to stand, and infants.
  - The **lateral chest radiograph** is taken with the patient's left side of chest held against the X-ray cassette (left instead of right to make the heart appear sharper and less magnified, since the heart is closer to the left side).
  - A **lateral decubitus view** is taken by making the patient lying down on the side. It helps to determine whether suspected fluid (pleural effusion) will layer out to the bottom, or suspected air (pneumothorax) will rise to the top.
- **Look for markers:** 'L' for Left, 'R' for Right, 'PA' for posteroanterior, 'AP' for anteroposterior, etc. Note the position of the patient: supine (lying flat), upright, lateral decubitus.
- **Note the technical quality of film.**
  - **Exposure (penetration):** Overexposed films look darker than normal, making fine details harder to see; underexposed films look whiter than normal, and cause the appearance of areas of opacification. Look for barely visible intervertebral bodies behind the heart in a properly penetrated chest X-ray. If detailed spine and pulmonary vessels are seen behind the heart, the exposure is correct. An under-penetrated chest X-ray cannot differentiate the vertebral bodies from the intervertebral spaces, while an over-penetrated film shows the intervertebral spaces very distinctly, but not the pulmonary vessels.
  - **Rotation:** Rotation means that the patient was not positioned flat on the X-ray film, with one plane of the chest rotated compared to the plane of the film. To assess rotation see if the medial ends of both clavicles are equidistant from the spinous process of the vertebrae.
  - **Inhalation:** Check for 9–10 posterior ribs or 6–7 anterior ribs in a properly inhaled radiograph.
- **External soft tissues:** Look at the soft tissues of neck, shoulders and axilla for any abnormalities, for example, enlarged lymph nodes, subcutaneous emphysema (air density below the skin), and other lesions.
- **Diaphragms:** Look for a flat or raised diaphragm. A flattened diaphragm may indicate emphysema. A raised diaphragm may indicate area of airspace consolidation (as in pneumonia). The right diaphragm is normally 2 cm higher than the left, due to the presence of the liver below the right diaphragm. Also look at the costophrenic angle for any blunting (normally sharp), which may indicate effusion.
- **Gas bubble:** Look for the presence of a gastric bubble, just below the left hemidiaphragm.
- **Free air:** Look for free air just beneath the diaphragm.
- **Bones:** Check the bones for any fractures, lesions and joint disease. Note the overall size, shape, and contour of each bone, cortical thickness in comparison to medullary cavity. At joints, look for joint spaces narrowing, widening, calcification in the cartilages, air in the joint space, abnormal fat pads, etc.
- **Spine:** Examine the spinous process, each vertebrae and intervertebral spaces.
- **Clavicle:** Examine both ends of the clavicle and the shaft.
- **Scapula:** Examine the coracoid process, acromioclavicular joint and glenoid fossa.
- **Humerus:** Examine the visible portion of the humerus.
- **Ribs:** Examine each and every visible rib.
- **Fields of the lungs:** Look for symmetry, vascularity, presence of any mass, nodules, infiltration, fluid, etc. in the upper, middle and lower zones of each lung.
- **Hila:** Look for nodes and masses in the hila of both lungs. On the frontal view, most of the hilar shadows represent the left and right pulmonary arteries. The left pulmonary artery is always more superior than the right, making the left hilum higher.
- **Airway:** Examine the trachea, carina (point of bifurcation of trachea) and main stem bronchi. Check to see if the airway is patent and midline. For example, in a tension pneumothorax, the airway is deviated away from the affected side.
- **Cardiac silhouette:** Look at the size of the cardiac silhouette (the bright white space between the lungs representing the outline of the heart). A normal cardiac silhouette occupies less than half the chest width. Look for abnormal shapes of heart on PA plain film, like water bottle shaped heart in pericardial effusion.

- **Edges of heart:** Look the edges of the heart for the silhouette sign (the loss of normal borders between thoracic structures, usually caused by intrathoracic masses).
- **Instrumentation:** Look for any tubes (e.g., tracheal, nasogastric), intravenous (IV) lines, ECG leads, pacemaker, surgical clips, drains, etc.

CONTRAST RADIOGRAPHY

- When the density of a structure is too similar to that of adjacent structures, it is more preferable to use a contrast media to enhance or outline its contours.
- Used to obtain more information about various soft tissues components and also various body cavities.
- Contrast media are classified as radiolucent (e.g., air) and radio-opaque (e.g., barium or iodinated contrast media).
- A contrast agent is being used here mainly consisting of salts of barium and iodine.
- These by utilization of photoelectric effect absorb X-rays completely resulting in white film where the beam has met a contrast agent.

BARIUM STUDIES

Used in mainly gastrointestinal (GI) tract evaluation.

Advantages	Disadvantages
➢ Inert, safe and no drug interaction	➢ Time consuming
➢ Coats the mucosal lining so allow detection of various diseases of mucosa from ulcers to cancers	➢ Difficulty of preparation of subjects for study

Types

Barium Swallow
- To visualize the region from hypopharynx to gastroesophageal junction.
- $BaSO_4$ suspension taken orally.

Barium Meal
- To visualize gastroesophageal junction to duodenojejunal flexure.
- Taken orally.

Barium Meal Follow Through
- To visualize from gastroesophageal junction to ileocecal junction.
- Taken orally.

Barium Follow Through
- To visualize from duodenojejunal flexure to ileocecal junction.
- Taken orally.

Small Bowel Enema
- To visualize from duodenojejunal junction to ileocecal junction.
- Done by using a tube placed at a duodenojejunal junction and barium given through it.

Barium Enema
- To visualize from rectum to ileocecal junction.
- Barium instilled through a catheter inserted per rectally.

BARIUM SWALLOW

- Barium studies are radiographic procedures used for visualization of the alimentary canal.
- **Principle:** Barium is a white, 'radio-opaque' powder (due to high molecular weight) that is not transparent to X-rays. The alimentary canal, like other soft-tissue structures, does not show clearly enough for diagnostic purposes on plain radiographs. But if a radiograph is taken after drinking a white liquid that consists of suspension of 5% barium sulfate in water, the outline of the upper parts of the gut (esophagus, stomach and small intestines) shows up clearly on radiographs. This is because X-rays do not pass through barium.

- The subject is restricted from eating or drinking for 6 hours prior to the examination.
- Subject is made to drink 5% barium sulfate solution.
- Subject should stand in front of an X-ray machine and X-ray pictures are taken as he swallows the solution.
- This test helps to check for problems in the esophagus, such as narrowing (stricture), hiatus hernias, tumors, reflux from the stomach, disorders of swallowing, etc.

BARIUM MEAL

- Similar to barium swallow.
- Help to check for problems in the stomach and duodenum.
- Subject is made to drink 5% barium sulfate solution (subject ingests gas pellets and citric acid to expand the stomach and duodenum and also pushes the barium to coat the lining of the stomach and duodenum, which makes the radiographs clearer).
- Subject is made to lie on a couch while the radiograph is being taken over the abdomen.
- Stomach and duodenum can be visualized immediately after barium drink.
- Barium is normally excreted within 24 hours.
- Barium meal mainly helps to detect problems like ulcers, polyps, tumors of stomach and duodenum.

BARIUM ENEMA

- This test helps to diagnose diseases and other problems that affect the large intestine.
- Subject is given mild laxative two nights before the examination to clean up the large intestine.
- About 2 liters of barium sulfate poured into the large intestine through a tube inserted into the anus.
- Enema is stopped when barium starts flowing into the terminal ileum through ileocecal valve and a radiograph is taken.
- Rectum and sigmoid colon appear much dilated and the colon also shows haustrations.
- There are two types of barium enemas:
  1. **Single-contrast study:** Barium outlines the intestine and reveals large abnormalities.
  2. **Double-contrast or air-contrast study:** The colon is first filled with barium and then the barium is evacuated, leaving only a thin layer of barium on the wall of the colon and air is injected through anus to distend the colon. This gives a detailed view of the inner surface of the colon, making it easy to point out narrowed areas (strictures), diverticula, or inflammation.
- Barium enema helps to find out intussusception, identify inflammation of the intestinal wall (inflammatory bowel diseases—ulcerative colitis or Crohn's disease) and its progress.

IODINE STUDIES

Used for both intravenous injection, intraluminal injection, etc.

Advantages	Disadvantages
➢ Bear no drug interaction	➢ Nausea*
➢ Pharmacologically inert	➢ Vomiting*
➢ Cause adequate contrast	

* Low risk

Types

- For urinary system studies:
  - Intravenous pyelography (IVP)
  - Retrograde pyelography (RGP)
  - Cystogram
- For biliary tree studies:
  - Endoscopic retrograde cholangiopancreatogram (ERCP)
- For arterial and venous system studies:
  - Angiogram
A. *Intravenous pyelography (IVP):* Visualization of urinary tract and functions though injection of contrast through the peripheral vein.
B. *Retrograde pyelography (RGP):* Contrast instilled through a tube placed in ureter for delineation of the ureteric abnormalities in a nonexcreting kidney.
C. *Cystogram:* Intracavitary instillation of contrast into urinary bladder enables morphological visualization.
D. *Endoscopic retrograde cholangiopancreatogram (ERCP):* Used in case of obstructive jaundice.

E. *Angiogram:* It is an imaging technique used to check the lumen and patency of blood vessels. Here, a catheter is introduced through a major blood vessel and then dye is injected near the blood vessel to be studied. Simultaneously, a series of X-ray images are taken and examined by the physician. One of the best examples is a coronary angiogram taken to examine coronary arteries.

INTRAVENOUS PYELOGRAPHY

- The IVP consists of a series of abdominal radiographs taken sequentially at 1, 5 and 15 minutes after injection of contrast (urografin, Conray 420).
- First a normal abdominal radiograph is taken, called as scout film. On scout film, kidney and bladder contours are normally visualized. Kidney stones are seen as white calcification over the kidney shadow and ureteric stones are seen as white calcification along the course of the ureters.
- In the contrast injected radiograph the urinary system becomes outlined by the white contrast material. The whitened kidney seen on radiograph is known as nephrogram.
- In addition we can also see renal calyces, renal pelvis, ureteropelvic junction (UPJ), the ureters, and the ureterovesical junction (UVJ).
- The scout film is compared with the contrast radiographs to check for abnormalities.
- No nephrogram means, kidney not functioning or absent.
- Dilated ureter indicates ureteric stone or a tumor encasing the ureter.

WATER-SOLUBLE CONTRAST STUDY

Water-soluble contrast media used:
- **Hysterosalpingography:**
  - Use of water-soluble iodinated contrast.
  - To delineate the uterus and fallopian tubes and assess tubal patency.
- **Myelography:**
  - Injection of contrast medium to subarachnoid space via lumbar puncture for evaluating abnormalities of the spinal cord and nerves which are not visible in plane X-ray.

HYSTEROSALPINGOGRAPHY

- The radiograph obtained is called a hysterosalpingogram (HSG).
- Investigations are done preferably in the first 5–10 days of the menstrual cycle.
- **Procedure:** A cannula is inserted into the internal os and is connected with a syringe. A dye (iodized oil, lipiodol) is passed through it into the uterus.
- Due to the anatomical continuation uterus with fallopian tube, the dye will flow into the fallopian tubes.
- Radiograph taken at this point shows the uterus and fallopian tube clearly.

Uses

- Determine the patency of the uterus and fallopian tube.
- To check the presence of polyps, fibroids, adhesions, or a foreign object in the uterus.
- To check the presence of an abnormal passage or fistula in the region.
- To check the success of tubal ligation post-surgery.

COMPUTED TOMOGRAPHY

- Here thin sections of body are achieved to create axial sections of the body:
- A CT scanner consists of an X-ray tube and a row of detectors, which rotate around the subject who is positioned in the center.
- The tube produces a fan shaped X-ray beam which passes the subject and hits the detector on the other side.
- Different tissues in a cross section are distinguished due to the difference in their atomic density and attenuation.

Commonly used CT's

- **Spiral CT**
- Here the scan is performed while the patient is continuously moving at a predefined speed through the scanner. This configuration reduces total scan time.
- **Multislice CT:** Here scanners are equipped with multiple and thinner detector rows and have faster rotation speeds.
- **High resolution CT (HRCT):** It allows detailed visualization of the tissue. It is commonly used to visualize lung parenchyma.

- **Noncontrast CT (NCCT):** Usually indicated for head injury, stroke, acute hemorrhage, etc.
- **Contrast enhanced CT (CECT):** Used for all cranial applications using iodinated contrast.

POSITRON EMISSION TOMOGRAPHY SCAN

- A positron emission tomography (PET) scan is a functional imaging technique.
- Here, radioactive substances known as radiotracers are given to patients by either oral, inhalation or intravenous route depending upon the site to be examined.
- With the help of a PET scanner, we can measure the blood flow, oxygen use, glucose utilization, etc., by tissues.
- These information gives a better idea about the metabolic activity of the tissue of interest. PET scan is used in cancer, heart diseases, nervous system disorders, etc.

IMAGING MODALITIES WITH NONIONIZING RADIATIONS

ULTRASONOGRAPHY

- Ultrasonography (USG) uses ultrasound waves. Here, a transducer containing numerous crystals with piezoelectric property converts electrical energy to ultrasound waves.
- The ultrasound waves sent from the transducer propagate through different tissues and then return reflected as echoes to the transducer.
- The returned echoes are converted back to the electrical impulses and are processed into ultrasound images.
- The waves are reflected at the surface between the tissues of different acoustic density and the reflections being proportional to the difference in the acoustic density.
- Homogeneous fluids like blood, bile, urine, contents of cysts, ascites and pleural effusion are seen as echo free structures.
- If the difference in acoustic density is very different, the sound is then completely reflected resulting in total acoustic shadowing and is seen behind bone structures, calculi and air (intestinal gas).
- They are very routinely used to examine heart, abdomen and related organs, prenatal scanning, etc.

DOPPLER STUDIES

- It is based on the Doppler effect theory which says there is a change in frequency of sound when it is being reflected from a moving target.
- An ultrasound wave is being bounced off from circulating red blood cells and with the help of computers, we can estimate the amount and direction of the blood flow.
- In color Doppler—the regions of blood flow is displayed as colors (blue away from the transducer, red towards transducer)
- In pulsed Doppler the exact velocity waveforms are obtained.
- Doppler is commonly indicated in peripheral vascular disease, portal hypertension, pregnancy-induced hypertension, intrauterine growth restriction, carotid atherosclerosis, etc.

MAGNETIC RESONANCE IMAGING

In magnetic resonance (MRI), a combination of radiowaves and strong magnetic fields are used. With the help of computers, cross-sectional images of internal organs and structures are generated.

It is based on the principle that hydrogen atoms when subjected to a magnetic field, they line up. If a radiofrequency is aimed at these atoms, it changes the alignment of their nuclei.

When the radio waves are turned off, the nuclei realign themselves and transmit a small electrical signal. With this, an image is generated from the returning pulses from the hydrogen atoms of the body.

In MRI, the tissues having higher water density appear brightest and vice versa. Hence this contrast in tissue based on the difference in water is used to differentiate different kinds of tissues in the body. For example, since teeth and bones contain low water, MRI helps in identifying tissues surrounded by bone such as the spinal cord. MRI can also be used to distinguish between brain white matter and gray matter, etc.

PLANE RADIOGRAPHS

A. UPPER LIMB

SHOULDER: ANTEROPOSTERIOR VIEW

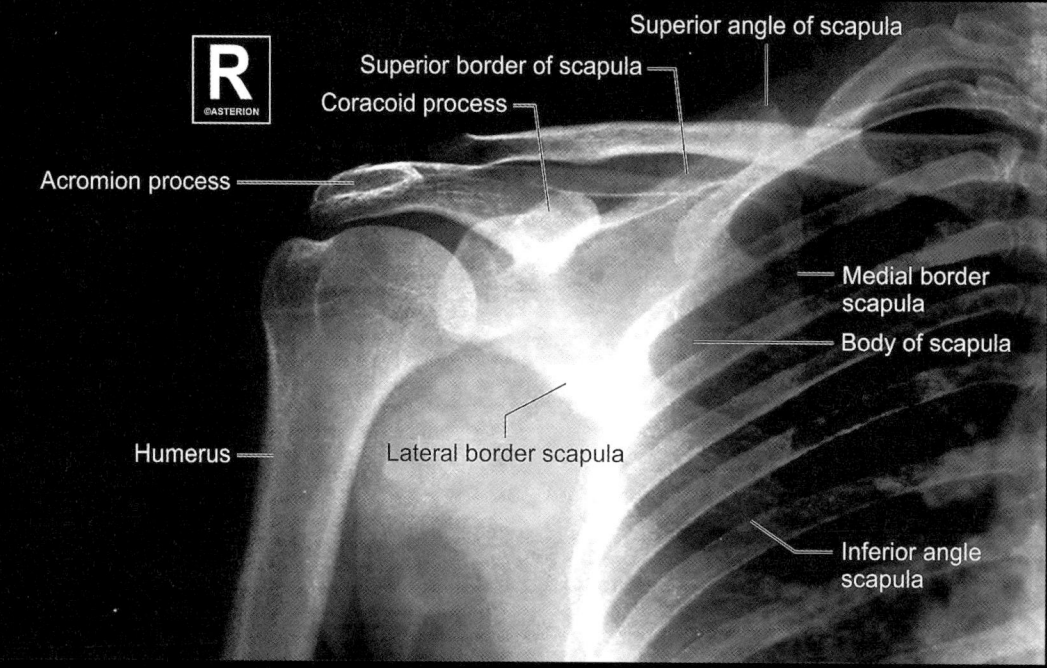

ARM: ANTEROPOSTERIOR VIEW

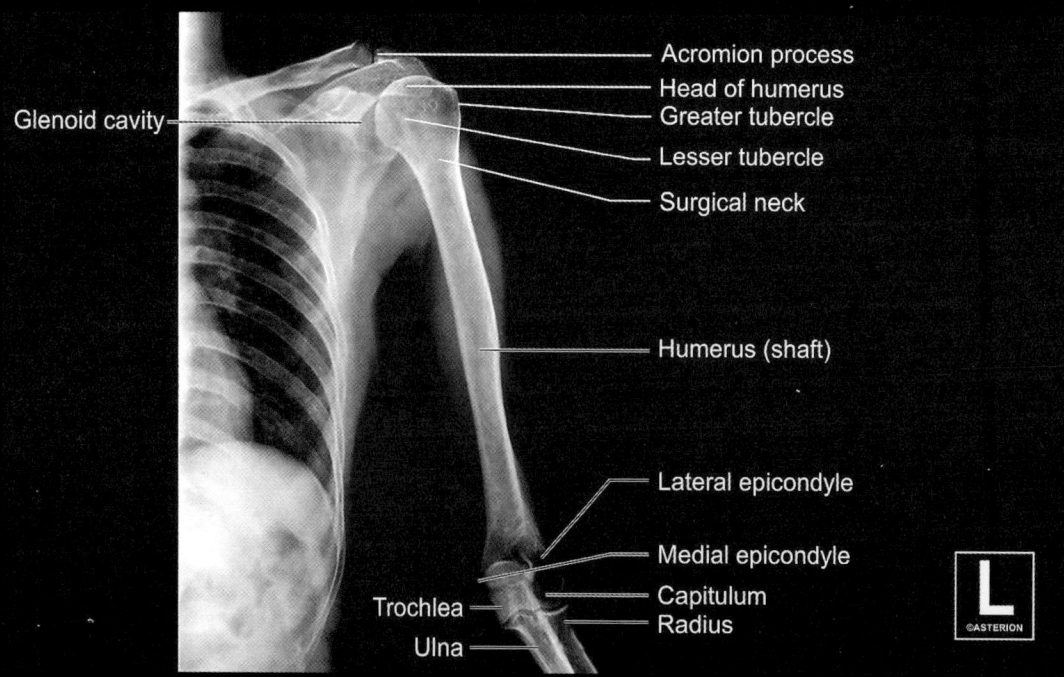

ELBOW: ANTEROPOSTERIOR VIEW

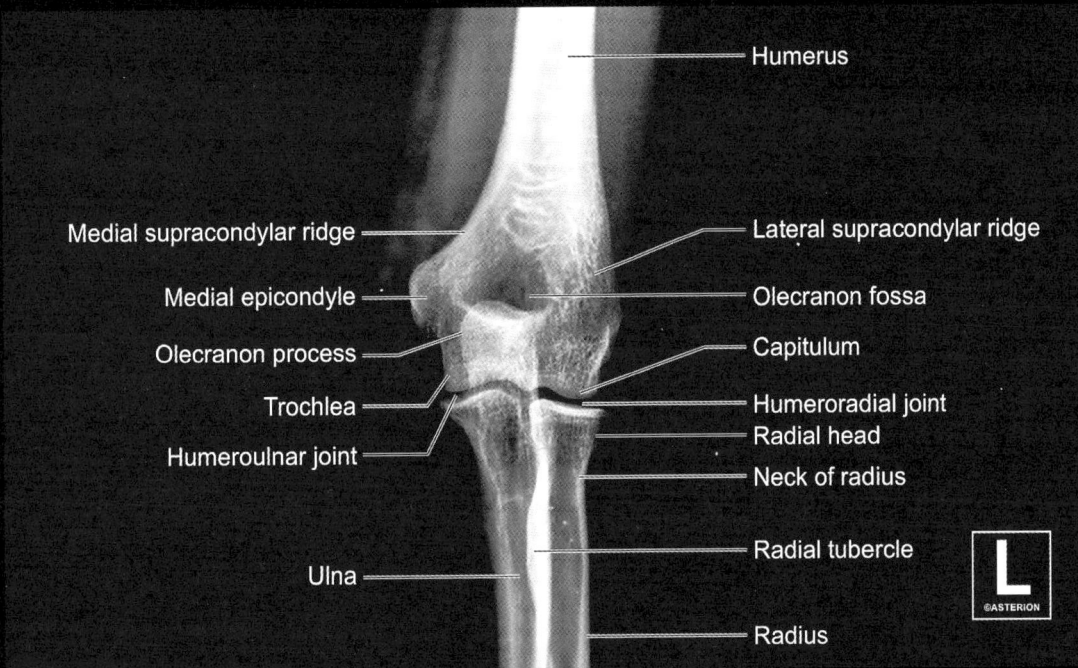

ELBOW: LATERAL VIEW

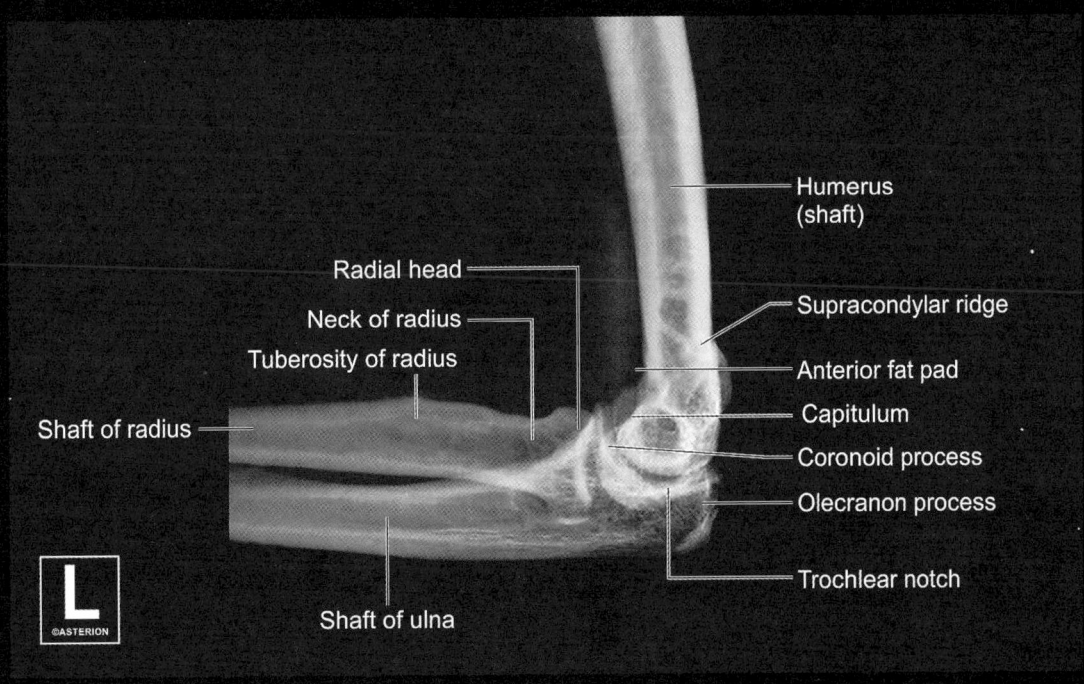

FOREARM: ANTEROPOSTERIOR VIEW

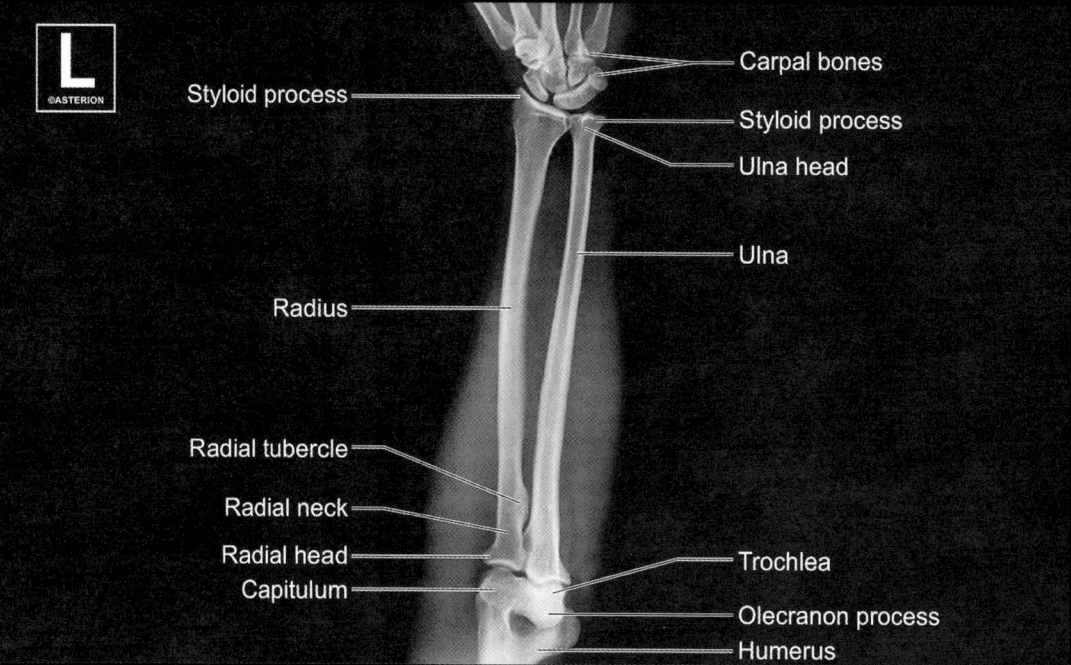

WRIST AND HAND: ANTEROPOSTERIOR VIEW

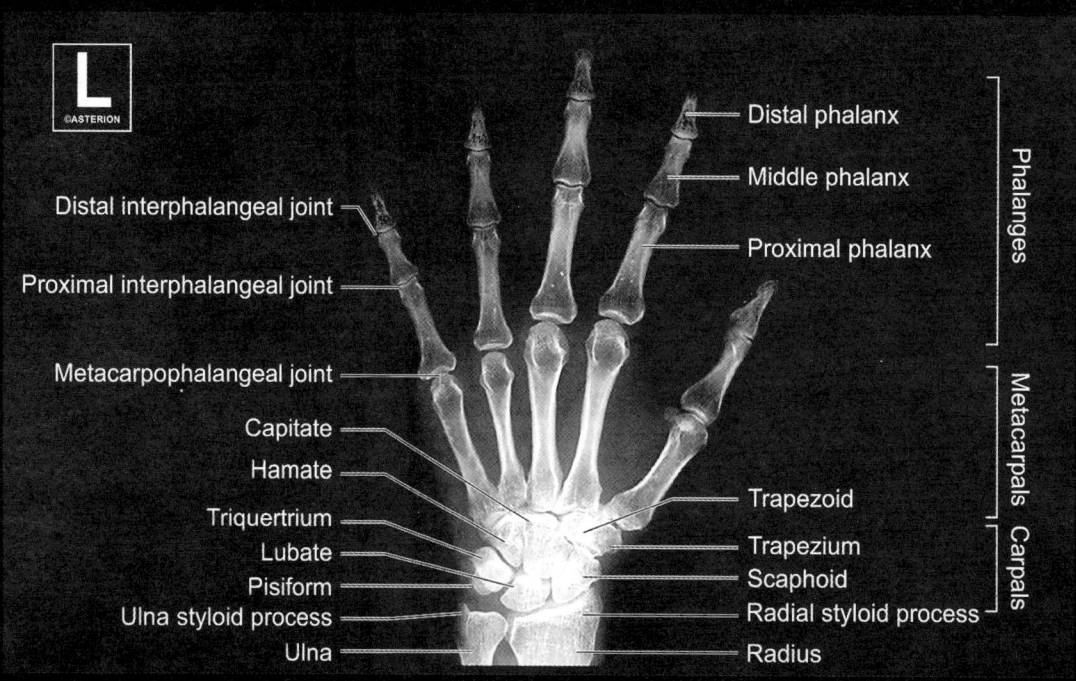

B. THORAX AND ABDOMEN

CHEST: POSTEROANTERIOR VIEW

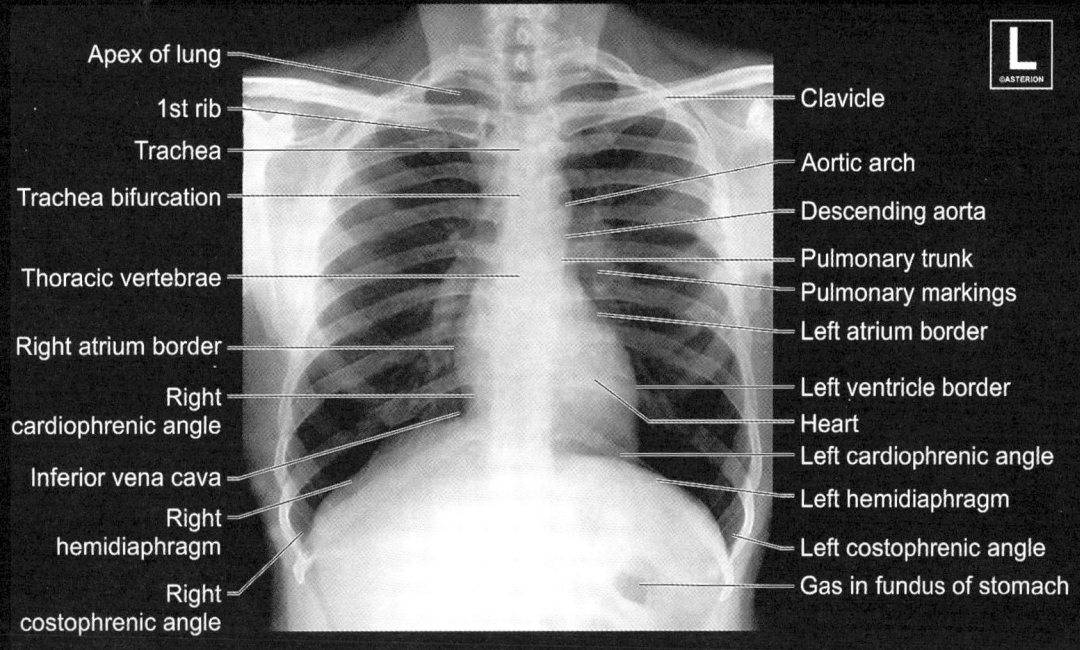

CHEST: LATERAL VIEW

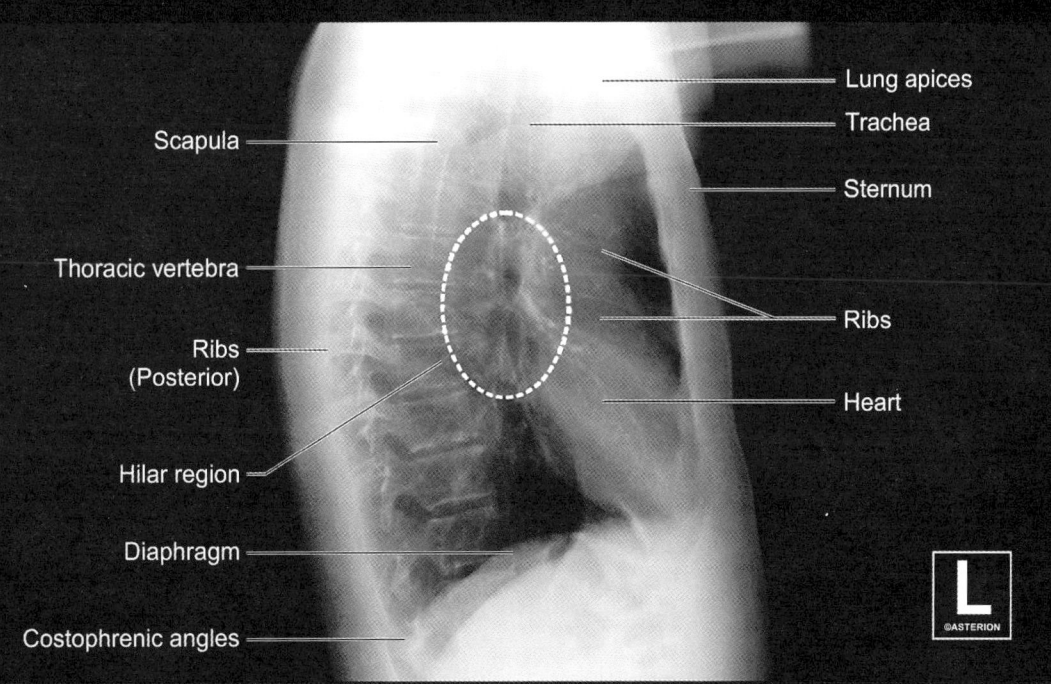

THORACIC VERTEBRAE: ANTEROPOSTERIOR VIEW

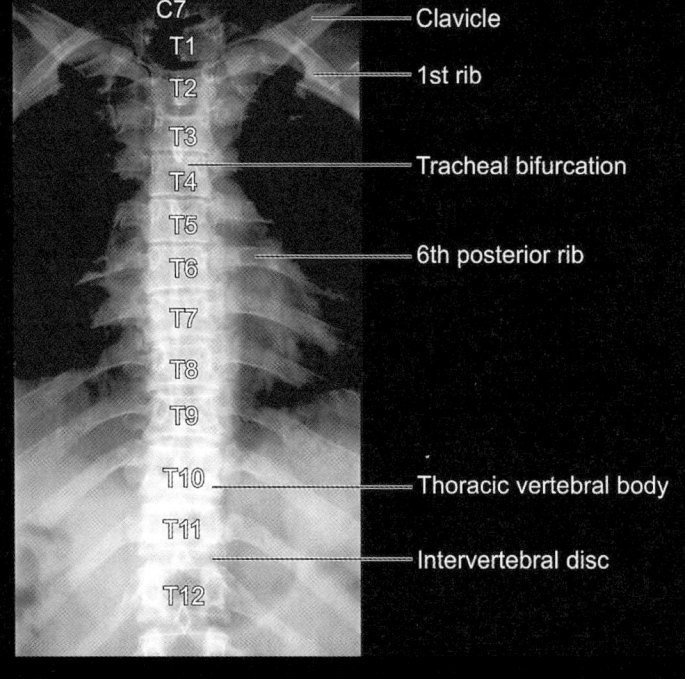

LUMBAR VERTEBRAE: ANTEROPOSTERIOR VIEW

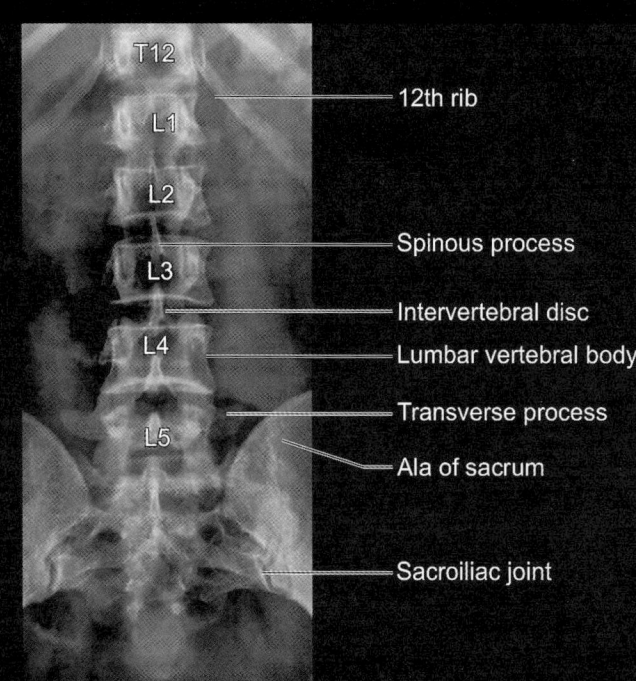

C. LOWER LIMB

PELVIS: ANTEROPOSTERIOR VIEW

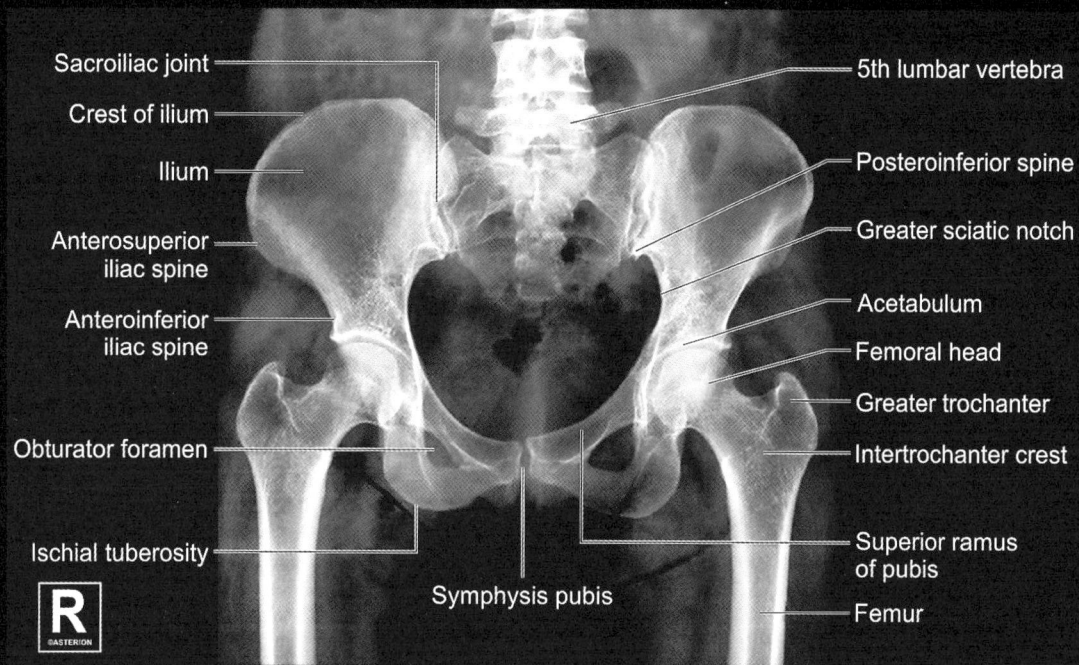

THIGH: ANTEROPOSTERIOR VIEW

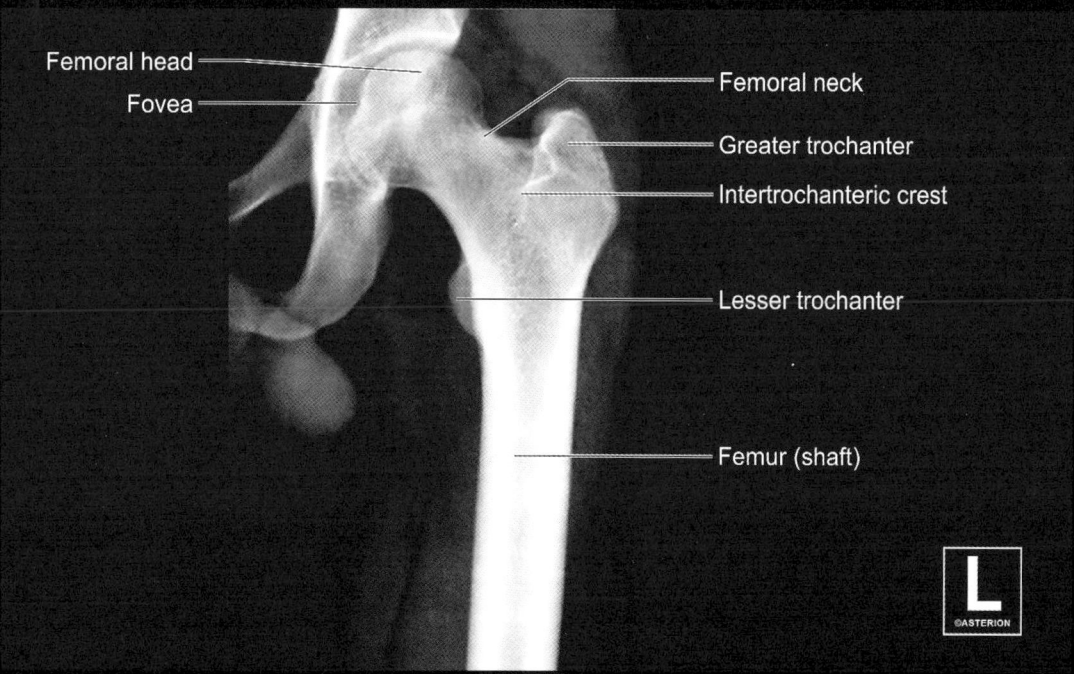

KNEE: ANTEROPOSTERIOR VIEW

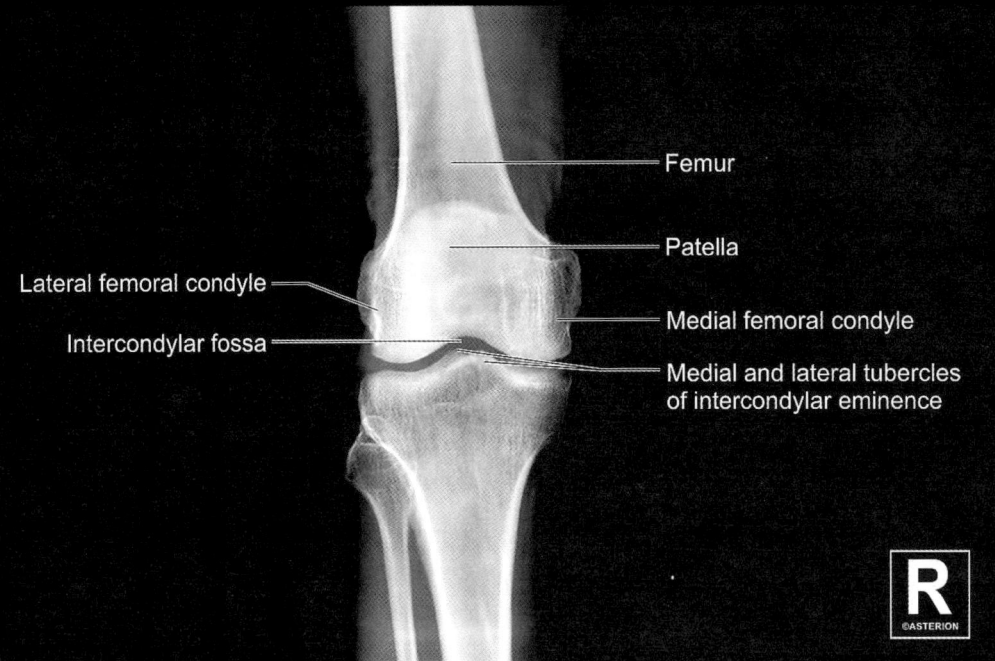

KNEE: LATERAL VIEW

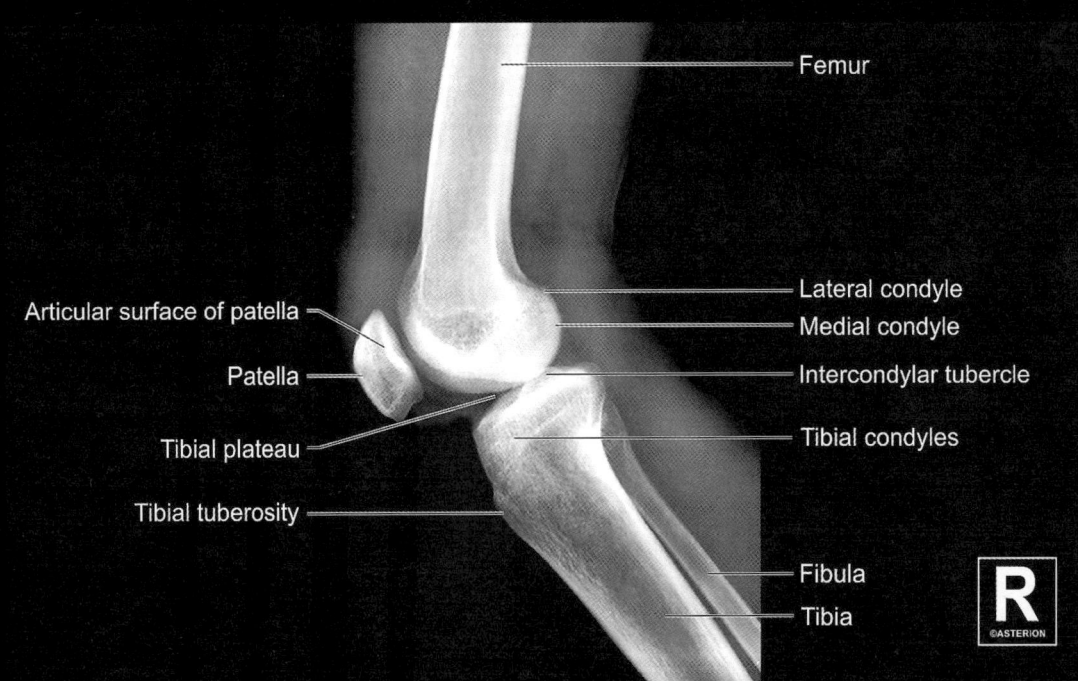

LEG: ANTEROPOSTERIOR VIEW

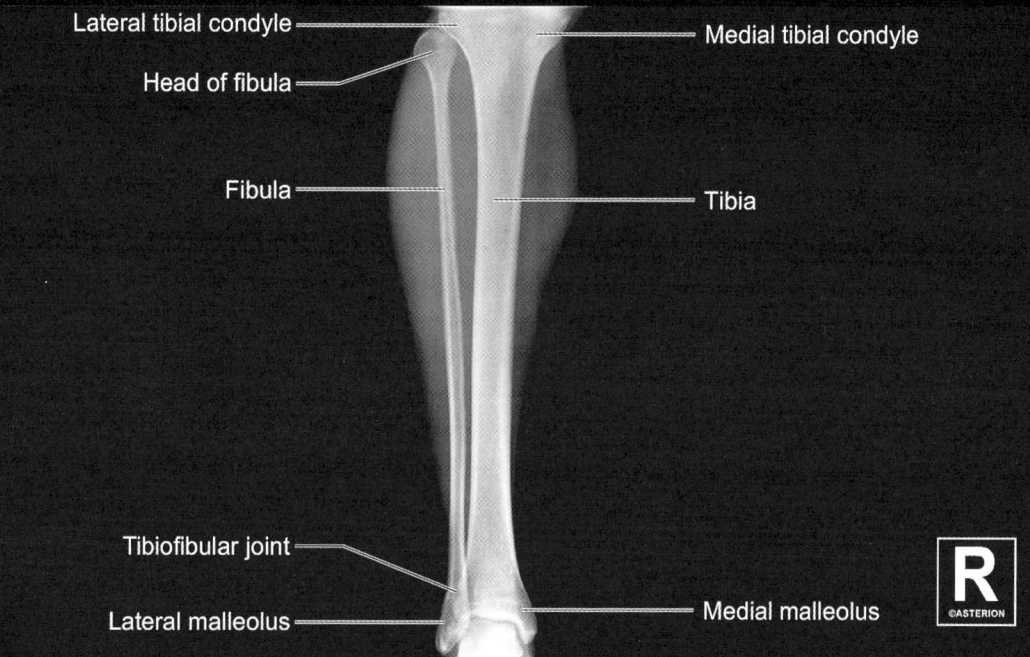

ANKLE: ANTEROPOSTERIOR VIEW

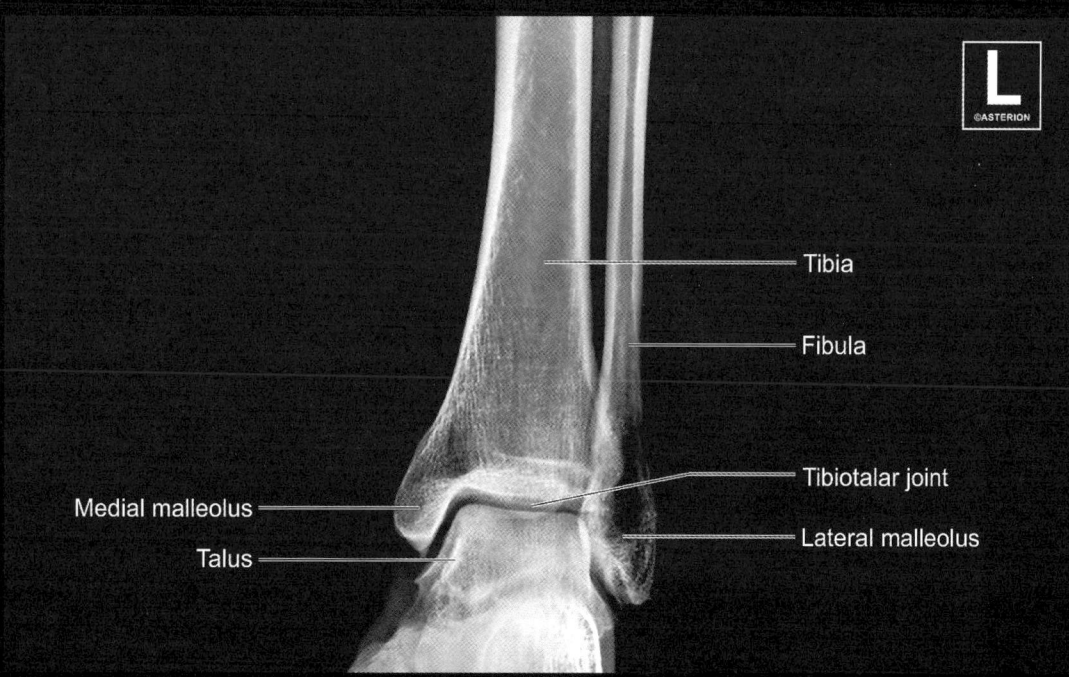

FOOT: LATERAL VIEW

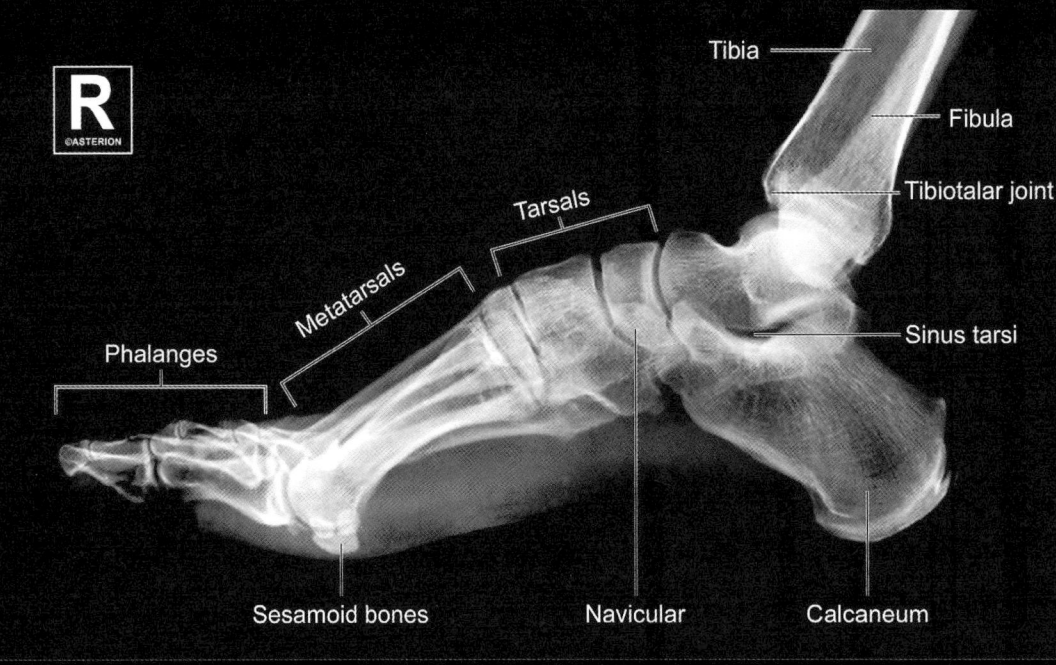

FOOT: OBLIQUE VIEW

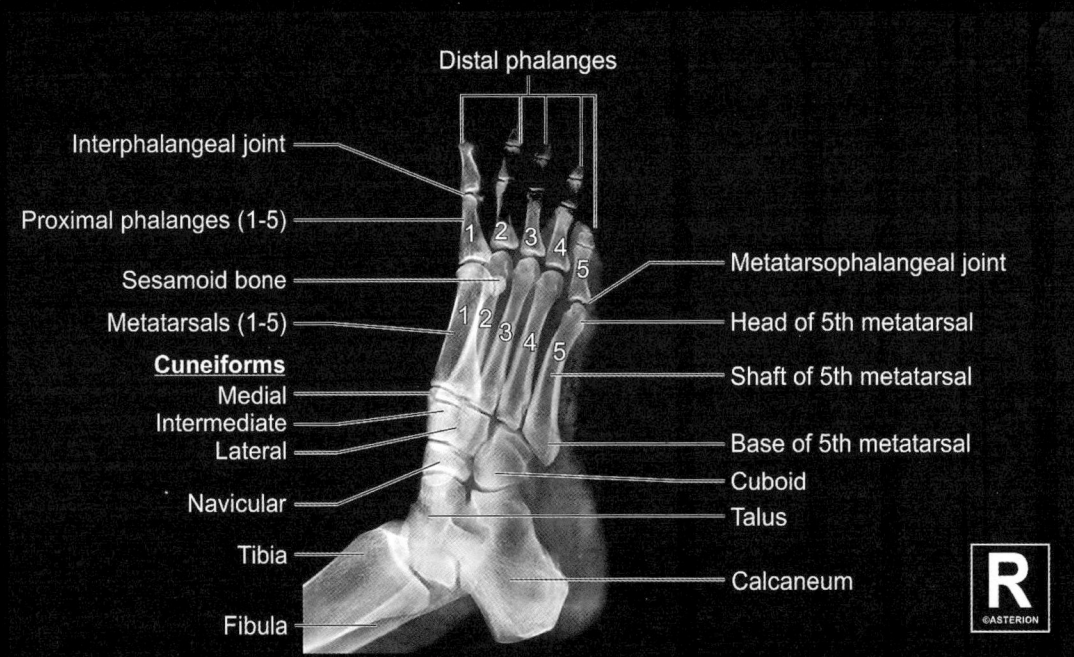

D. HEAD AND NECK

SKULL: ANTEROPOSTERIOR VIEW

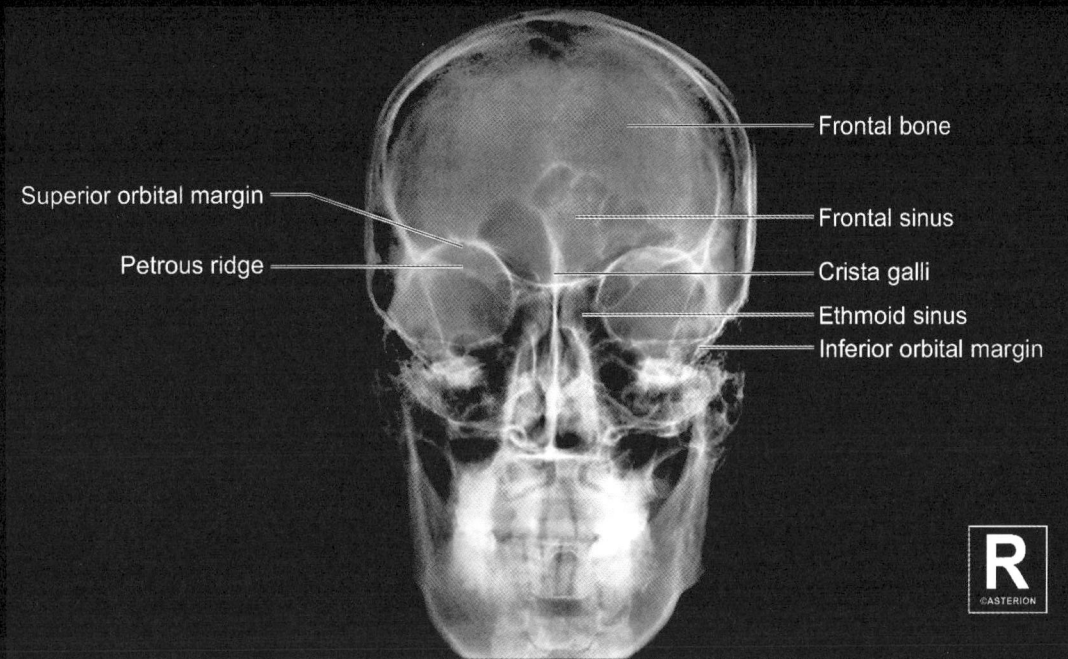

SKULL: OCCIPITOMENTAL VIEW

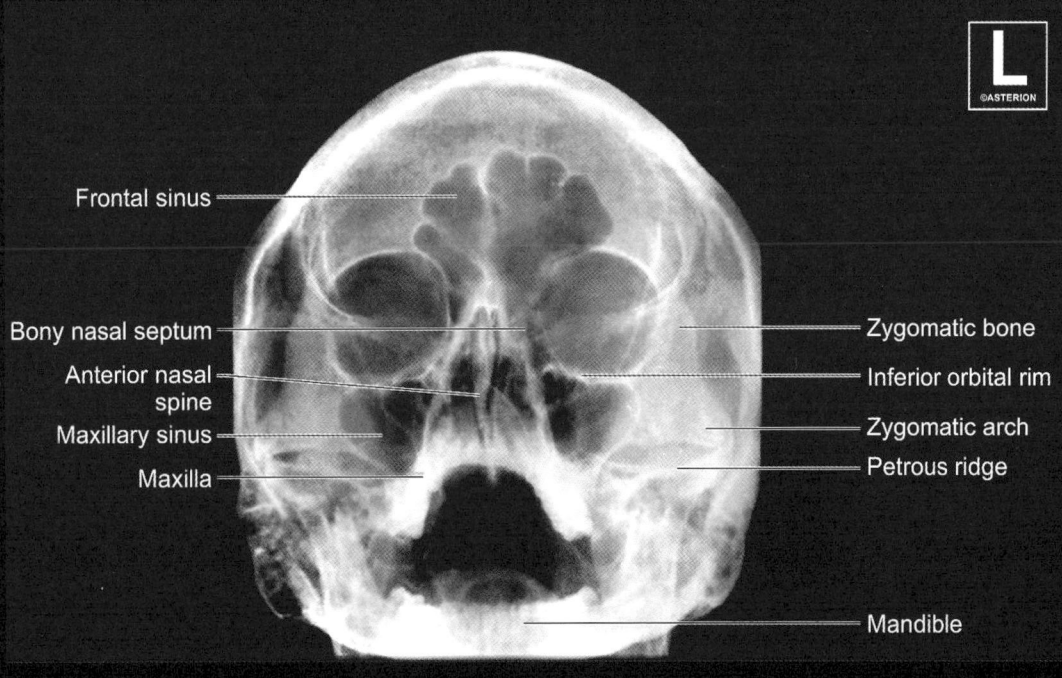

SKULL: LATERAL VIEW

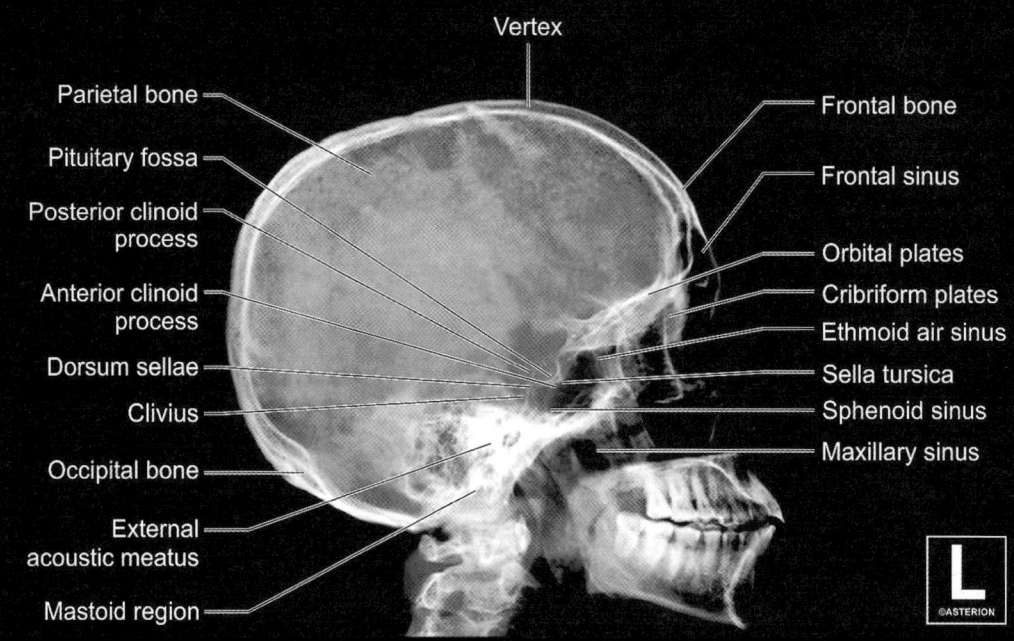

NECK: LATERAL VIEW

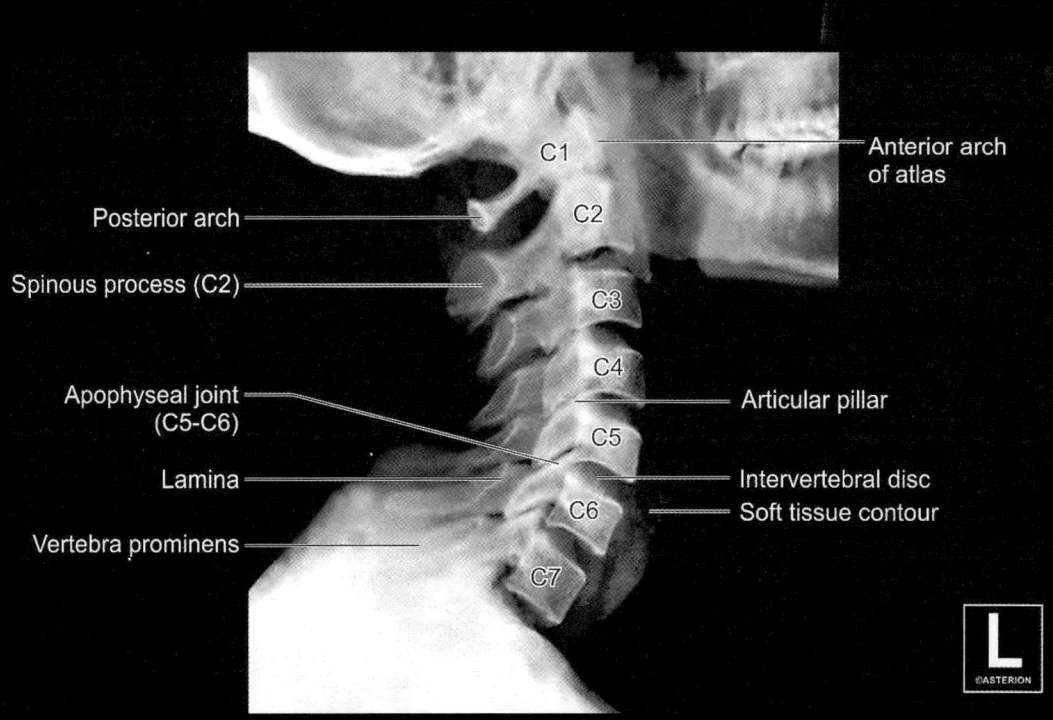

CONTRAST RADIOGRAPHS

BARIUM SWALLOW

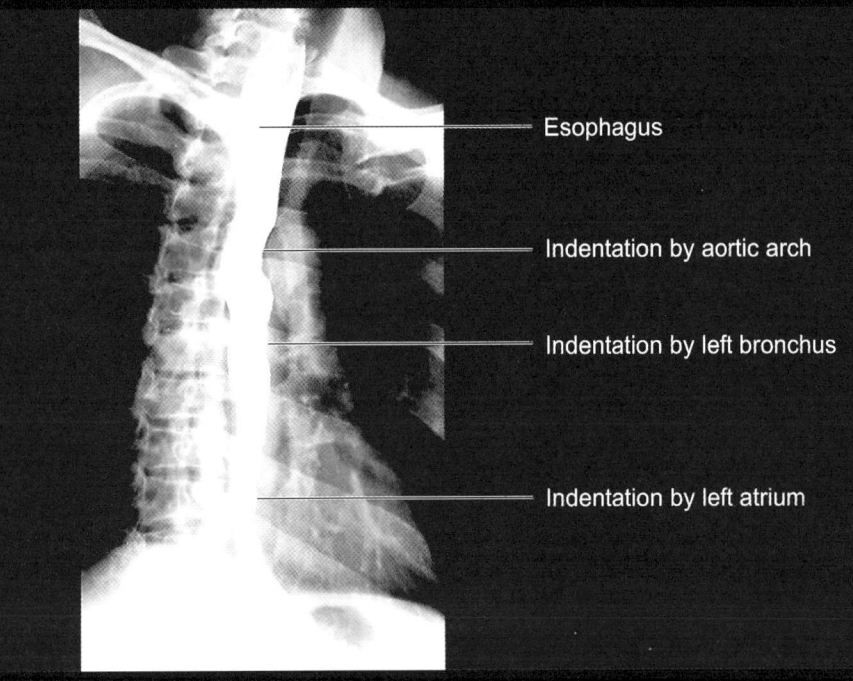

BARIUM MEAL

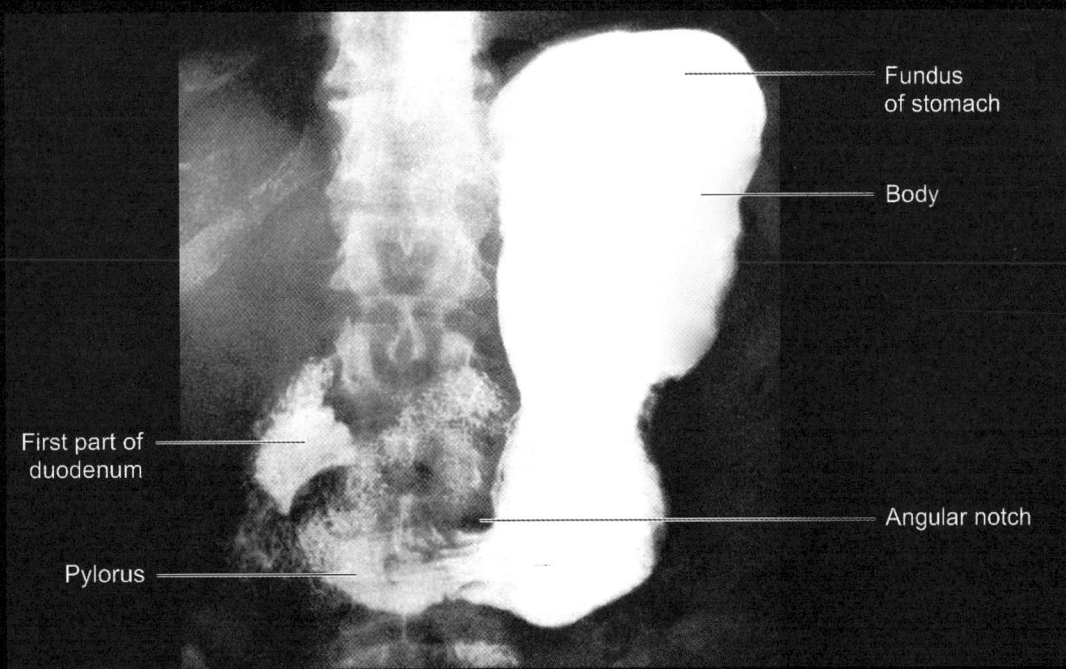

BARIUM MEAL FOLLOW THROUGH

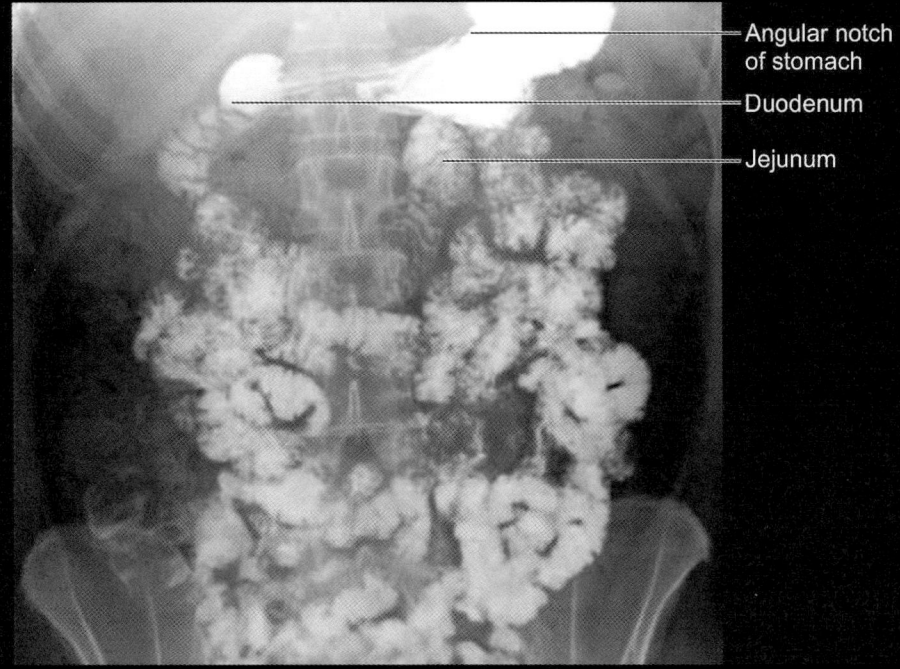

BARIUM ENEMA (DOUBLE CONTRAST)

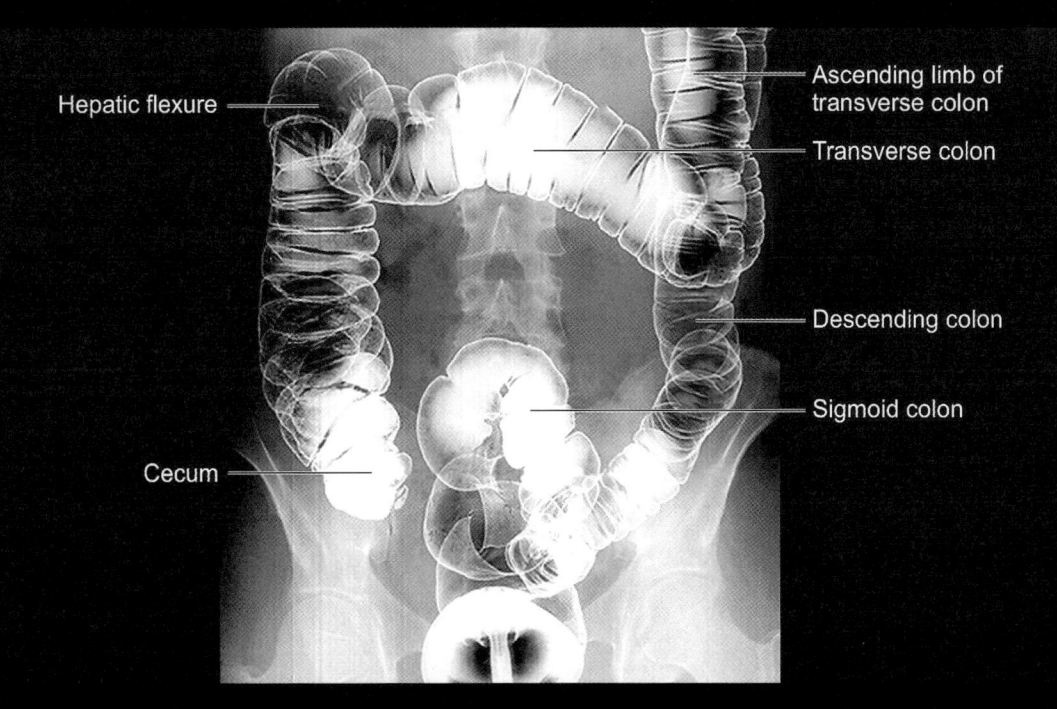

INTRAVENOUS PYELOGRAM

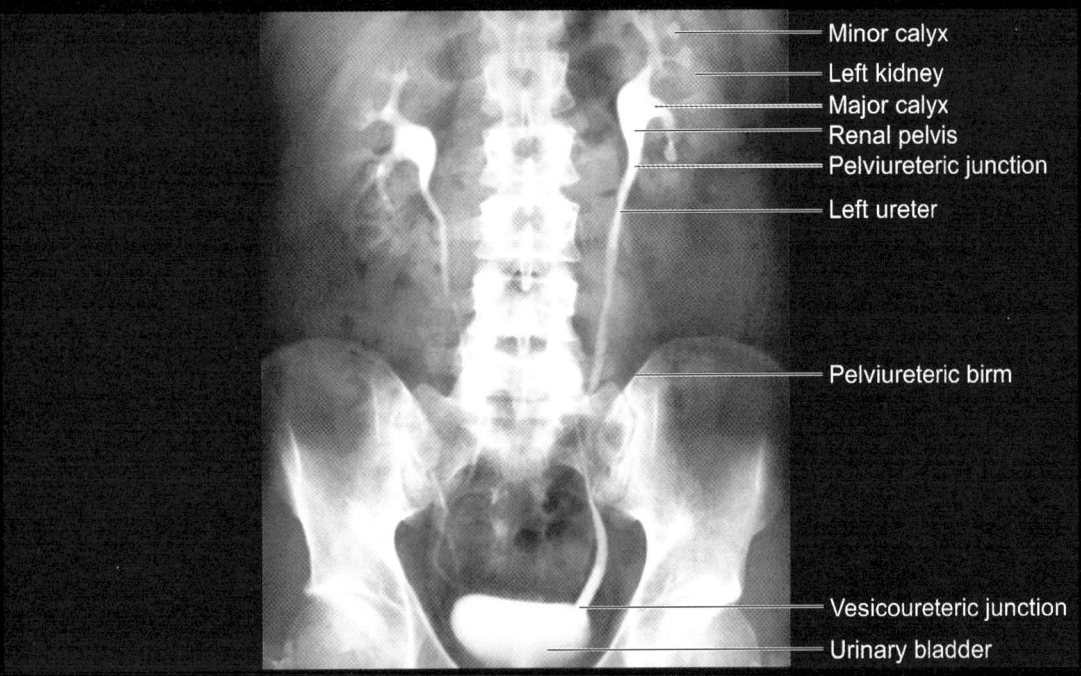

HYSTEROSALPINGOGRAM

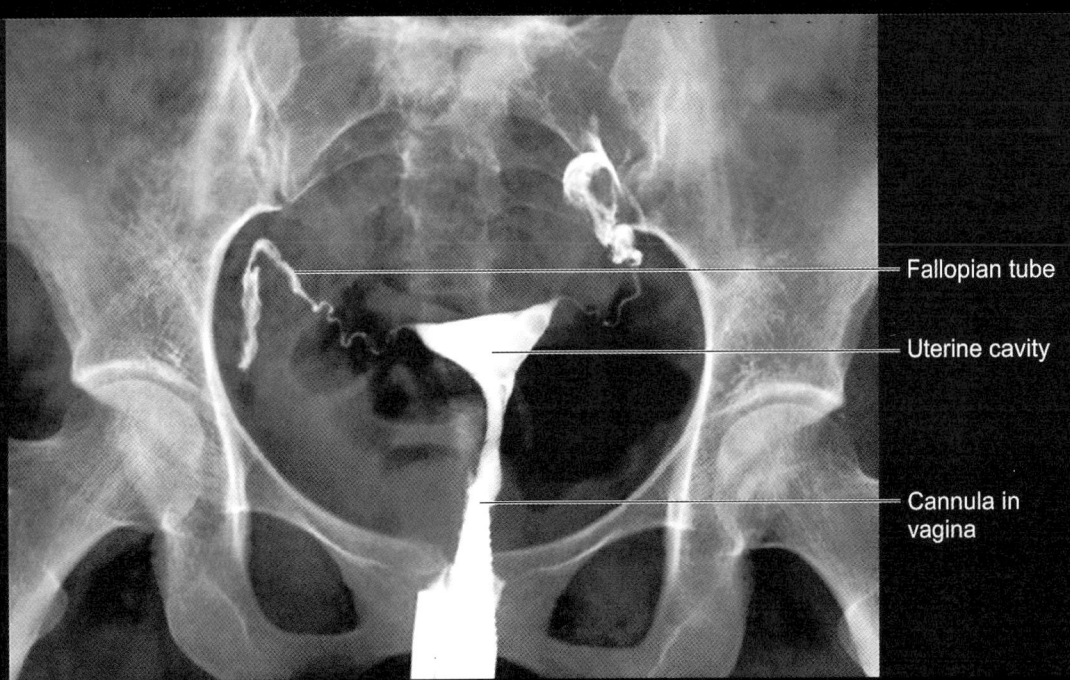

OTHER IMAGING MODALITIES

ULTRASONOGRAPH: ANTENATAL SCANNING

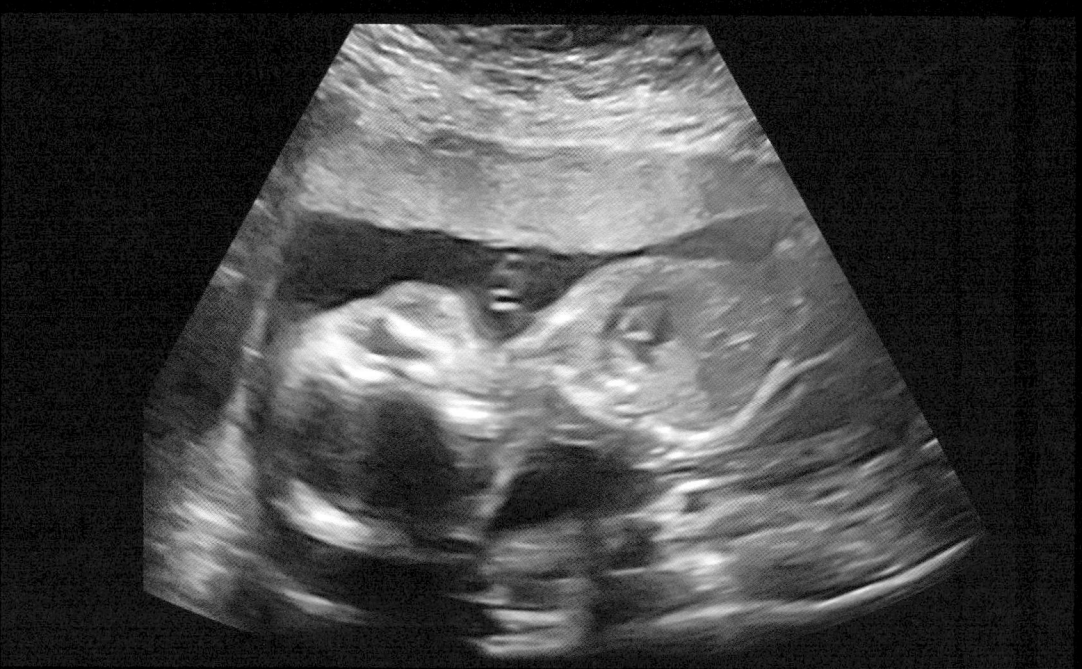

COMPUTERIZED TOMOGRAPHIC SCAN (BRAIN)

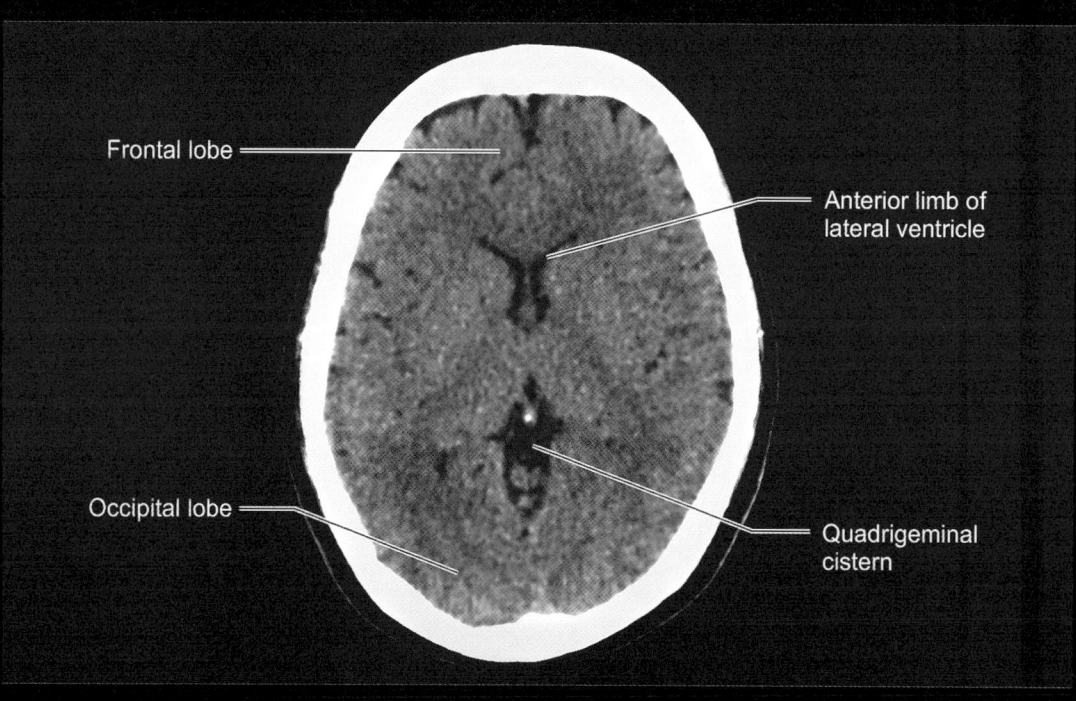

MAGNETIC RESONANCE CHOLANGIOPANCREATOGRAPHY (MRCP) SCAN

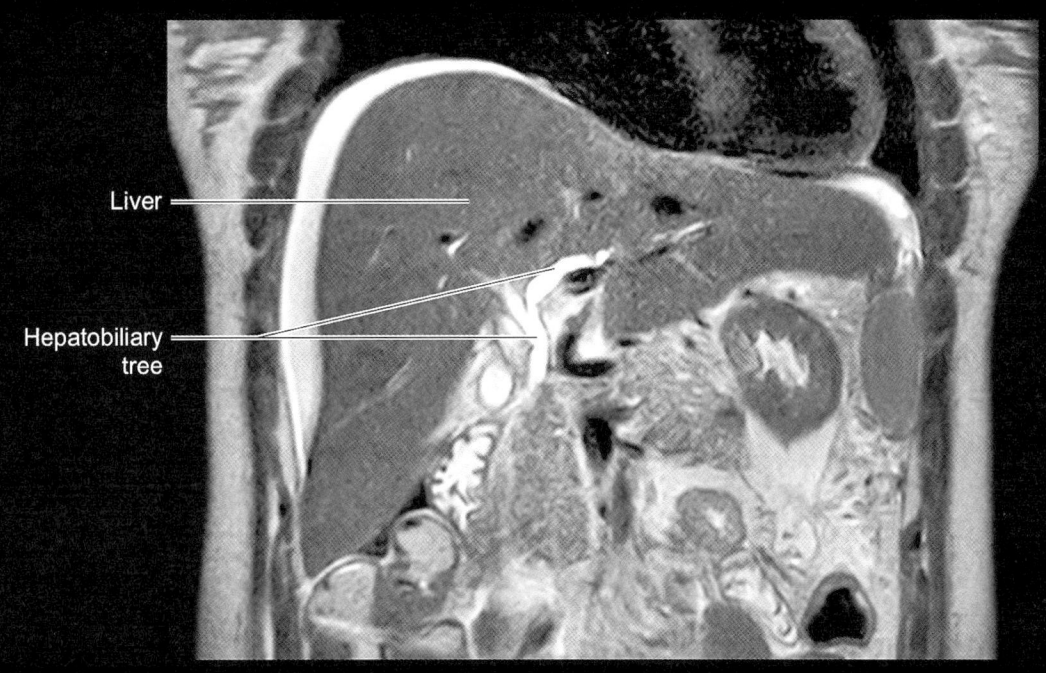

MRI SCAN (BRAIN)

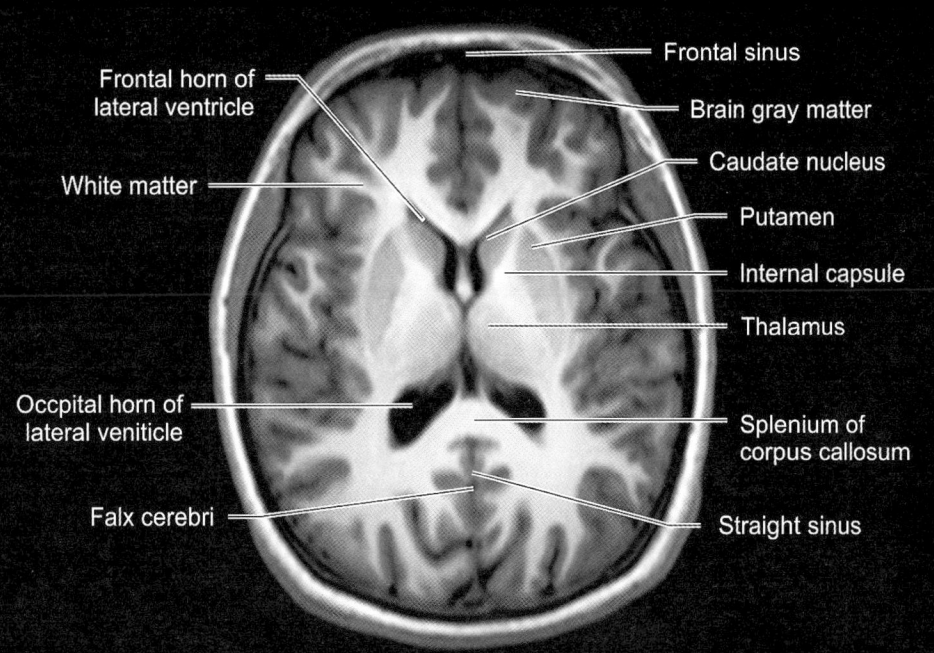

CHAPTER 4

Osteology

OUTLINE

- Introduction to Bones
- Markings on the Bones
- Age and Sex Determination with Bones
- Clinical Aspects of Osteology
- Atlas of Bones

INTRODUCTION TO BONES

- An adult's skeleton contains 206 bones.
- Babies have more bones than adults. When a baby grows up, some of the bones fuse together to form one bone.
- A matured adult skeleton can be divided into axial and the appendicular skeleton.

Axial Skeleton

It consists of the bones that form the vertical axis of the body. Axial skeleton has 80 bones.
- Skull bones—22
- Auditory ossilcles—malleous, incus and stapes one each in both ears—6
- Hyoid bone
- Vertebral column—cervical, thoracic and lumbar vertebrae, sacrum and coccyx.
- 12 pairs of ribs and sternum.

Appendicular Skeleton

It consists of all the bones of the arms and legs and those bones that attach them to the axial skeleton.
- Appendicular skeleton has 126 bones.
- Each upper limb have 30 bones: Humerus, radius, ulna, carpals—8, metacarpals—5, phalanges—14
- Each lower limb have 30 bones: Femur, patella, tibia, fibula, tarsals—7, metatarsals—5, phalanges—14
- Pectoral girdle has both scapula and clavicle each side.
- Pelvic girdle is made of two hip bones from both sides. Each pelvic bone is made of ilium, ischium and pubis.

MARKINGS ON THE BONES

Parts of a Bone

Long bones are composed of four distinct parts:
1. Head—epiphysis
2. Neck—metaphysis
3. Body—diaphysis
4. Articular surface—making joints

Projections and Parts

- *Condyle* is a rounded knob that form articulation with other bones.
- *Epicondyle* is a bony area on or above a condyle. It provides area for a muscle or ligament to attach.
- *Process* is a bulging bony outgrowth of a larger bone.
- *Protuberances* are similar to processes. Appears as swelling, bulging or protruding parts of bone.
- *Tubercle* is a small rounded prominence, usually give site for tendon or ligament to attach.
- *Tuberosity* is larger comapred to tubercle. They are found in varying shapes and texture.
- *Trochanter* is a very large, blunt, irregularly shaped process of the femur that serves as an attachment point for a couple of muscles and ligaments.
- S*pine/spinous process* is a sharp, slender projection of the bone in which muscles or ligaments attach.
- *Linea* refers to a subtle, long, and narrow marking which distinguishes itself in elevation, color or texture from surrounding tissues.
- *Facet* is a flat smooth area which serves as an articular surface.
- *Crests* are prominent, raised edges of a bone.
- *Ridges* are linear elevations, margins or borders.

Depressions and Openings

- *Foramina* are holes or openings in a bone through which nerves and blood vessels pass.
- *Fissures* are open slits/grooves/depressions in a bone, housing nerves and blood vessels.
- *Meatus* is a short, tube-like passage extending into the bone.
- *Fossa* is a depression on a bone surface which is often broad and shallow. It is seen supporting brain structures or receiving another bone for articulation.
- *Fovea* refers to a pit or depression on bone. Compared with fossa, it is much smaller.
- *Notch* is an indentation at the edge of a bone.
- *Sulci* are groove-like areas and can be traced through the bone where nerves or vessels runs safely from outside compression forces.
- A *sinus* is a cavity or hollow space.

Osteology

AGE AND SEX DETERMINATION WITH BONES

Anthropologists often rely upon bones to determine the age and sex.

Age Determination
- As a child grows to an adult, the epiphyses of different bones fuse at known ages.
- By examining which epiphyses are closed and which are open, we can determine the age of an adolescent.
- But, once an individual reaches adulthood, all epiphyses have fused and this method becomes of no use other than to indicate the individual was an adult.
- In adults, age estimation is usually done by assessing the degree of degenerative changes in the bone.
- The pubic symphysis and the auricular surface of sacroiliac joints undergo erosive and degenerative changes throughout the life of an individual. Similarly, the articular surface of the sternal end of the fourth rib is also examined for edge thinning and increased surface porosity. Accordingly, adult age is often categorized as young (20–35 years); middle (35–50 years) or old (50+ years) by anthropologists.

Sex Determination
- Anthropologists study a number of morphological features on the bones to determine whether the individual is male or female.
- Skull bone, mandible and pelvis gives better light to sex determination.
- On the skull, the nuchal crest is more pronounced and rougher in males than females.
- Mastoid process is longer and wider with respect to the external auditory meatus in males than females.
- Supraorbital margin appears sharper and thinner in females. But in males, it is blunt and thick. Supraorbital ridge and glabella are larger in males.
- Compared to females, males have more pronounced mental eminence, squarer chin, and jaw has more acute angle.
- We accordingly score cranial traits on a scale from 1 to 5; 1 being minimal (female) expression and 5 maximal (male) expression.
- Child bearing in females demands mechanical adjustments in female plevis compared to that of males.
- Generally, the female pelvis is wider and more angled.
- Subpubic angle is greater, and sciatic notch is broader in females.
- There is subpubic concavity in females, but it is absent or minimal in males.
- A sharp ridge runs down the medial aspect of the ischiopubic ramus in females, which is absent in males.
- Preauricular sulcus is more commonly seen on a female pelvis.

CLINICAL ASPECTS OF OSTEOLOGY

- Common distal radius fractures.
- Distal radius fractures are most commonly caused by a fall on an outstretched hand.
    - A *Colles' fracture* is an extra-articular fracture of the distal end of radius with dorsal angulation and dorsal displacement, near to the articular surface. This type of fracture typically occurs as a "fragility fracture" in osteoporotic bone. It happens when a person falls forwards and plants their outstretched hand in front of them.
    - A *Smiths fracture* is an extra-articular fracture of the distal end of radius with the volar angulation of the distal fragment with or without volar displacement (reverse of a Colles fracture). This usually happens when a person falls backwards and plants the outstretched hand behind the body.
    - A *Bartons* is an intra-articular fracture of the distal radius with associated dislocation of the radiocarpal joint.
- Surgical neck of the humerus is a constriction distal to the tubercles where the shaft begins. The surgical neck is a common site for fractures, while fractures of the anatomical neck are rare.
- *March fracture* is a type of a stress fracture of the metatarsals, named because the injury is sometimes sustained by soldiers during prolonged periods of marching.
- *Undertaker's fracture* is an artifact related to poor handling of the corpse characterized by subluxation of the lower cervical spine from tearing of the intervertebral disc at C6-C7 vertebral level.
- A *hangman's fracture* is traumatic spondylolisthesis of axis vertebra. Here, traumatic fracture of the bilateral pars interarticularis of C2 occurs. Injury occurs due to impacts of high force causing hyperextension of the neck and great axial load onto the C2 vertebrae. It usually occurs in case of judicial hanging, during falls usually in older adults and motor accidents.
- Clavicle usually breaks at the junction of medial 2/3rd and lateral 1/3rd and a 'figure of eight' bandage may be used to manage the condition.
- Secondary ossification centers at the lower end of femur appear almost at the time of birth, only if the newborn is viable. This feature is made used in medicolegal cases to know whether the a newborn was born viable or not.
- Scaphoid fracture is common during falling on outstretched hand; since scaphoid has very low blood supply. As a result, fracture of scaphoid (especially proximal part) is vulnerable to loss of the blood supply to that part, leading to avascular necrosis. Referred to as scaphoid nonunion.

SKULL

SKULL: ANTERIOR VIEW

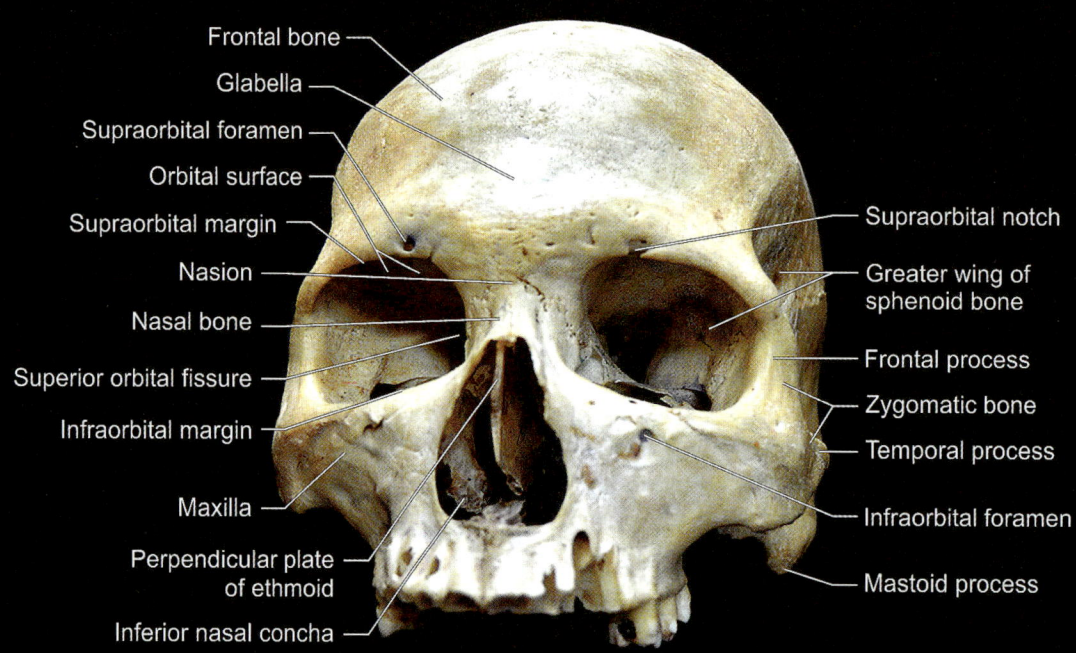

SKULL: POSTERIOR VIEW

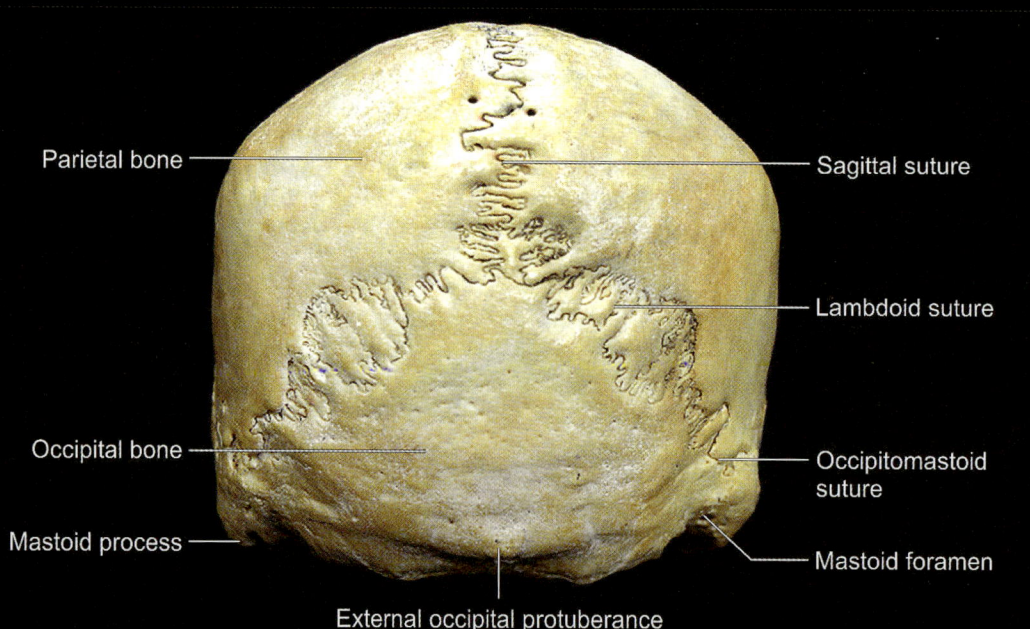

SKULL: LATERAL VIEW

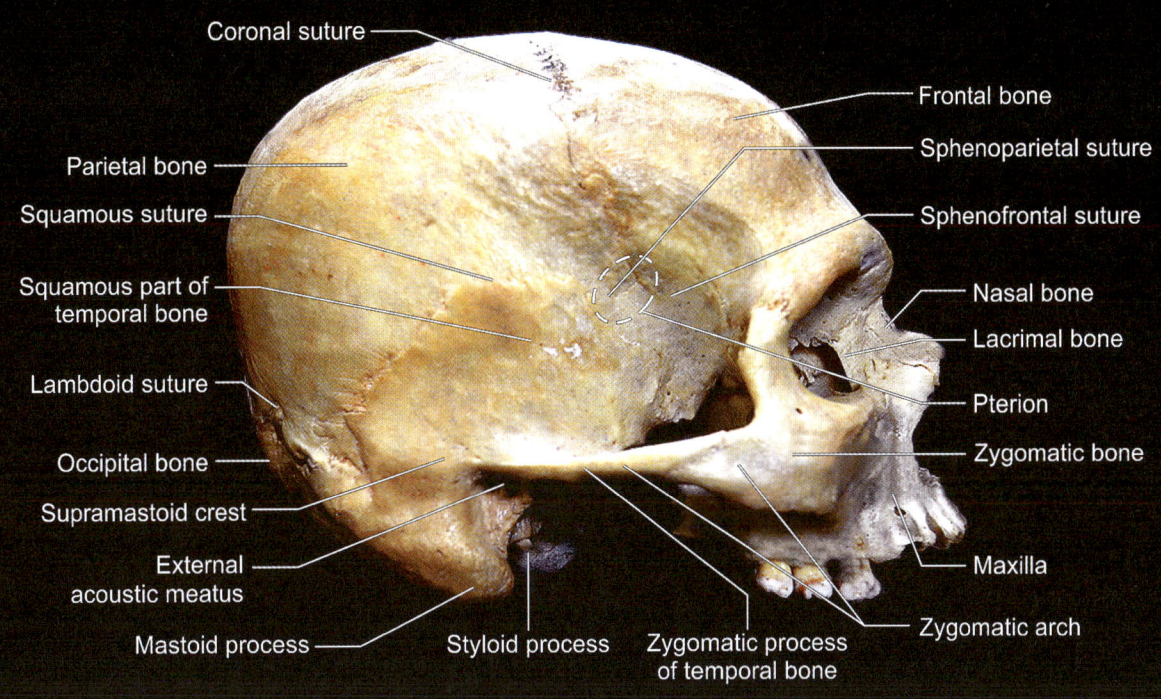

SKULL: INFERIOR VIEW

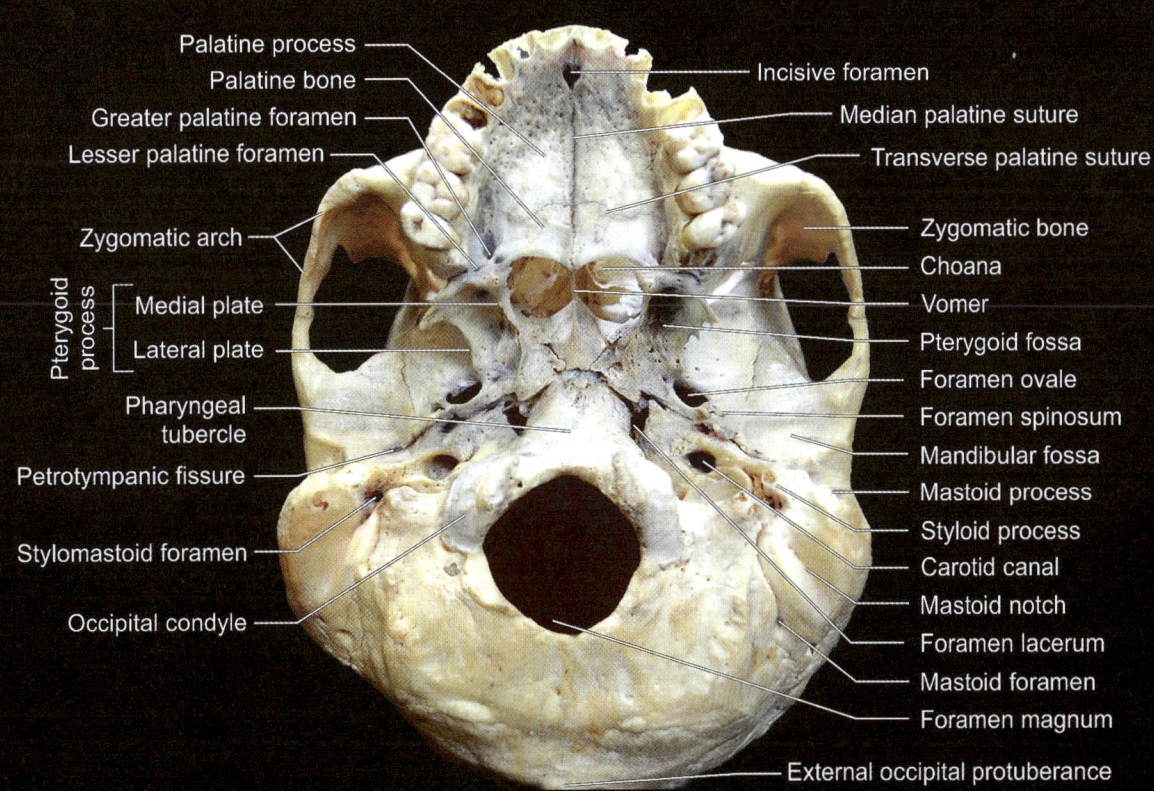

Structures Passing Through Foramina

- *Incisive fossa*: Nasopalatine nerve, sphenopalatine vessels
- *Greater palatine foramen*: Greater palatine nerve and vessels
- *Lesser palatine foramen*: Lesser palatine nerve and vessels
- *Foramen lacerum*: Greater petrosal nerve
- *Foramen ovale*: Lesser petrosal nerve, mandibular nerve, accessory meningeal artery
- *Foramen spinosum*: Middle meningeal vessels, meningeal branch of mandibular nerve
- *Carotid canal*: Internal carotid artery, carotid autonomic plexus
- *Petrotympanic fissure*: Chorda tympani of facial nerve
- *Tympanic canaliculus*: Tympanic branch of glossopharyngeal nerve
- *Mastoid canaliculus*: Auricular branch of vagus nerve
- *Stylomastoid foramen*: Facial nerve
- *Jugular fossa*: Glossopharyngeal nerve, vagus nerve, accessory nerve, superior bulb, internal jugular vein
- *Mastoid foramen*: Mastoid emisary vein, posterior meningeal artey
- *Hypoglossal canal*: Hypoglossal nerve
- *Foramen magnum*: Medulla oblongata, vertebral arteries and venous plexus, spinal accessory nerves.

FLOOR OF CRANIAL CAVITY: POSTEROSUPERIOR VIEW

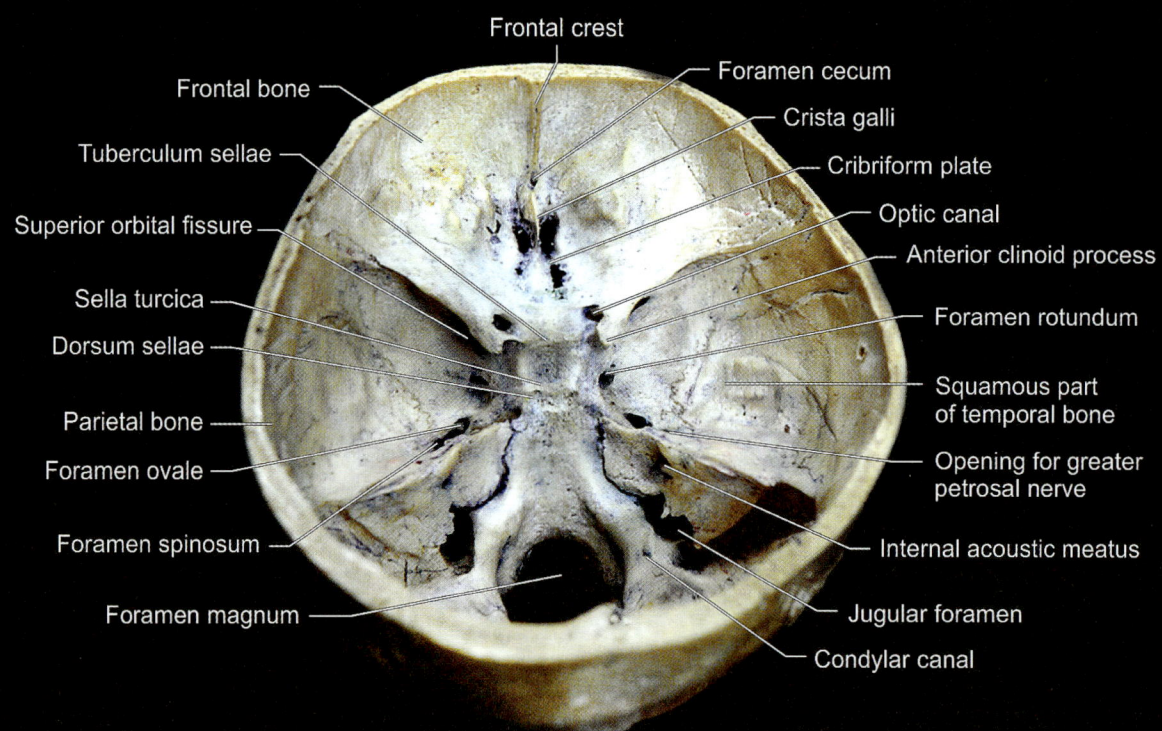

FLOOR OF CRANIAL CAVITY: SUPERIOR VIEW

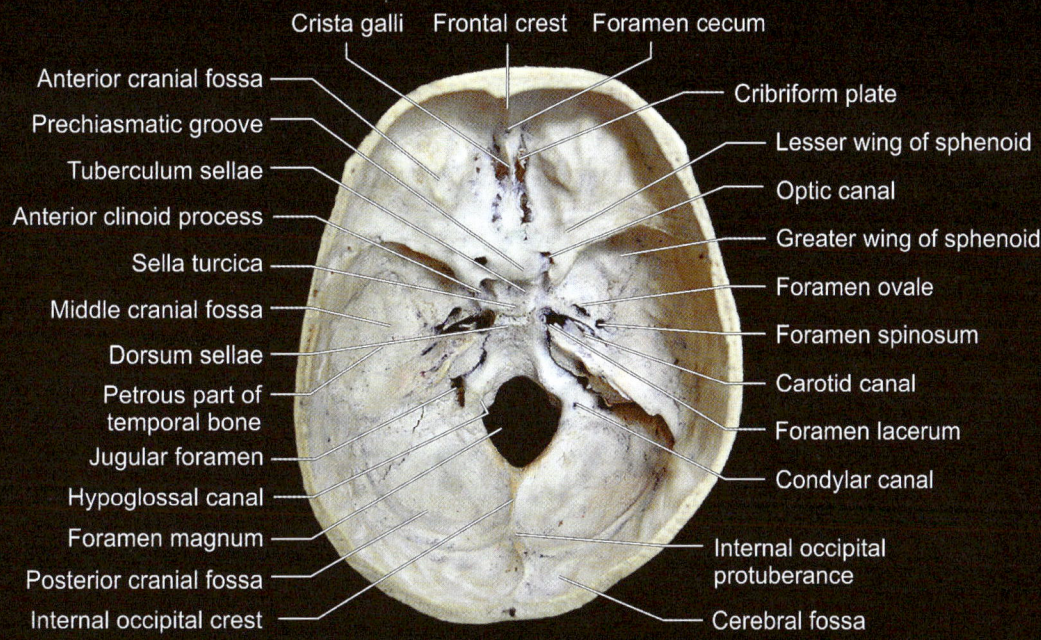

Structures Passing Through Foramina

- *Foramen cecum*: Emissary vein to superior sagittal sinus
- *Nasal slit and anterior ethmoidal foramen*: Anterior ethmoidal artery, vein and nerve
- *Foramina of cribriform plate*: Olfactory nerves
- *Posterior ethmoidal foramen*: Posterior ethmoidal artery, vein, and nerve
- *Optic canal*: Optic nerve, ophthalmic artery
- *Superior orbital fissure*: Oculomotor nerve, trochlear nerve, lacrimal, frontal, and nasociliary branches of ophthalmic nerve, abducent nerve, superior ophthalmic vein
- *Foramen rotundum*: Maxillary nerve
- *Foramen ovale*: Mandibular nerve, accessory meningeal artery, lesser petrosal nerve
- *Foramen spinosum*: Middle meningeal artery and vein, meningeal branch of mandibular nerve
- Sphenoidal emissary foramen (of Vesalius) (inconstant)
- *Carotid canal*: Internal carotid artery, internal carotid nerve plexus
- *Foramen lacerum*: Greater petrosal nerve
- Hiatus for lesser petrosal nerve
- Hiatus for greater petrosal nerve
- *Internal acoustic meatus:* Facial nerve, vestibulocochlear nerve, labyrinthine artery
- *Opening of vestibular aqueduct*: Endolymphatic duct
- *Mastoid foramen*: Emissary vein and occasional branch of occipital artery
- *Jugular foramen*: Inferior petrosal sinus, glossopharyngeal nerve, vagus nerve, accessory nerve, sigmoid sinus, posterior meningeal artery
- *Hypoglossal canal*: Hypoglossal nerve
- *Foramen magnum*: Medulla oblongata, meninges, vertebral arteries, meningeal branches of vertebral arteries, spinal roots of accessory nerves.

MANDIBLE: ANTERIOR VIEW

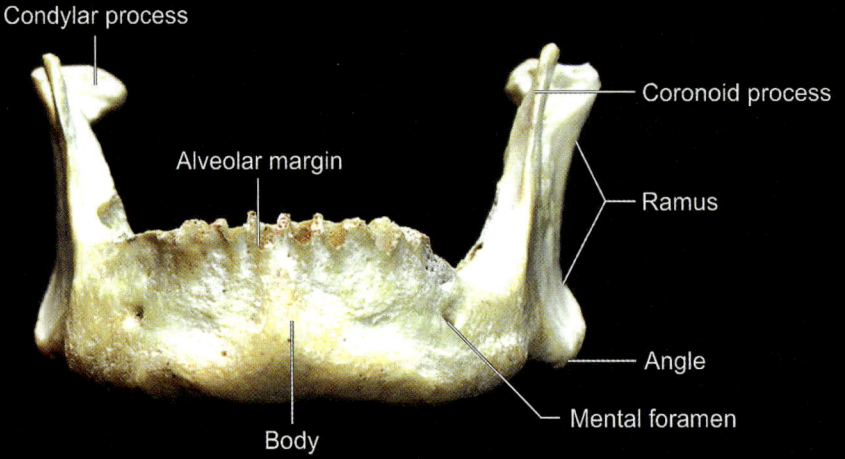

MANDIBLE: LATERAL VIEW

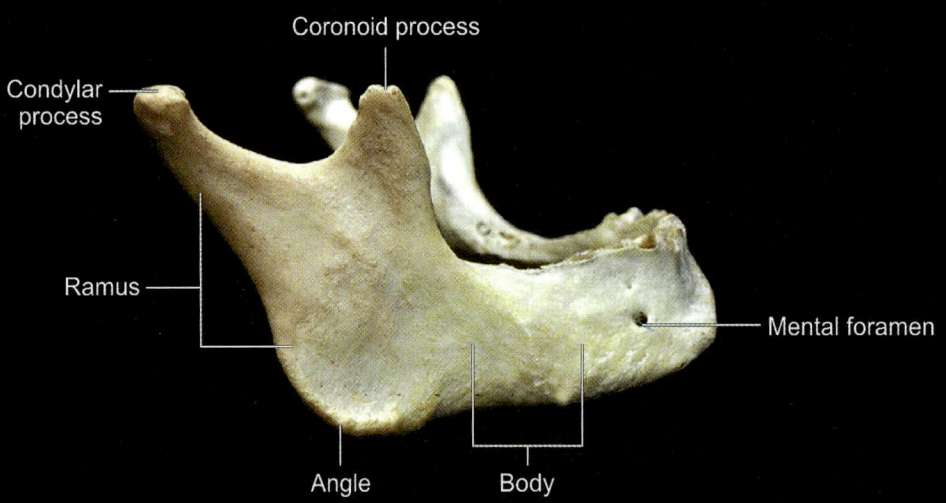

MANDIBLE: POSTERIOR VIEW

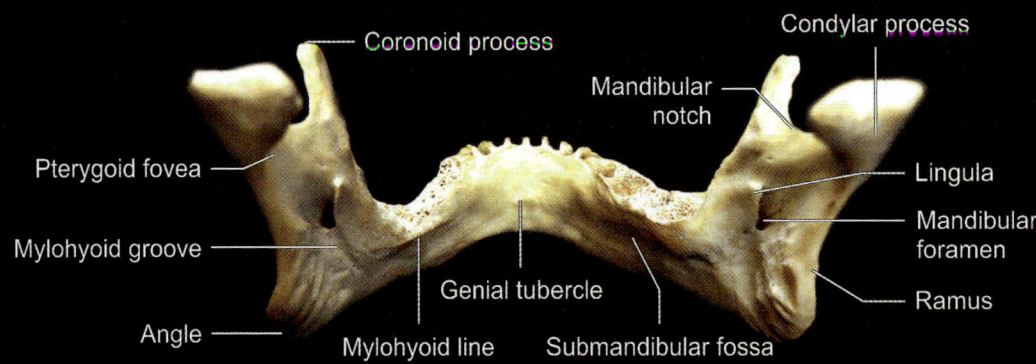

UPPER LIMB

CLAVICLE: SUPERIOR VIEW

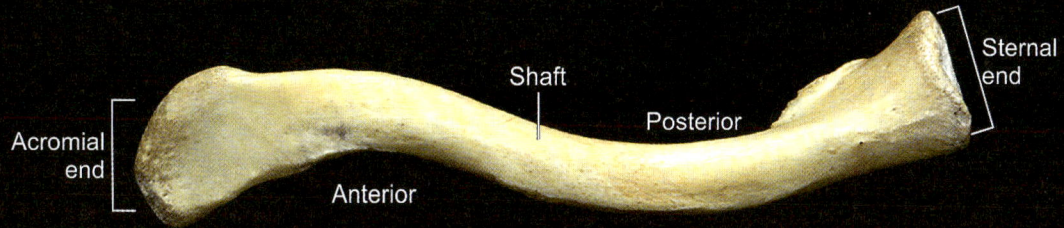

CLAVICLE: INFERIOR VIEW

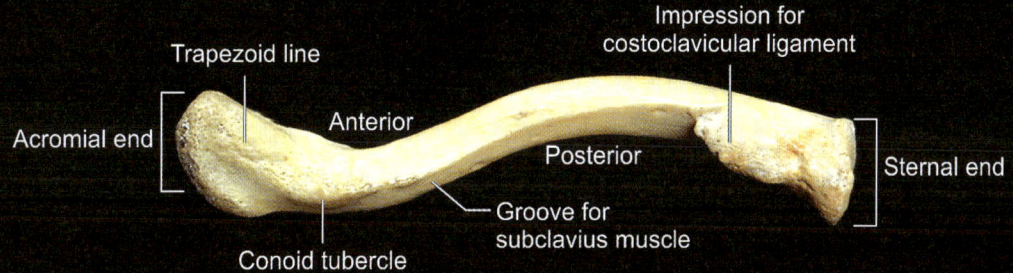

SCAPULA: ANTERIOR VIEW

Left Scapula Anterior View

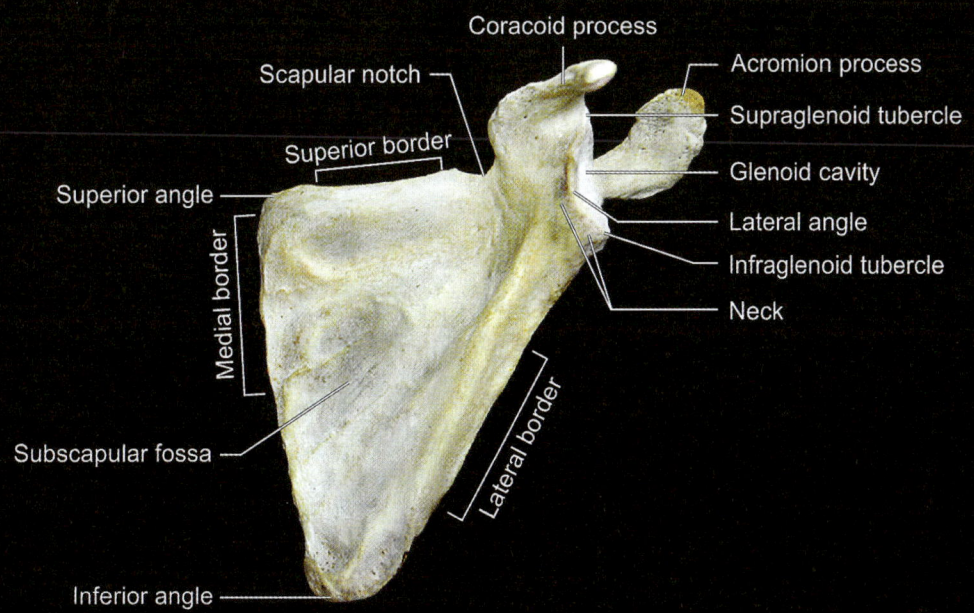

SCAPULA: POSTERIOR VIEW

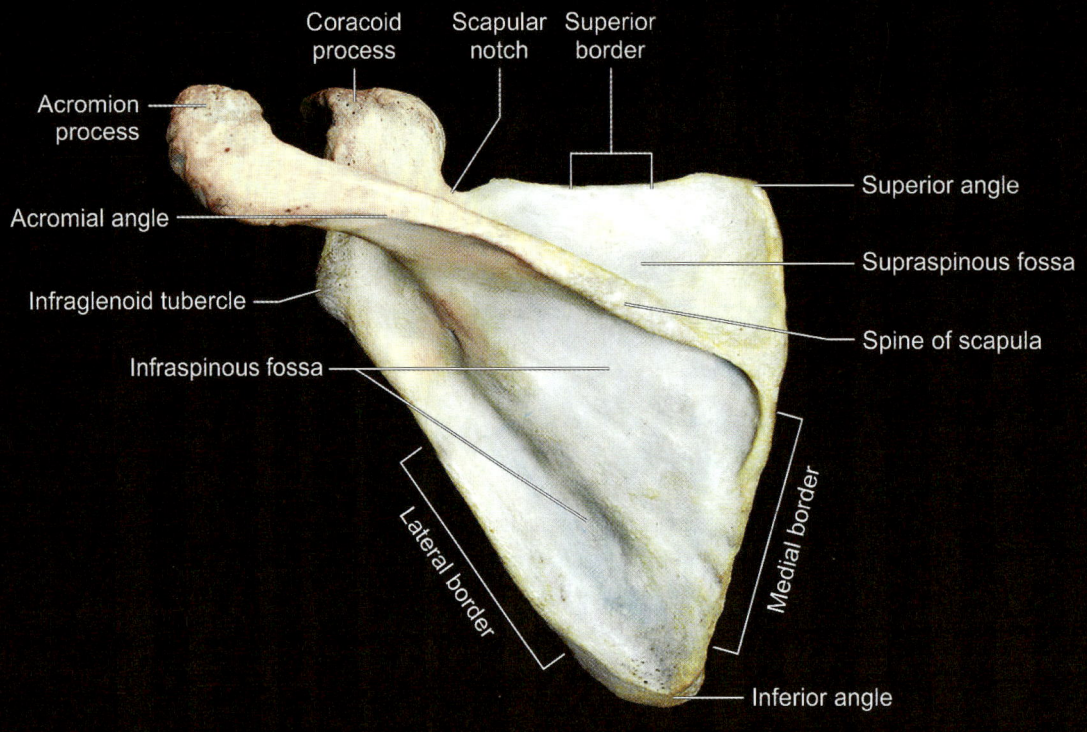

SCAPULA: LATERAL VIEW

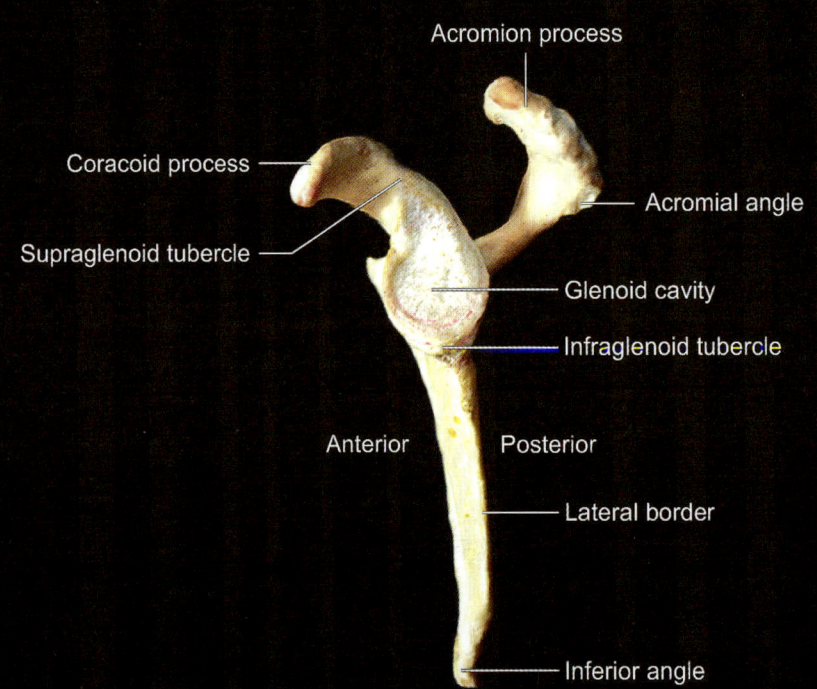

HUMERUS

ANTERIOR VIEW

POSTERIOR VIEW

PROXIMAL VIEW

DISTAL VIEW

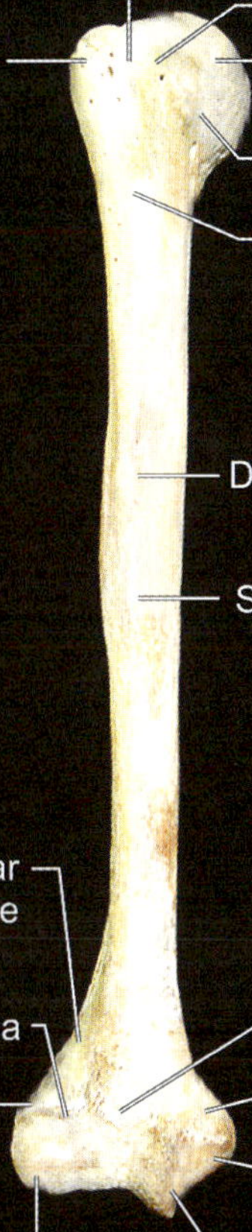

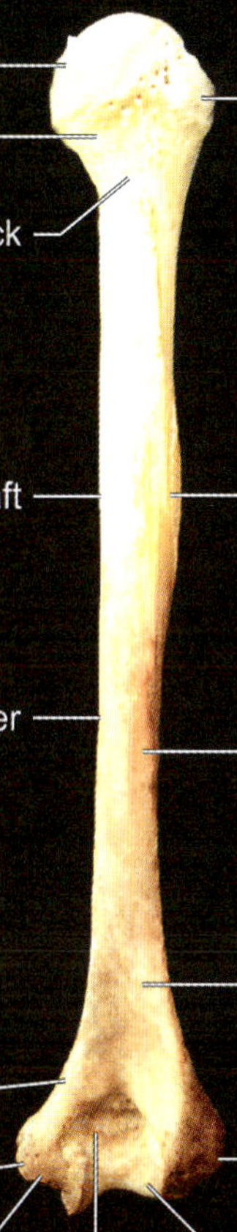

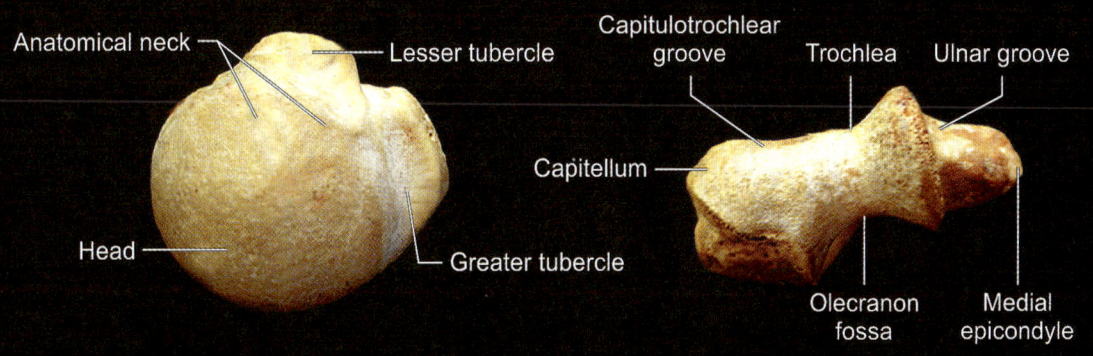

RADIUS AND ULNA

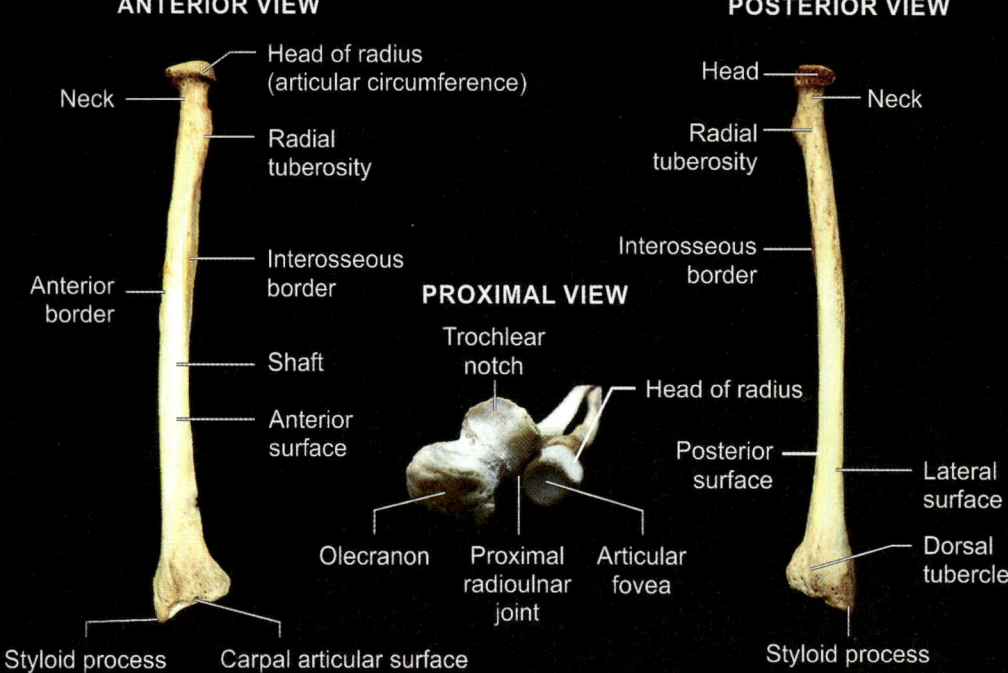

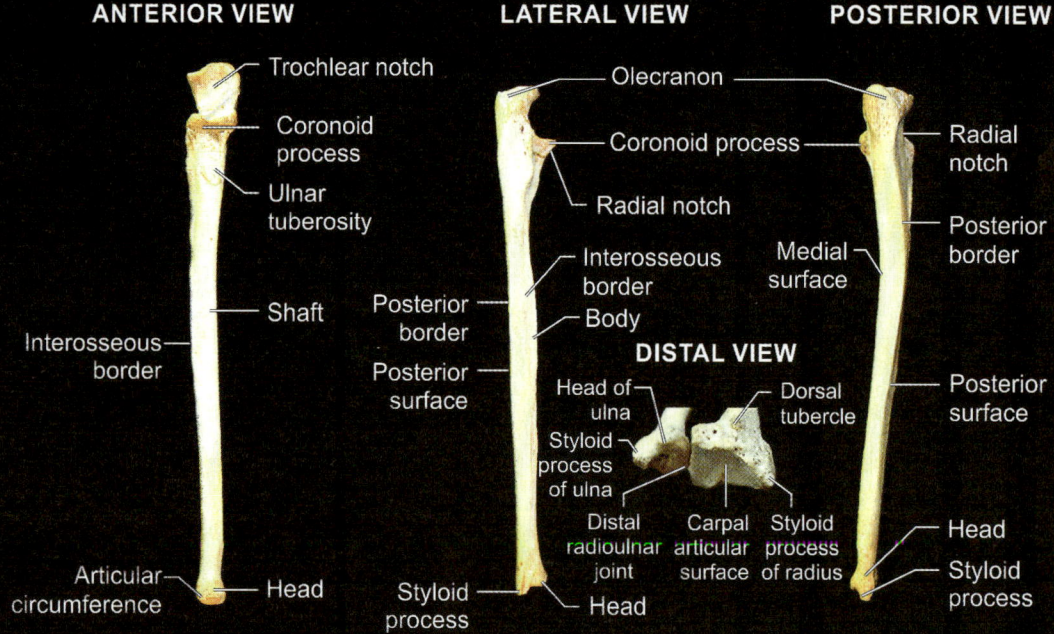

HAND: DORSAL VIEW

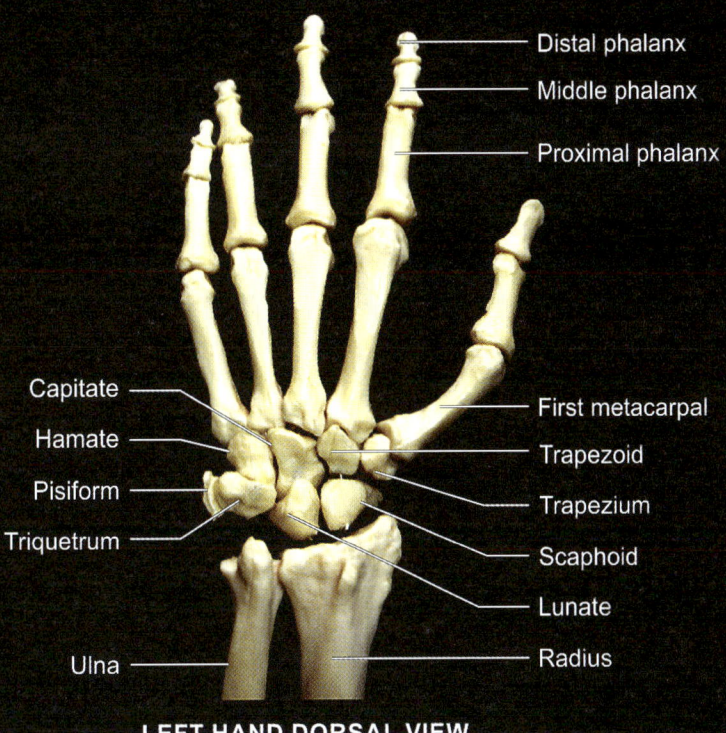

LEFT HAND DORSAL VIEW

LOWER LIMB

PELVIS: ANTERIOR VIEW

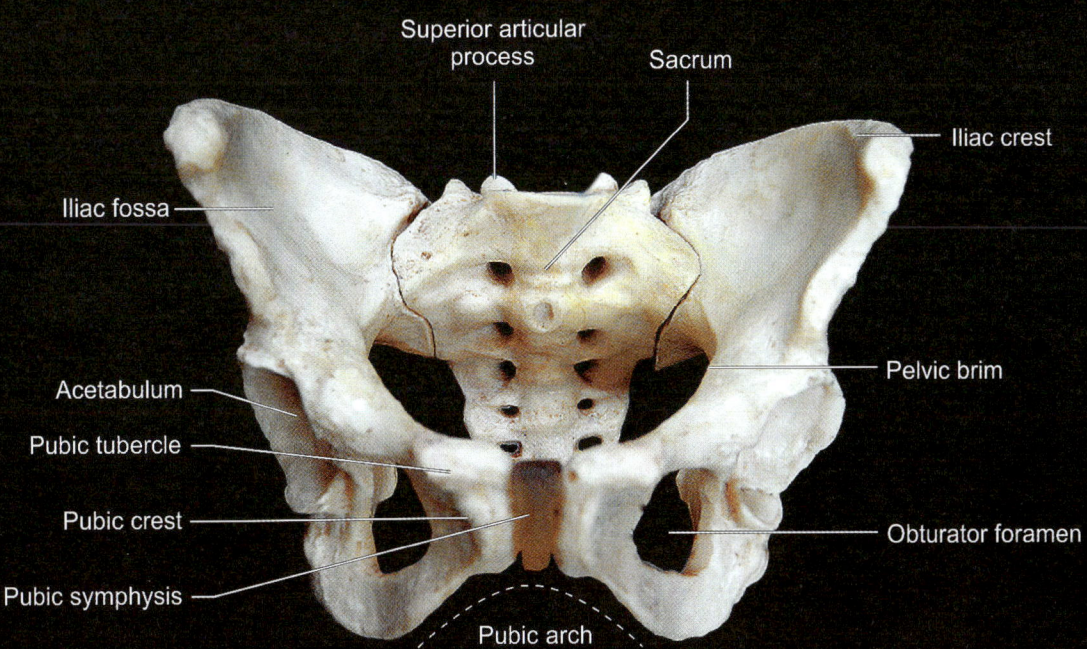

PELVIS: POSTERIOR VIEW

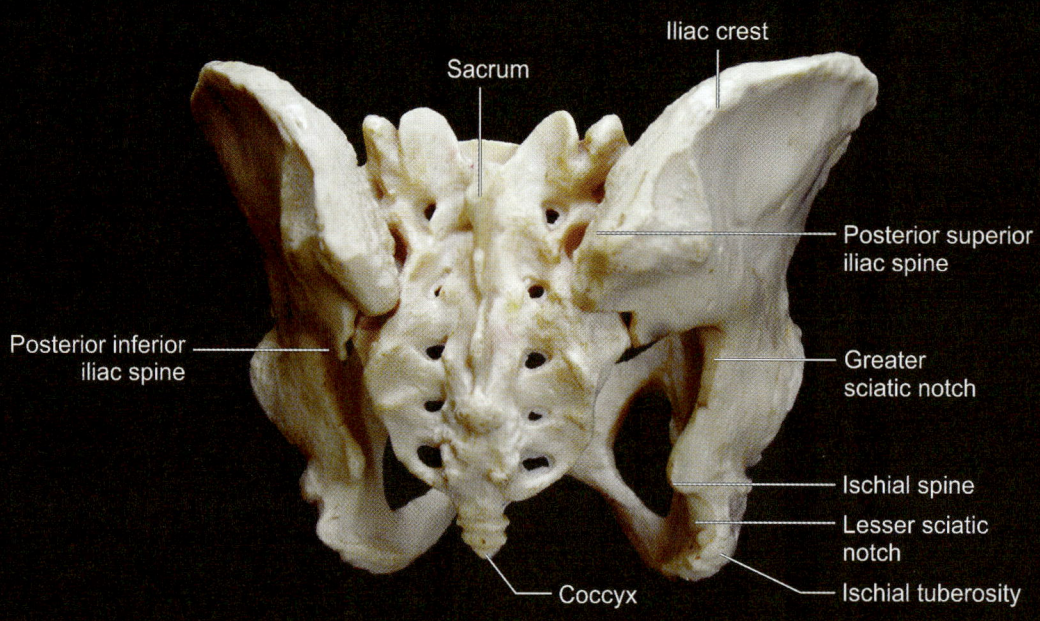

HIP BONE: MEDIAL VIEW

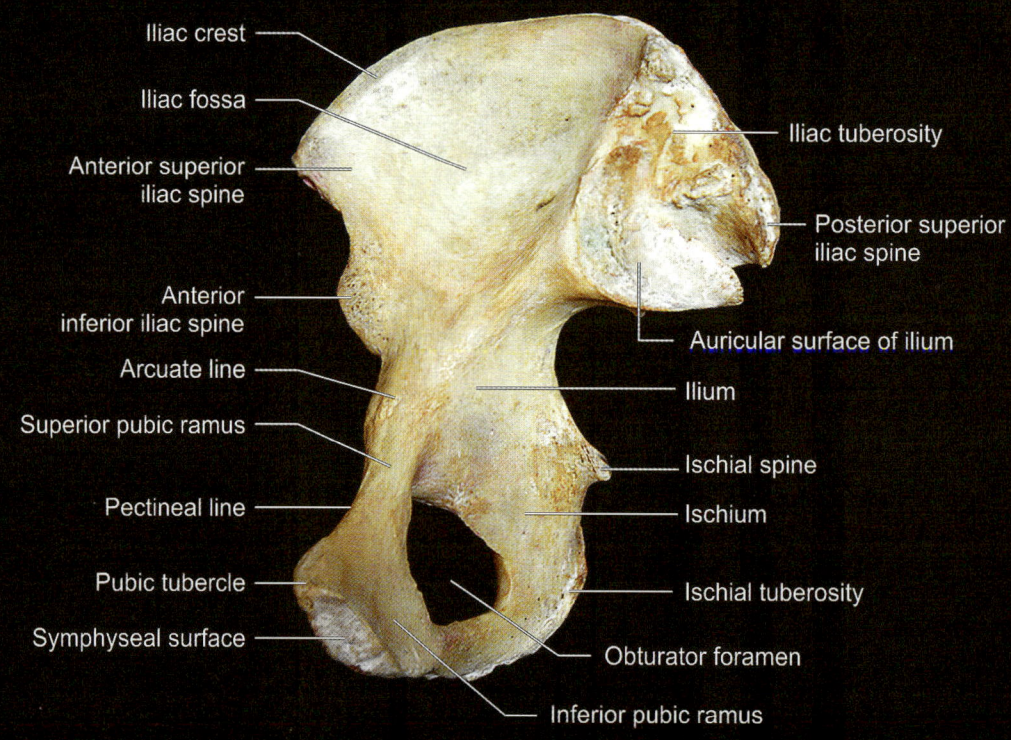

HIP BONE: LATERAL VIEW

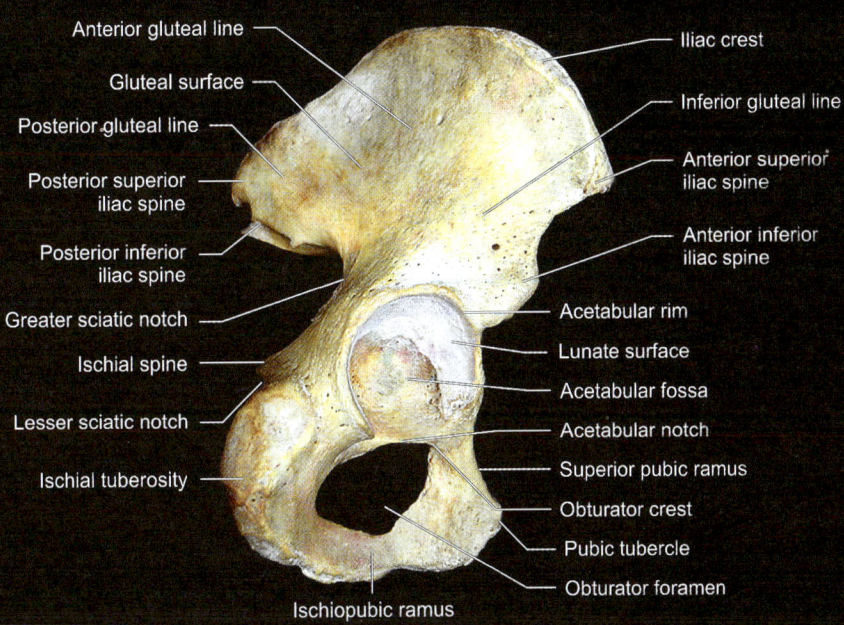

PATELLA

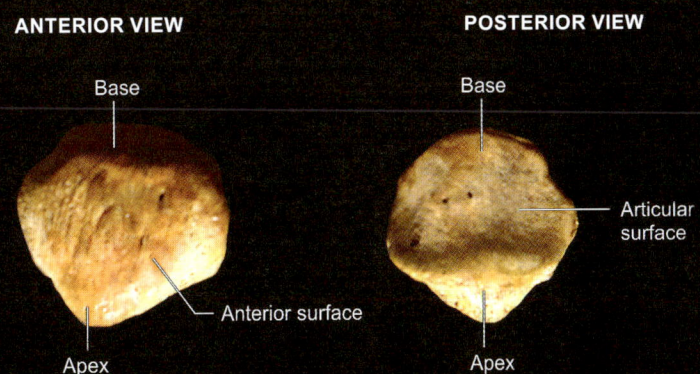

FEMUR

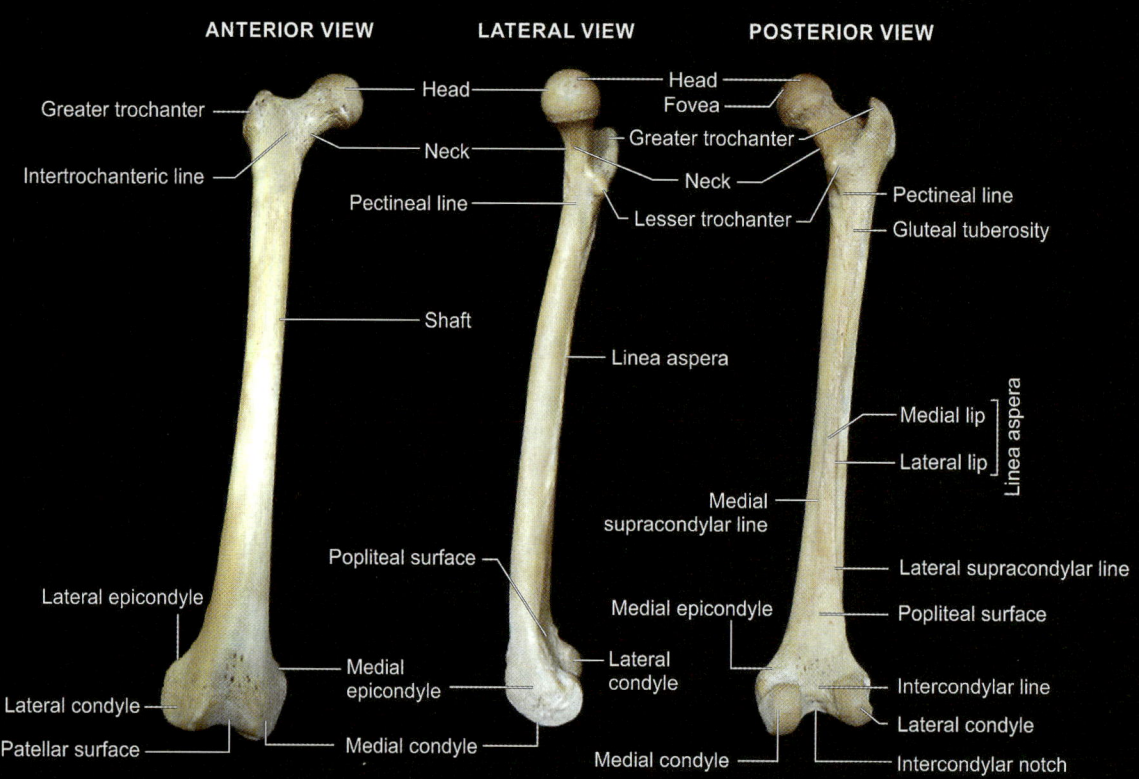

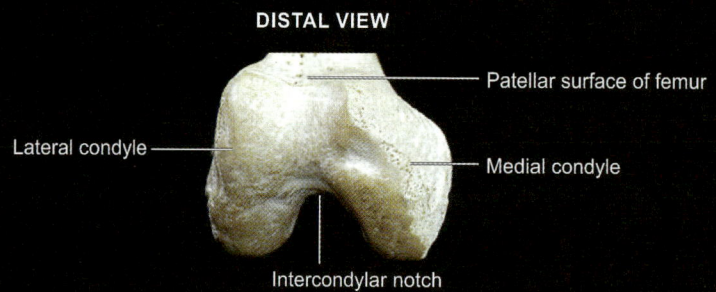

TIBIA AND FIBULA

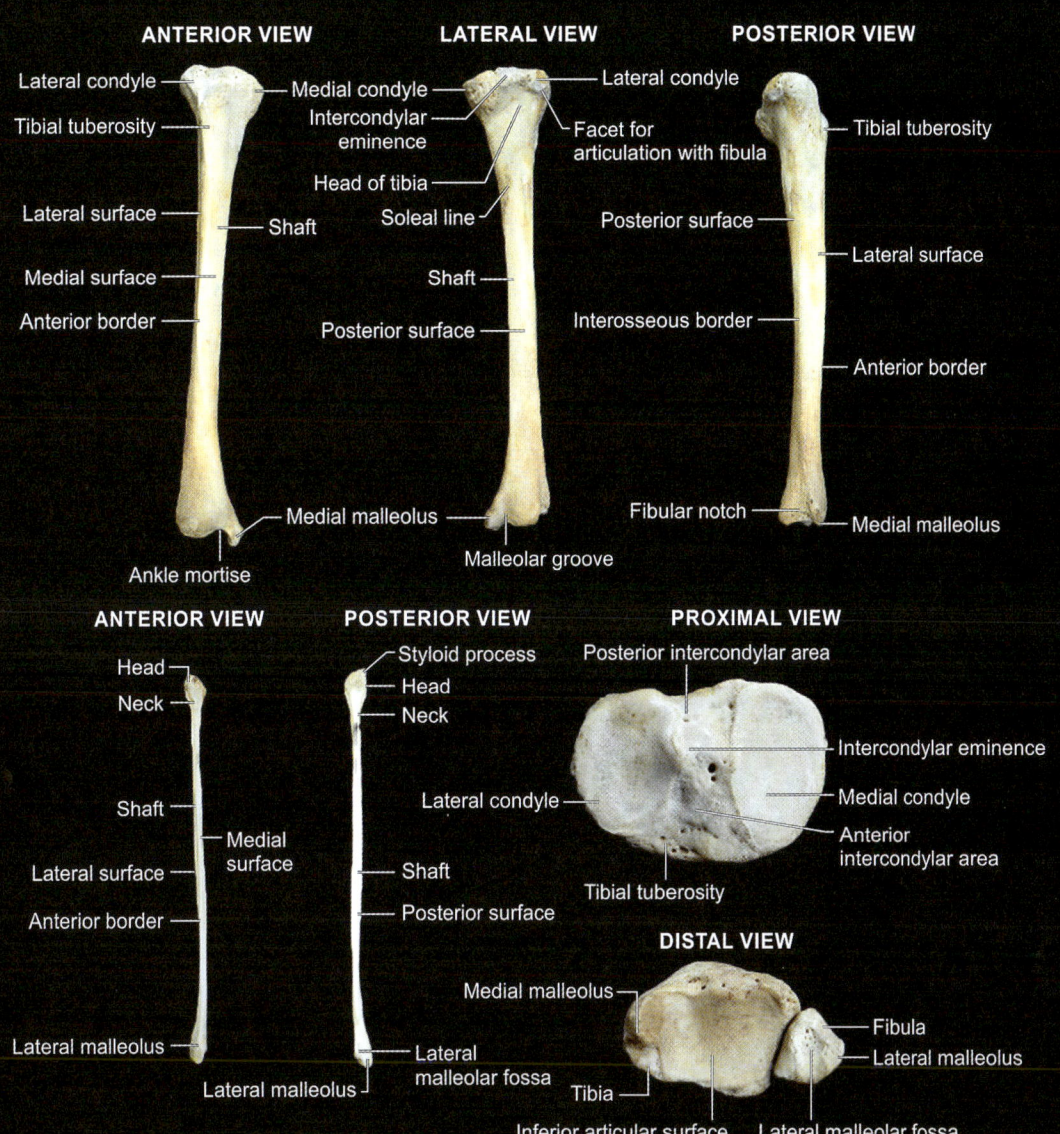

FOOT: LATERAL VIEW

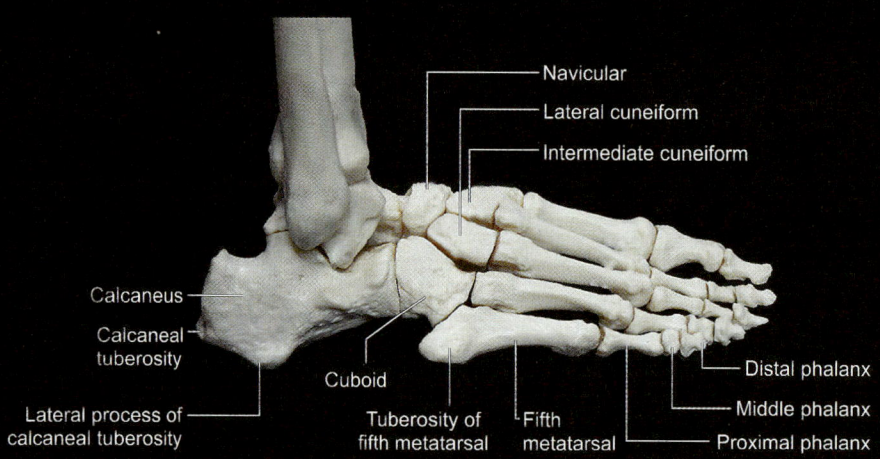

FOOT: MEDIAL VIEW

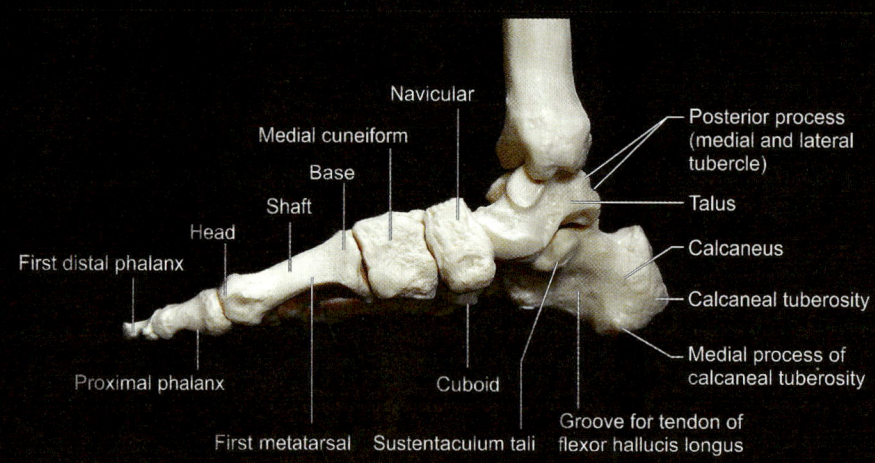

THORAX

STERNUM: ANTERIOR VIEW

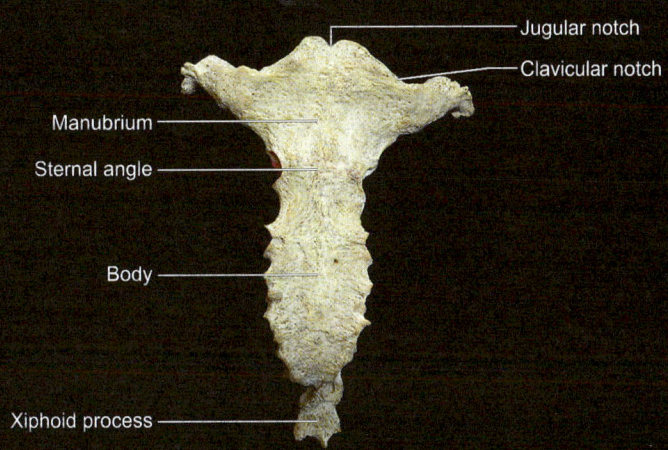

STERNUM: LATERAL VIEW

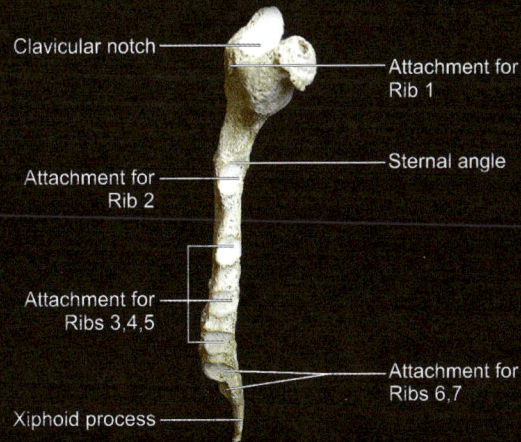

RIB 1: SUPERIOR VIEW

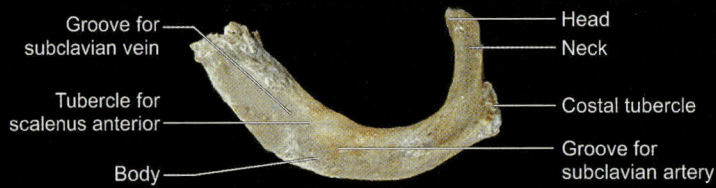

RIB 5 : MEDIAL VIEW

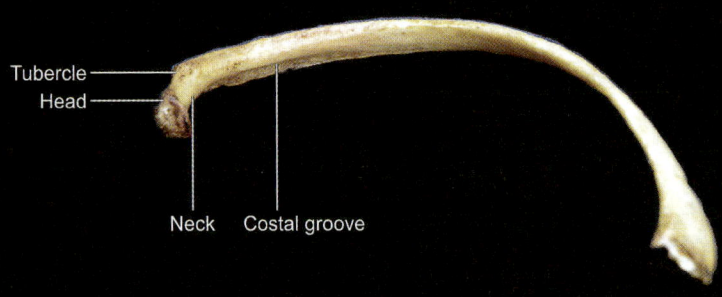

RIB 5 : LATERAL VIEW

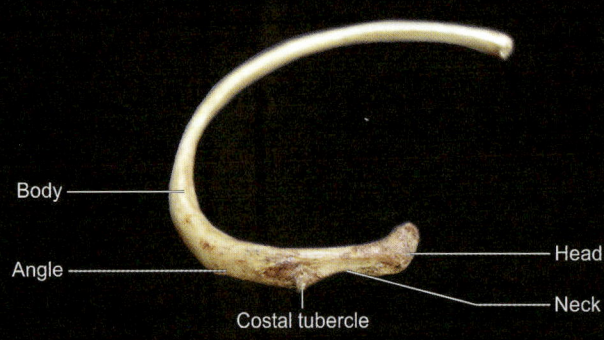

VERTEBRAE

ATLAS: SUPERIOR VIEW

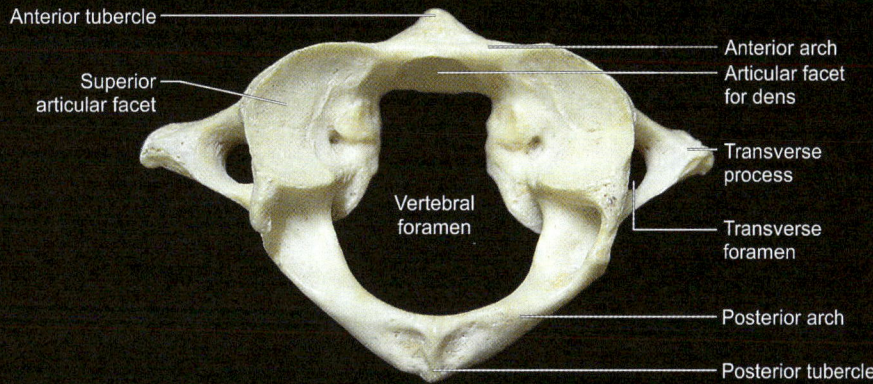

ATLAS: INFERIOR VIEW

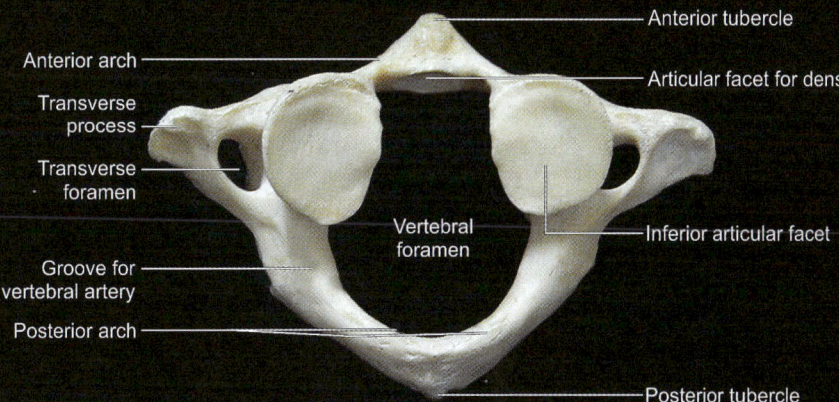

AXIS: ANTERIOR VIEW

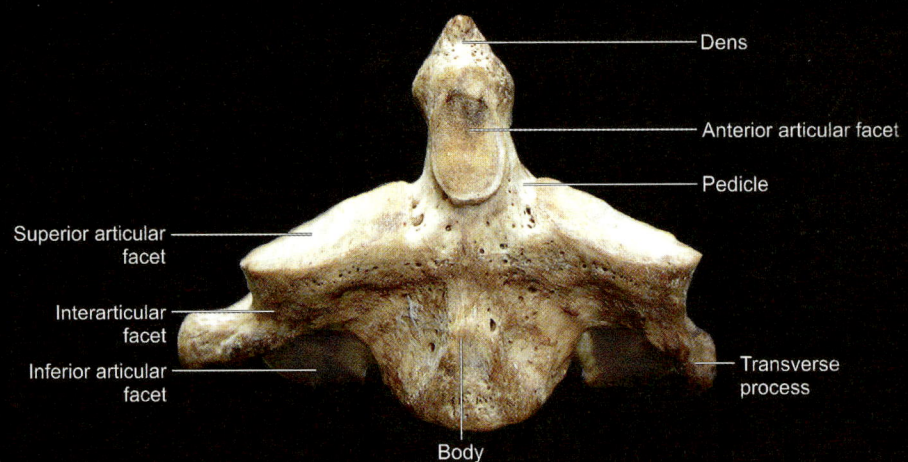

AXIS: POSTERIOR VIEW

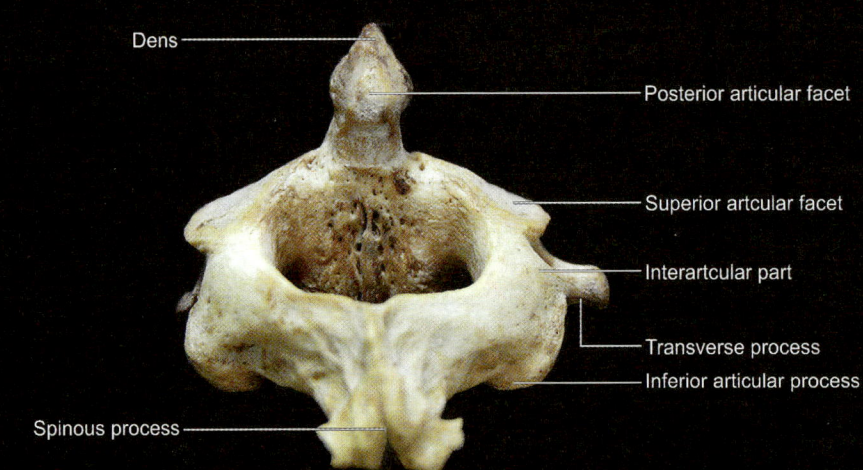

CERVICAL VERTEBRAE: ANTERIOR VIEW

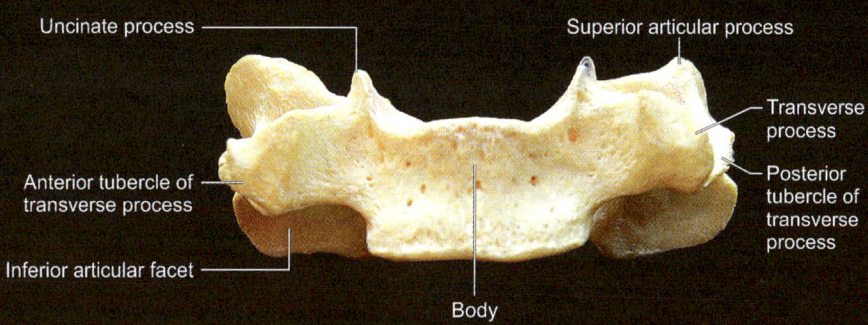

CERVICAL VERTEBRAE: POSTEROLATERAL OBLIQUE VIEW

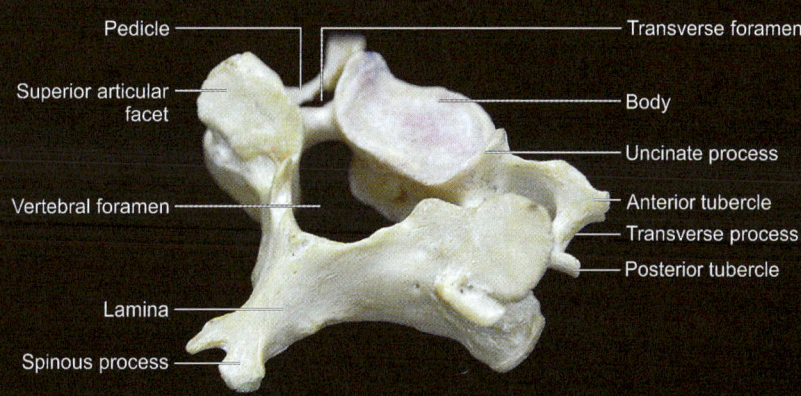

CERVICAL VERTEBRAE: SUPERIOR VIEW

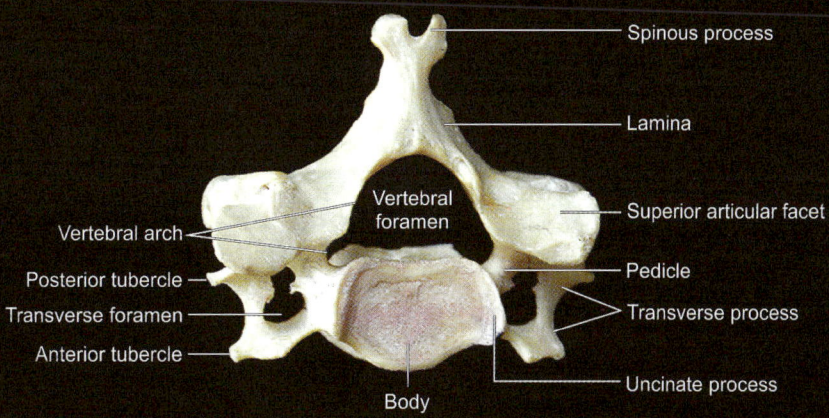

THORACIC VERTEBRAE: SUPERIOR VIEW

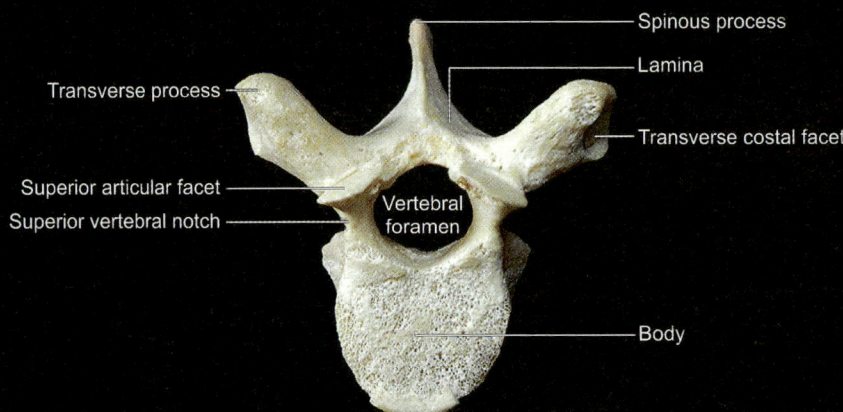

THORACIC VERTEBRAE: LATERAL VIEW

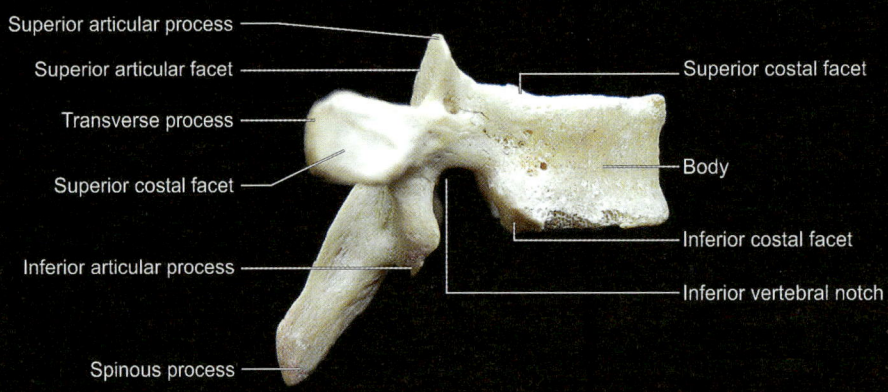

THORACIC VERTEBRAE: POSTERIOR VIEW

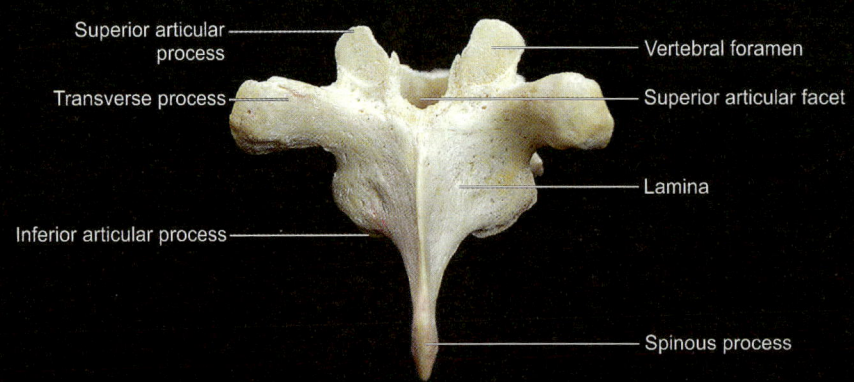

LUMBAR VERTEBRAE: SUPERIOR VIEW

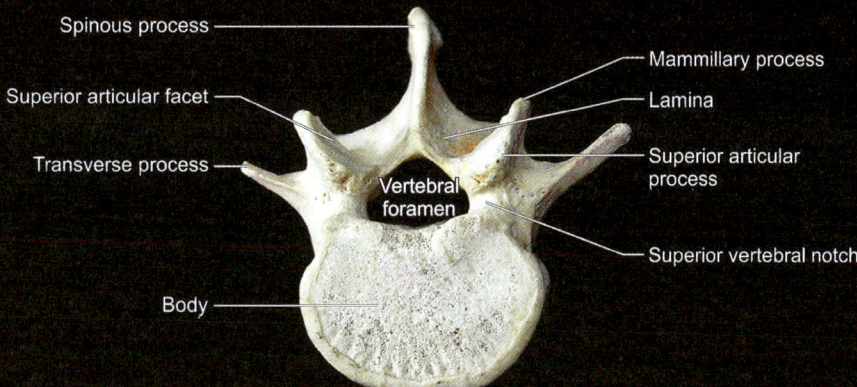

LUMBAR VERTEBRAE: LATERAL VIEW

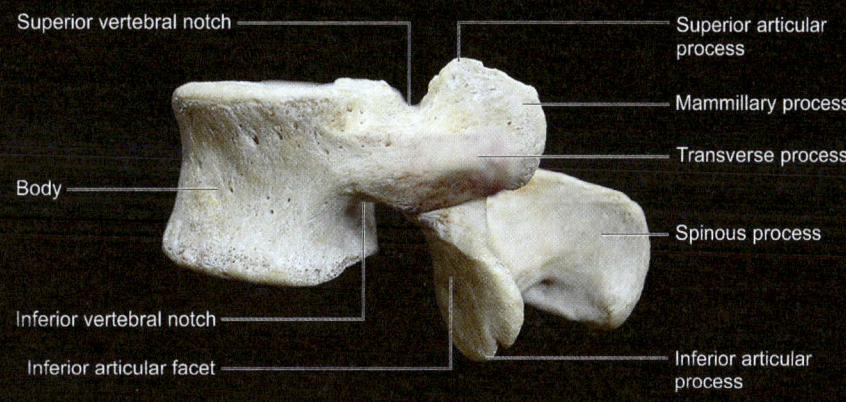

LUMBAR VERTEBRAE: POSTERIOR VIEW

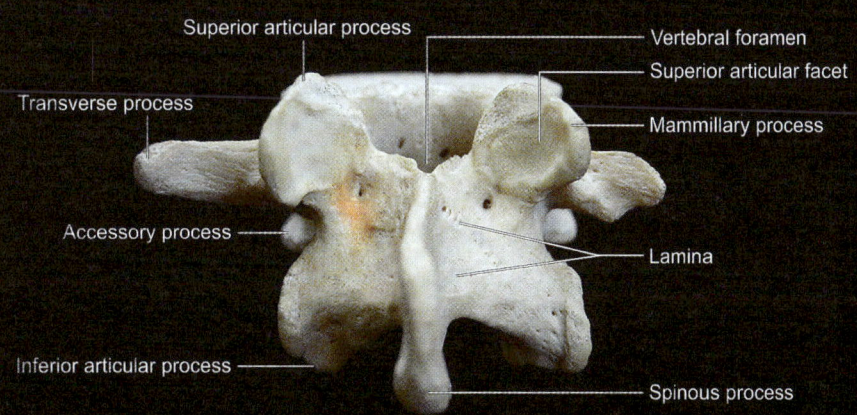

SACRUM: ANTERIOR VIEW

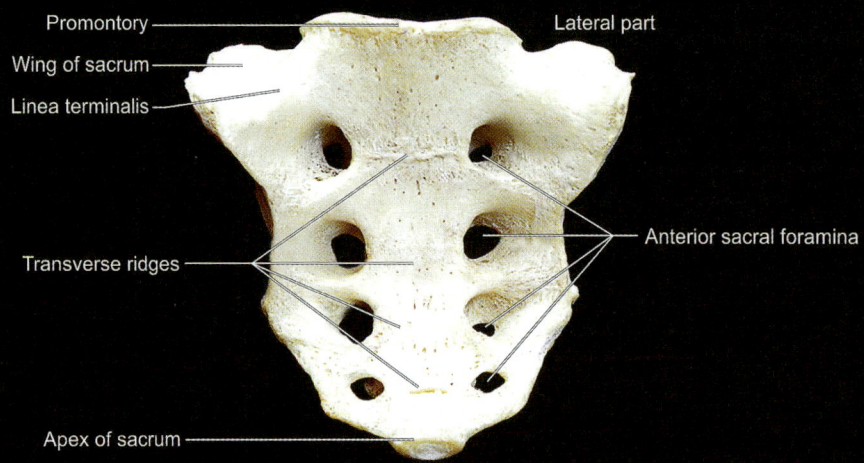

SACRUM: POSTERIOR VIEW

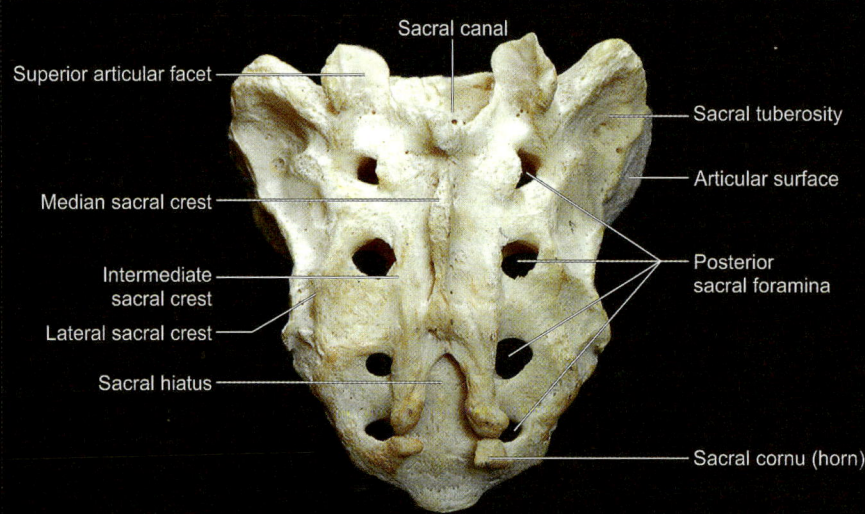

CHAPTER 5: Surface Marking

OUTLINE

- Upper Limb
- Lower Limb
- Thorax
- Abdomen and Pelvis
- Head and Neck

UPPER LIMB

AXILLARY ARTERY

- Abduct the arm at 90 degrees.
- Mark the midpoint of clavicle.
- Mark a point at the anterior 1/3rd and posterior 2/3rd of lateral wall of axilla at its lower limit
- Join these points by a broad line to get the surface marking.

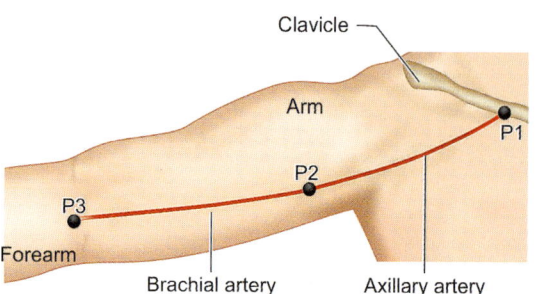

BRACHIAL ARTERY

- Mark a point at the anterior 1/3rd and posterior 2/3rd of lateral wall of axilla at its lower limit.
- Mark another point at the level of neck of radius in the elbow medial to the tendon of biceps.
- Join these points.

RADIAL ARTERY

- Mark a point at level of neck of radius in the elbow medial to tendon of biceps.
- Mark a point at wrist in the interval between tendon of flexi carpi radialis medially and anterior border of radius laterally.
- Join the points with curved line having convexity to lateral side to get surface marking.

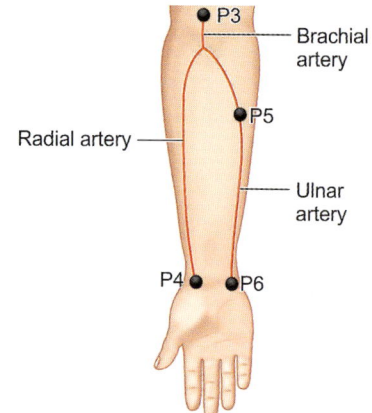

ULNAR ARTERY

- Mark a point in the middle line of forearm opposite to the neck of the radius.
- Mark another point at the junction of upper 1/3rd and lower 2/3rd of the forearm near its medial border.
- Mark the third point at the lateral edge of pisiform.
- Join the first two points by a curved line which passes downwards and medially.
- Then join the second point with third one to get the surface marking.

AXILLARY NERVE

- Mark the midpoint of the line joining the tip of the acromion to the deltoid tuberosity.
- Mark another point 2 cm above the midpoint of the above line.
- Draw a transverse line from the second point across the deltoid muscle to get the surface marking.

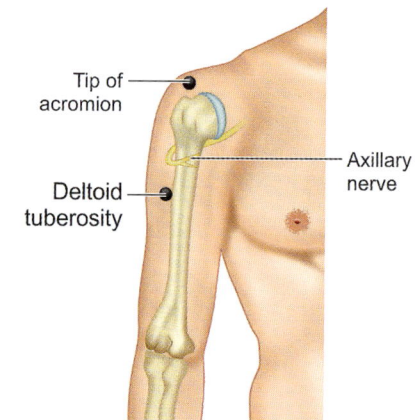

MEDIAN NERVE

Arm

- Mark brachial artery first.
- Median nerve lies lateral to artery in the upper half, medial to the artery in the lower half.
- It crosses the vessel ventrally in the middle of the arm.

Forearm

- Mark the first point at the level of neck of the radius in the middle line of the forearm.
- Mark second point at the wrist 1 cm medial to the flexor carpi radialis tendon.
- Join the two points.
- At wrist nerve runs laterally from undercover of palmaris longus tendon.

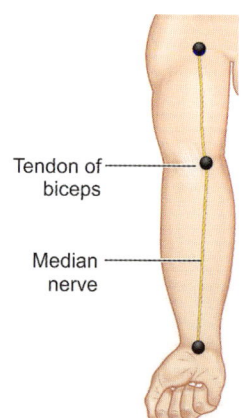

Surface Marking

MUSCULOCUTANEOUS NERVE
- Mark a point 5 cm below the coracoid process.
- Mark the midpoint of elevation caused by the biceps.
- Third point is marked just lateral to tendon of biceps.
- Join these points.

RADIAL NERVE

Arm
- Mark a point at the lower end of axillary artery.
- Mark the junction between the upper 1/3rd and lower 2/3rd of the line joining insertion of deltoid to the lateral epicondyle.
- Mark a point 1 cm lateral to the tendon of biceps at the level of lateral epicondyle.
- Join these points.

Forearm
- Mark a point 1 cm lateral to tendon of biceps at the level of lateral epicondyle of humerus.
- Mark a point at the junction of middle and lower 1/3rd of lateral border of forearm.
- Mark a point in the anatomical snuff box.
- Join these three points.

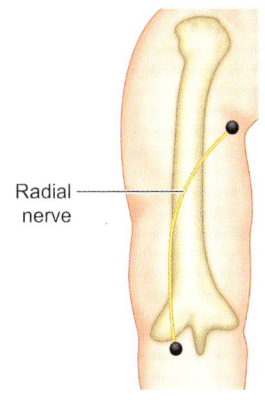

Radial nerve

ULNAR NERVE

Arm
- Mark a point medial to lower end of axillary artery.
- Mark another point just medial to midpoint of brachial artery.
- Mark a point on the posterior aspect of the medial epicondyle of humerus.
- Join these 3 points.

Forearm
- Mark a mark on the base of medial epicondyle of humerus.
- Mark a point at the lateral edge of pisiform bone.
- Join these points by a line which should follow the lateral side of the tendon of flexor carpi ulnaris in the lower part of the forearm.

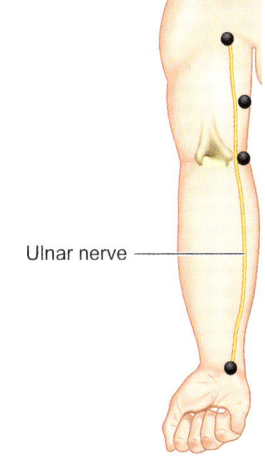

Ulnar nerve

FLEXOR RETINACULUM
- Mark the hook of hamate.
- Mark the crest of trapezium.
- Mark a point on the pisiform bone.
- Mark the tubercle of scaphoid.
- Join first two points by a line concave downwards.
- And last two points by a line concave upwards.
- Wide band between these two lines represent the flexor retinaculum.

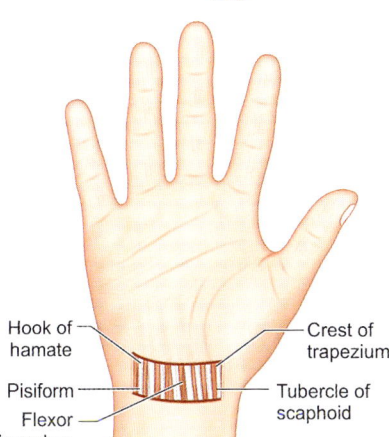

Hook of hamate — Crest of trapezium
Pisiform — Tubercle of scaphoid
Flexor retinaculum

EXTENSOR RETINACULUM
- Mark a point on the anterior border of radius above its styloid process.
- Mark a point on the styloid process of ulna.
- Mark the lower border of anterior end of radius.
- Mark a point on the triquetral bone.
- Join first two points to get upper border.
- Draw a line by joining the last two points parallel to upper border to get lower border.

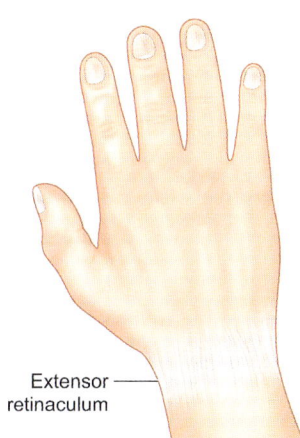

Extensor retinaculum

Surface Marking

SUPERFICIAL PALMAR ARCH
- Mark a point just lateral and distal side to the pisiform bone.
- Mark the hook of hamate.
- Mark a point on the center of the palm, at the level of distal margin of extended thumb.
- Superficial palmar arch is marked as a curved line with convexity towards fingers on joining these points.

DEEP PALMAR ARCH
- Mark a point near the proximal end of first intermetacarpal space.
- Mark another point just distal to hook of hamate.
- Join these points by a 4 cm horizontal line with a slight distal convexity (towards fingers) about one finger's breadth above the level of superficial palmar arch.

LOWER LIMB

Midinguinal point: Midpoint between anterosuperior iliac spine and symphysis pubis.

Midpoint of inguinal ligament: Midpoint of anterosuperior iliac spine and pubic tubercle.

FEMORAL ARTERY
- Mark the midinguinal point.
- Mark another point at adductor tubercle.
- Join the two points to obtain a line.
- Artery lies at upper 2/3rd of the line obtained.

POPLITEAL ARTERY
- First point is marked at junction of middle and lower 1/3rd of thigh, 2.5 cm medial to midline on the back of lower limb.
- Mark the second point in the midline of back of knee.
- Mark the third point at level of tibial tuberosity in the midline of back of leg.
- Join the three points.

POSTERIOR TIBIAL ARTERY
- Mark a point in the middle line of the leg at the level of neck of fibula.
- Mark another point midway between medial malleolus and tendocalcaneous.
- Join these points.

DORSALIS PEDIS ARTERY
- Mark a point midway between two malleoli.
- Mark another point at the proximal end of first intermetatarsal space.
- Join these points.

SAPHENOUS OPENING
- Mark a point 4 cm lateral and 4 cm below the pubic tubercle.
- It gives the center of saphenous opening.
- It is 2.5 cm long and 2 cm broad.

GREAT SAPHENOUS VEIN
- Mark a point on dorsum of foot at medial end of dorsal venous arch.
- Mark the next point at the anterior surface of medial malleolus.
- Third point on the medial border of tibia at the junction of upper 2/3rd and lower 1/3rd of the leg.

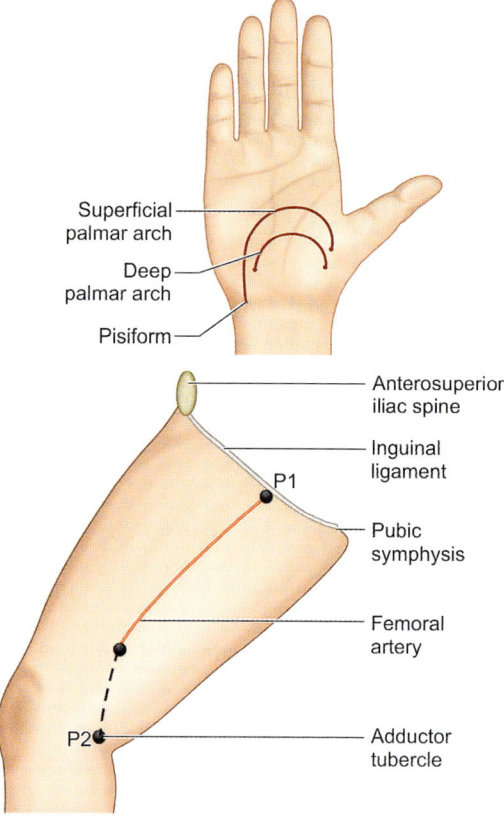

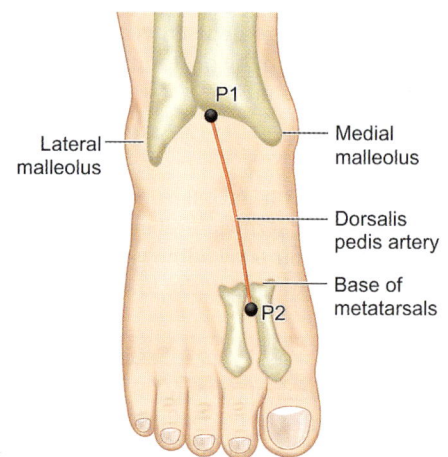

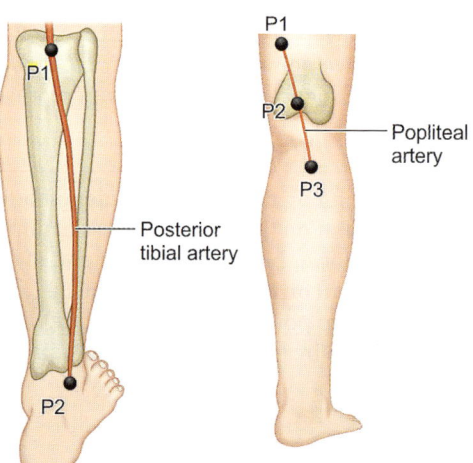

Surface Marking

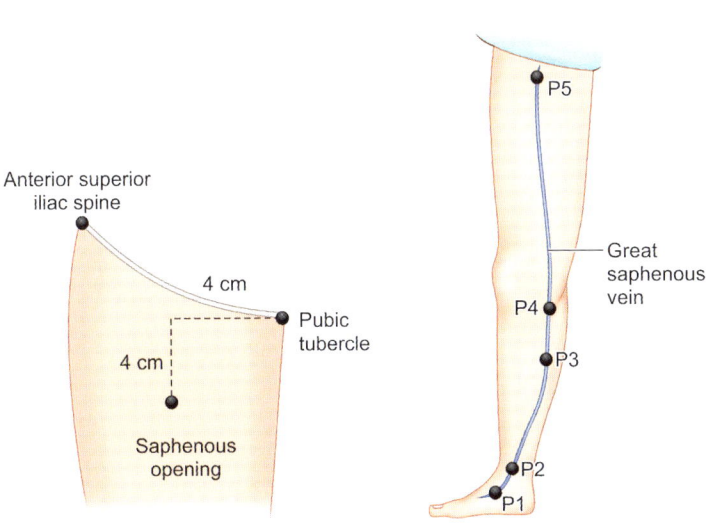
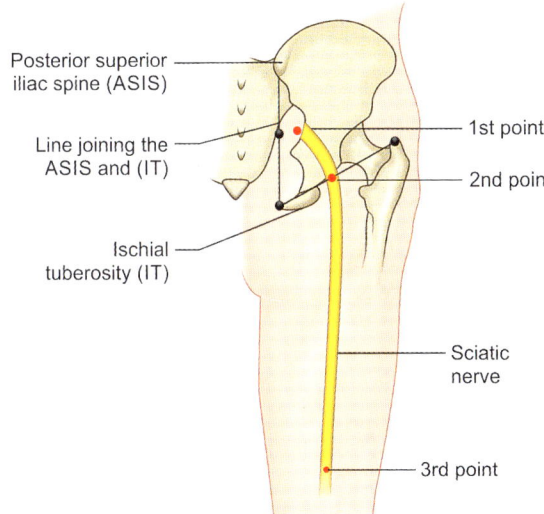

- Next point at the adductor tubercle and mark 5th point below the center of saphenous opening.
- Join these points.

SCIATIC NERVE

- Draw a line joining the posterosuperior iliac spine and ischial tuberosity.
- Mark a point 2.5 cm lateral to midpoint of above line.
- Second point is marked just medial to midpoint between ischial tuberosity and greater trochanter.
- Third point is marked at junction of upper 1/3rd and lower 1/3rd in the midline of back of thigh.
- Join the 3 points.

SUPERIOR EXTENSOR RETINACULUM

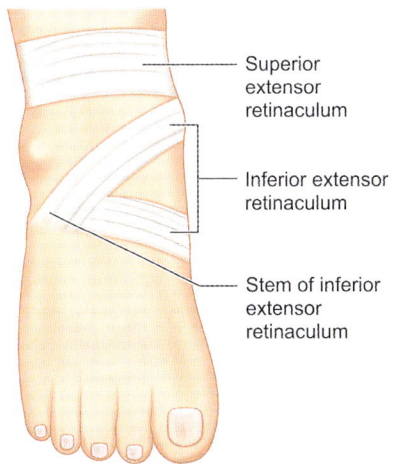

- Draw a 3 cm wide band, running medially and little upwards.
- From anterior border of triangular subcutaneous area of fibula.
- To lower part of anterior borders of tibia.

INFERIOR EXTENSOR RETINACULUM

- Draw a band passing medially on the dorsum of the foot.
- Band should be 1.5 cm wide and the band is the stem.
- Extend the band from anterior part of the upper surface of calcaneum to a point on the medial side of the tendons of extensor digitorum longus.
- At the second point, band divides into two limbs.
- Upper limb passes to medial malleolus.
- Lower limb passes round the medial aspect of foot.

FLEXOR RETINACULUM

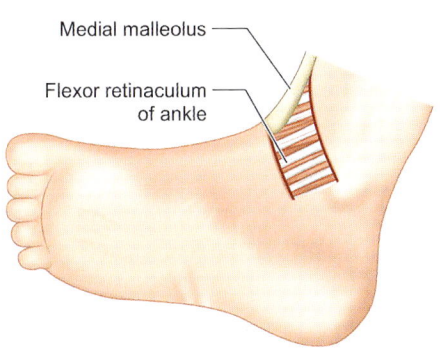

Draw a band 2.5 cm thick passing downwards and backwards from the medial malleolus to the medial side of the heel.

THORAX

■ HEART

Upper Border

- Mark a point at the lower border of the second left costal cartilage about 1.3 cm from sternal margin.
- Mark another point at the upper border of third right costal cartilage, 0.8 cm from sternal margin.
- Join these two points by a straight line to mark the upper border.

Lower Border

- Mark a point at the lower border of the sixth right costal cartilage 2 cm from the sternal margin.
- Mark another point in the fifth left intercostal space 9 cm from midsternal line (point represents apex of heart).
- Join these points by a straight line to mark the lower border.

Right Border

- Join the right ends of upper and lower borders.
- Line should be slightly convex to the right.
- Maximum convexity is marked 3.7 cm lateral to median plane in the right fourth intercostal space.

Left Border

Draw a line showing convexity towards left by joining the left ends of upper and lower borders of heart.

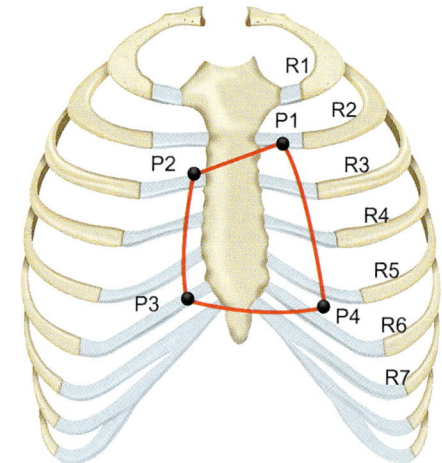

■ ARCH OF AORTA

- Mark the right extremity of the sternal angle.
- Mark the second point on the center of manubrium.
- Mark the third point at sternal extremity of second left costal cartilage.
- Draw a convex (directed upwards) line through these points.
- *Note:* The beginning and end of the arch lie at same level.

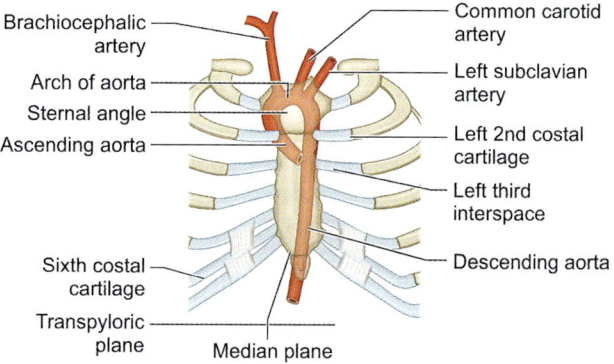

■ LUNGS

Apex

- Mark a point in the neck 2.5 cm above medial 1/3rd of clavicle.
- Draw a convex line directed upwards through this point.

Anterior Border

Right Lung

- *First point*: At the right sternoclavicular joint.
- *Second point*: At the midpoint of sternal angle.
- *Third point*: On the sixth right chondrosternal junction.
- Join these points to get anterior border of right lung.

Left Lung

- *First point*: At the left sternoclavicular joint.
- *Second point*: In the midpoint of the sternal angle.
- *Third point*: On the fourth left chondrosternal junction.

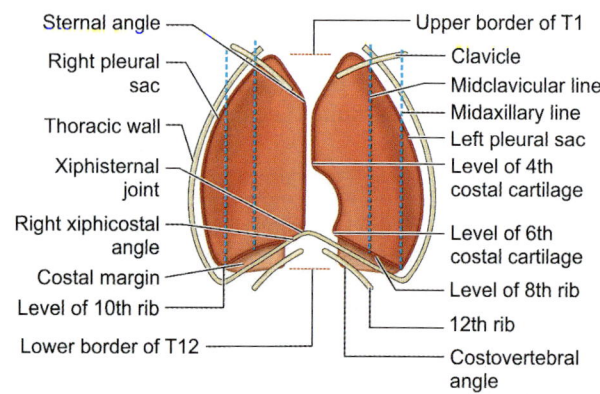

- *Fourth point*: On the sixth costal cartilage 3.5 cm from the left margin of sternum.
- Join these points to get a line representing anterior border of left lung.
- Line becomes concave (directed medially) between last two points, represents cardiac notch.

Posterior Border
- *First point*: 2 cm from midline at level of spinous process of tenth thoracic vertebrae.
- *Second point*: 2 cm lateral to second thoracic spine.
- Join these points by a vertical line to get the posterior border.

Inferior Border
- *First point*:
  - *Right lung*: Mark a point on sixth chondrosternal junction.
  - *Left lung*: Mark a point on sixth costal cartilage 2.5 cm from left margin of sternum.
- *Second point*: Where midclavicular line cuts with sixth rib.
- *Third point*: Where midaxillary line cuts the eight rib.
- *Fourth point*: 2 cm lateral to T10 spine.
- Join these points by a line which goes a little upwards posteriorly.

PLEURAL REFLECTION

Right Costomediastinal Reflection
- *First point*: At sternoclavicular joint.
- *Second point*: On the midpoint of sternal angle.
- *Third point*: At midpoint of xiphisternal joint.
- Draw a line joining these points.

Left Costomediastinal Reflection
- *First point*: At sternoclavicular joint.
- *Second point*: Midpoint of sternal angle.
- *Third point* in midline at the level of left fourth costal cartilage.
- *Fourth point*: At left extremity of xiphisternal joint.
- Draw a line by joining the first three points and extend it to the left sternal margin.
- Follow the margin to reach the fourth point.

Cervical Pleura
- *First point*: At sternoclavicular joint.
- *Second point*: On the junction of medial and middle third of clavicle.
- *Third point*: Between the above two points, about 2.5 cm above clavicle.
- Draw a line joining these points.

Costodiaphragmatic Reflection
- *First point*: Xiphisternal joint.
- *Second point*: Where the midclavicular line passes over 8th rib.
- *Third point*: Where midaxillary line passes over 10th rib.
- *Fourth point*: At the tip of 12th costal cartilage.
- *Fifth point*: 2 cm lateral to upper border of T12 spine.
- Draw a line joining these points.

ESOPHAGUS
- Mark two points 2.5 cm apart.
- First at the lower border of cricoid cartilage across median plane.
- Second in the root of the neck a little to the left of the median plane.
- Third at sternal angle across the median plane.
- Fourth on the left 7th costal cartilage 2.5 cm from the median plane.
- Esophagus is marked by two parallel lines formed by joining these points.

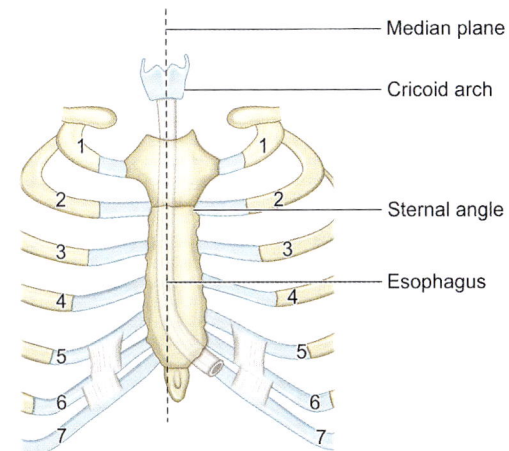

THORACIC DUCT

- Mark a point 2 cm above transpyloric plane and just 2 cm right of median plane.
- Mark midpoint of sternal angle (approx 5 cm below suprasternal notch).
- Mark another point 2 cm lateral to median plane and 2.5 cm above left clavicle.
- Mark a point 1.2 cm lateral to previous point. Join these points and end it behind clavicle.

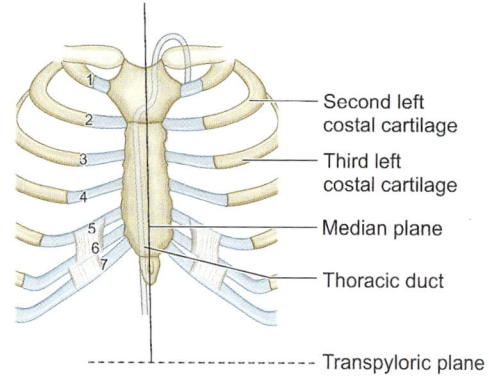

ABDOMEN AND PELVIS

ABDOMEN PLANES AND QUADRANTS

Median Vertical Plane

Plane passing through suprasternal notch and pubic symphysis.

Lateral Vertical Planes

- Plane passing midway between midinguinal point and middle of clavicle.
- There are left and right lateral vertical plane.

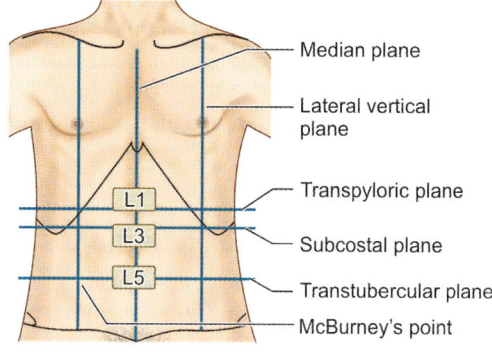

Transpyloric Plane of Addison

- Plane passing through the tip of 9th costal cartilage and midway between median vertical plane.
- Anteriorly, it passes through tip of 9th costal cartilage and posteriorly, it passes through lower part of body of L1 vertebra.
- Pylorus, inferior margin of liver, neck of gallbladder, anterior end of spleen, hilum of kidney, portal vein, etc., lie at this level.

Subcostal Plane

- Transverse plane passing just below 10th rib.
- Lies at the upper border of L3 vertebra.

Transtubercular Plane

- Transverse passing through the level of tubercle on iliac crest.
- Lies at the upper border of L5 vertebra.

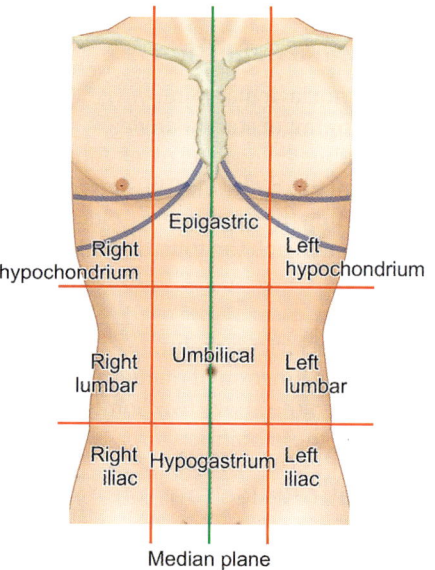

All these planes divide the abdomen into 9 quadrants.
1. Right hypochondriac region
2. Left hypochondriac region
3. Epigastric region
4. Right lumbar region
5. Left lumbar region
6. Umbilical region
7. Right iliac region
8. Left iliac region
9. Hypogastric region

INGUINAL CANAL

- *First point*: 1.25 cm above midpoint of the inguinal ligament, it corresponds to deep inguinal ring.
- *Second point*: Mark immediately above the pubic tubercle, it corresponds to superficial inguinal ring.

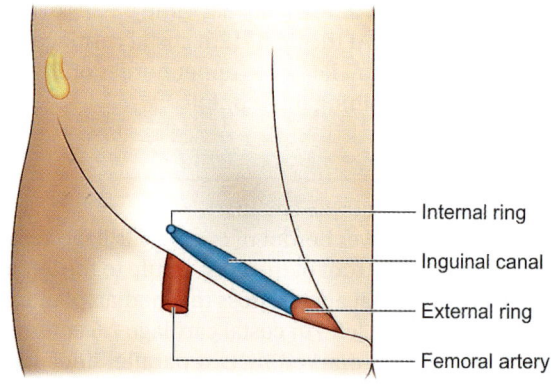

- Join these points by two parallel lines 1 cm apart and 3.7 cm long above the medial half of inguinal ligament to surface mark the inguinal canal.

STOMACH

Cardiac Orifice
- Draw the median vertical plane.
- Mark a point 2.5 cm to the left of median plane on the 7th costal cartilage.
- Draw a band 2 cm thick, from the above point inclining downwards to the left.

Pylorus
- Draw the transpyloric plane.
- Mark a point on the above plane 1.2 cm to the right of the median plane.
- Draw a band 2 cm thick, directed to upwards and right.

Fundus
- Mark a point at the left 5th intercostal space just below the nipple.
- Draw an upward convex line from the above point to the left margin of cardiac orifice.

Greater Curvature
- Draw the subcostal plane.
- Mark a point between the tips of left 9th and 10th costal cartilages.
- Draw a curved line convex to the left and downwards from fundus to above point which extends to the subcostal plane and lower margin of pylorus orifice.

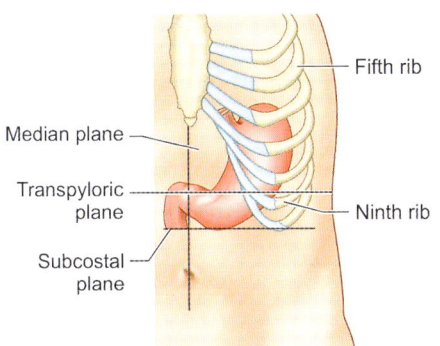

LIVER

Upper Border
- *First point*: In left 5th intercostal space 9 cm from median plane.
- *Second point*: At the xiphisternal joint.
- *Third point*: At 6th rib in midaxillary line.
- Join the first 2 points by a convex line and the 2nd and 3rd points by another convex line (both directed upwards and laterally).

Right Border
- *First point*: A little below right nipple.
- *Second point*: At 1 cm below the tip of right 10th costal cartilage.
- Draw a convex line (directed laterally) joining the above points.

Lower Border
- Draw median and transpyloric planes.
- Mark a point at the tip of right 9th costal cartilage.
- Join the lower end of the right border to left end of upper border by a line crossing the median plane at transpyloric plane.

FUNDUS OF GALLBLADDER

It is marked at the angle between right costal margin and outer border of rectus abdominis.

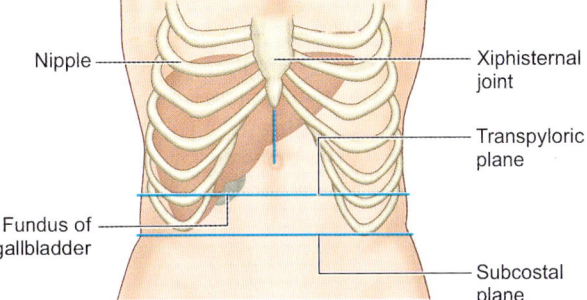

ABDOMINAL AORTA

- Mark a point 2.5 cm above transpyloric plane.
- Mark another point 1.2 cm below and left of umbilicus (at L4 vertebra level).
- Join these points by parallel lines 2 cm apart.

SPLEEN

- First point marked 4 cm lateral to spine of T10 vertebra, represents upper pole.
- Second point it is marked where the left 11th rib is crossed by the midaxillary line, represents lower pole.
- Join 2 points by 2 convex lines passing along the upper border of 9th (convexity directed upwards) and lower border of 11th rib (convexity directed downwards).
- Width of spleen corresponds to width of 9th and 10th intercostal spaces and width of 9th, 10th and 11th ribs.

ROOT OF MESENTERY

- Mark a point 1 cm below transpyloric plane and 3 cm to left of the median plane.
- Mark second point on the junction between right lateral and transtubercular plane.
- Join these two points by 2 parallel lines close together.

McBURNEY'S POINT

Point at the junction of lateral 1/3rd and medial 2/3rd of the line joining anterosuperior iliac spine and umbilicus.

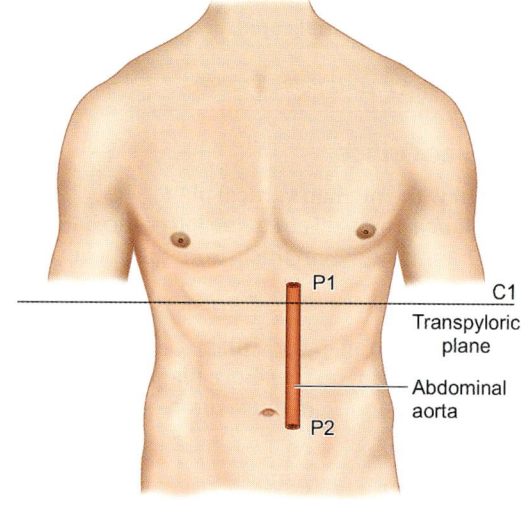

KIDNEY

On Back

Marked within Morris parallelogram drawn in following way:
- Two horizontal lines are drawn, one at level of the 11th thoracic spine and other at the level of 3rd lumbar spine.
- Then two vertical lines are drawn, one 2.5 cm and other 9 cm from median plane.
- Hilum lies opposite the lower border of 1st lumbar spine. Lower on right side.

On Front

- On right side the center of hilum lies 5 cm from median plane a little below the transpyloric plane.
- On left side it lies 5 cm from median plane a little above transpyloric plane, just medial to tip of 9th costal cartilage.
- Upper pole 4–5 cm from midline, midway between xiphisternum and transpyloric plane. Right one little lower.
- Lower pole lies 6–7 cm from the midline on right side at umbilical plane and on left side subcostal plane.

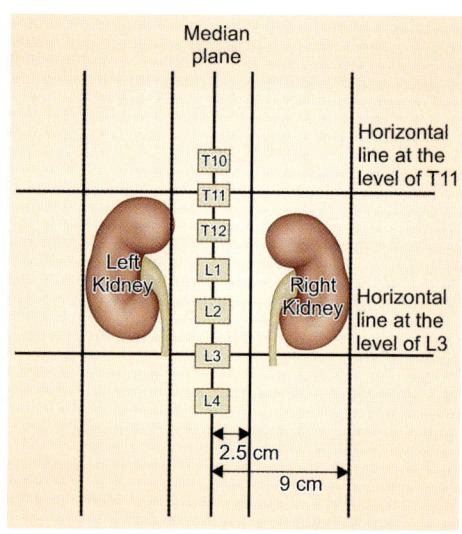

URETER

On Front

- Mark a point slightly medial to tip of 9th costal cartilage.
- Mark a point on pubic tubercle.
- Join these 2 points, the upper 5 cm represents renal pelvis.

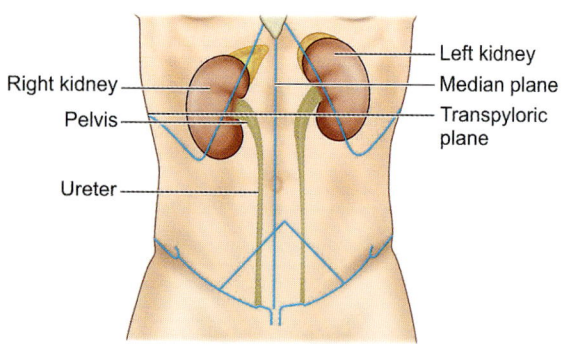

Surface Marking

On Back
- Mark a point 4 cm from median plane at the level of L2 vertebrae.
- Mark a point on posterosuperior iliac spine.
- Join these lines.

HEAD AND NECK

COMMON CAROTID ARTERY
- Mark the first point at sternoclavicular joint.
- Second point marked on the anterior border of the sternocleidomastoid at the level of upper border of thyroid cartilage.
- Join the points by a broad line along anterior border of sternocleidomastoid.

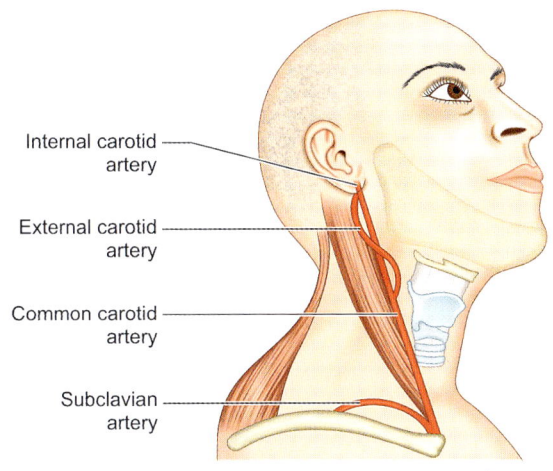

EXTERNAL CAROTID ARTERY
- Mark a point on the anterior border of sternocleidomastoid at the level of upper border of thyroid cartilage.
- Mark the second point on the posterior border of the neck of mandible.
- Join the points with a line which is convex forwards in lower half and concave forwards in upper half.

FACIAL ARTERY
- Mark a point on the base of mandible at the anterior border of the masseter muscle.
- Mark another point 1.5 cm lateral to angle of the mouth.
- Third point is given at the medial angle of the eye.
- Join these points.

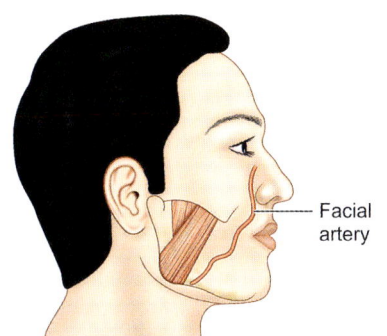

FACIAL VEIN
Represented by a line drawn just behind the facial artery.

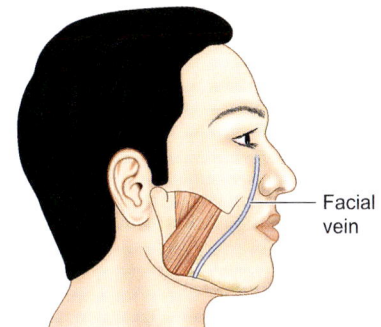

INTERNAL JUGULAR VEIN
- Mark a point on the neck medial to lobule of the ear.
- Mark the medial end of the clavicle.
- Join these points by a broad line to mark the internal jugular vein.

EXTERNAL JUGULAR VEIN
- Mark a point little below and behind the angle of mandible.
- Mark the next point on the clavicle lateral to posterior border of sternocleidomastoid.
- Join these points.

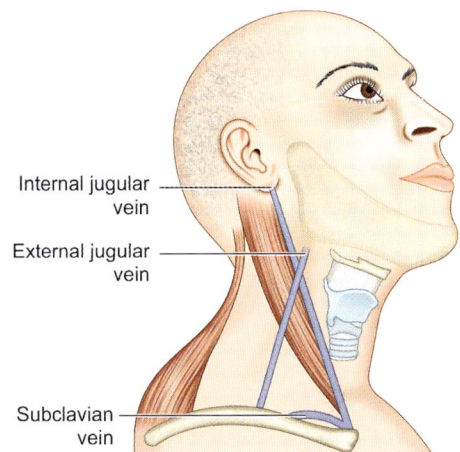

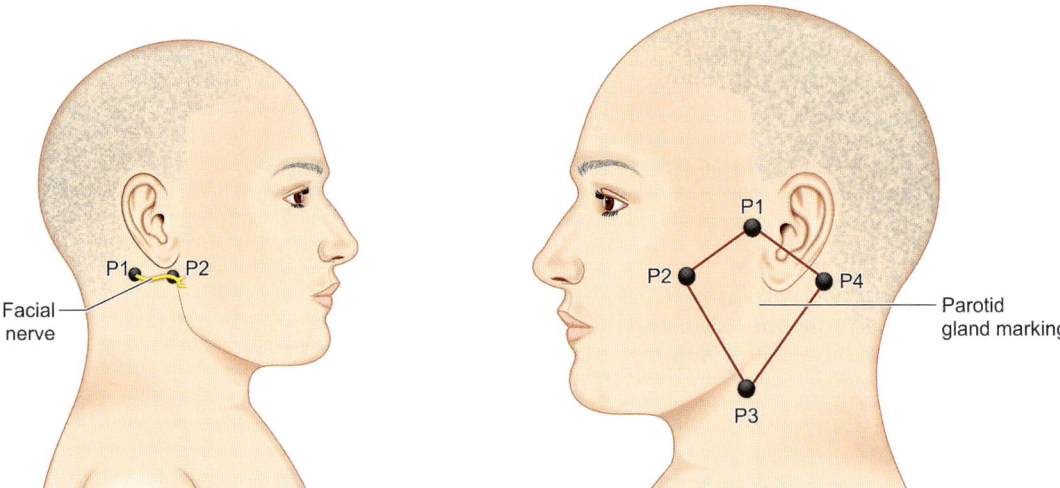

FACIAL NERVE

- Mark a point on the middle of the anterior border of the mastoid process.
- Second point given behind neck of mandible.
- Facial nerve is marked by a short horizontal line joining these two points.

PAROTID GLAND

- Point 1 is head of mandible in front of the tragus of the ear.
- Point 2 is center of masseter muscle.
- Point 3 is a point posteroinferior to angle of mandible.
- Point 4 is upper end of anterior margin of mastoid process.
- Anterior border is marked by joining points 1,2 and 3. Posterior border is marked by joining points 3 to 4. Upper surface/base is marked by joining 1 and 4.

PAROTID DUCT

- First point at the lower border of tragus.
- Second point it is marked midway between ala of nose and the red margin of the upper lip.
- Draw a line by joining these two points.
- Middle third of the line represents the parotid duct (see **Figure** below).

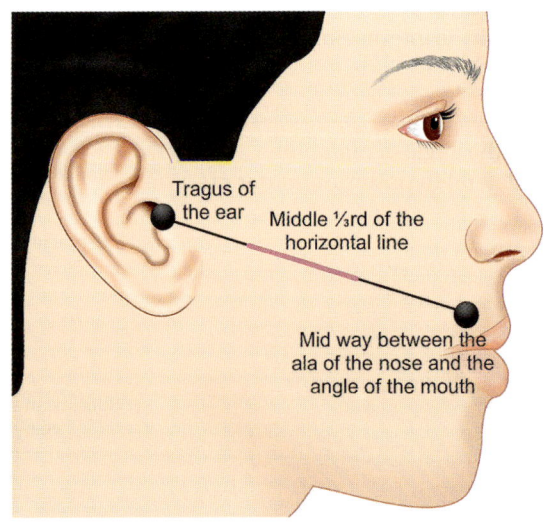

CHAPTER 6
Spotters and Discussion Topics

OUTLINE

- Spotters
- Discussion Topics

- Study the important attachments and side identification of the bones.
- For a nerve study the formation, root value, branches and supply.
- For an artery study the origin and main branches.
- For a vein study the formation, tributaries and termination.
- For a muscle study origin, insertion, nerve supply and actions.
- For every paired organ, study side identification and relevant applied anatomy.

SPOTTERS

UPPER LIMB

1. Anatomical snuff box
2. Articular capsule of shoulder joint
3. Cubital fossa
4. Palmar aponeurosis
5. Flexor retinaculum
6. Extensor retinaculum
7. Clavicle
8. Scapula
9. Humerus
10. Radius
11. Ulna
12. Carpal bones
13. Quadrangular and triangular spaces
14. Axillary nerve and artery
15. Musculocutaneous nerve
16. Radial nerve (in radial groove imp)
17. Median nerve
18. Ulnar nerve
19. Median cubital vein
20. Cephalic vein
21. Posterior interosseous artery and nerve
22. Anterior interosseous artery
23. Brachial artery
24. Dorsal venous arch
25. Radial artery and deep palmar arch
26. Ulnar artery and superficial palmar arch
27. Biceps brachii
28. Deltoid
29. Coracobrachialis
30. Brachialis
31. Brachioradialis
32. Triceps
33. Anconeus
34. Pronator teres
35. Supinator
36. Palmaris longus
37. Pronator quadratus
38. Interossei and lumbricals

LOWER LIMB

1. Hip bone (attachments on iliac crest)
2. Femur (attachments on linea aspera)
3. Tibia and fibula
4. Patella

5. Talus and calcaneum
6. Femoral artery
7. Profunda femoris artery
8. Obturator artery
9. Popliteal artery
10. Internal pudendal artery
11. Anterior tibial artery
12. Dorsalis pedis artery
13. Great saphenous vein
14. Femoral vein
15. Femoral nerve
16. Obturator nerve
17. Pudendal nerve and nerve to obturator internus
18. Tibial nerve
19. Sciatic nerve
20. Common peroneal nerve
21. Deep peroneal nerve
22. Iliotibial tract
23. Femoral sheath
24. Flexor, extensor and peroneal retinaculum
25. Tendocalcaneous
26. Plantar aponeurosis
27. Ligamentum patellae
28. Tibial and fibular collateral ligament
29. Cruciate ligaments and menisci of knee joint
30. Spring ligament
31. Adductor canal
32. Sartorius
33. Vastus medialis and lateralis
34. Adductor magnus
35. Gluteus maximus, medius and minimus
36. Piriformis
37. Peroneus longus and brevis
38. Plantaris
39. Popliteus
40. Tibialis posterior

THORAX

1. 1st rib
2. Typical and nontypical rib
3. Sternum
4. Thoracic vertebrae
5. Internal thoracic artery
6. Aorta
7. Subclavian artery
8. Coronary arteries
9. Azygos vein
10. Great cardiac vein
11. Superior vena cava
12. Coronary sinus
13. Thoracic duct
14. Recurrent laryngeal nerve
15. Phrenic nerve
16. Pulmonary ligament
17. Fossa ovalis
18. Ligamentum arteriosum
19. Atrioventricular valves

20. Interventricular septum
21. Pleura
22. Intercostal muscles (direction-fibers)
23. Root of lung
24. Sinuses of pericardium
25. Fissures of lung
26. Right atrium

ABDOMEN AND PELVIS

1. Superior mesenteric artery
2. Inferior mesenteric artery
3. Abdominal aorta
4. Common iliac artery
5. Internal iliac artery
6. Inferior vena cava
7. Portal vein
8. Obturator nerve
9. Rectus sheath and rectus abdominis
10. Inguinal canal
11. Ligaments of liver
12. Broad ligament
13. Epiploic foramen
14. Anterior abdominal wall muscles
15. Diaphragm (openings)
16. Greater omentum
17. Stomach
18. Duodenum (both papilla)
19. Pancreas (parts)
20. Liver (impressions, bare area)
21. Spleen (splenic ridge)
22. Gallbladder
23. Sigmoid colon
24. Appendix
25. Cecum
26. Kidney (structures at hilum)
27. Suprarenal gland
28. Ureters
29. Urinary bladder (trigone)
30. Testis (sinus)
31. Spermatic cord (contents)
32. Vas deferens
33. Prostate
34. Ovary
35. Fallopian tube
36. Psoas major
37. Hip bone (sex differences)

HEAD AND NECK

1. Parietal bone
2. Temporal bone
3. Frontal bone
4. Palatine bone
5. Occipital bone
6. Sphenoid bone
7. Atlas, axis
8. Mandible

9. Hyoid bone
10. Hard and soft palate
11. Styloid process
12. Mastoid process
13. Crista galli
14. Tentorium cerebelli
15. Falx cerebri
16. Foramen ovale
17. Styloid foramen, foramen spinosum
18. Jugular foramen
19. Hypoglossal canal
20. Frontal air sinuses
21. Constrictors of pharynx
22. Facial artery
23. Basilar artery
24. Vertebral artery
25. External carotid artery
26. Middle meningeal artery
27. Maxillary artery
28. Greater palatine artery
29. Jugular vein
30. Internal and external jugular vein
31. Cranial nerves
32. Facial nerve
33. Glossopharyngeal nerve
34. Hypoglossal nerve
35. Greater auricular nerve
36. Vagus
37. Spinal root of accessory nerve
38. Ansa cervicalis
39. Vocal folds
40. Conchae and meatuses
41. Temporalis muscle
42. Masseter
43. Buccinator
44. Sternocleidomastoid
45. Scalenus anterior
46. Posterior belly of digastric
47. Posterior cricoarytenoid
48. Cricothyroid
49. Genioglossus
50. Hyoglossus
51. Stylohyoid
52. Mylohyoid
53. Extraocular muscles
54. Auditory tube
55. Infrahyoid membrane
56. Internal acoustic meatus
57. Maxillary sinus
58. Superior sagittal sinus
59. Nasal septum
60. Submandibular gland and duct
61. Parotid gland and duct

BRAIN

1. Dura mater
2. Superior colliculus
3. Cerebral peduncle
4. Cerebral aqueduct
5. Flocculus and lingula of cerebellum
6. Horizontal fissure of cerebellum
7. Corpus callosum
8. Fornix
9. Anterior commissure
10. Mammillary body
11. Optic chiasma
12. Interthalamic adhesion
13. Lateral ventricle
14. Fourth ventricle
15. Internal capsule
16. Caudate and lentiform nuclei

DISCUSSION TOPICS

DISCUSSION TOPICS

1. Arm, forearm—flexor and extensor compartment
2. Triangular and quadrangular spaces
3. Cubital and popliteal fossa
4. Palm and sole
5. Femoral triangle and adductor canal, knee joint
6. Structures under cover of gluteus maximus
7. Thigh and leg (all compartments)
8. Lungs (root, pleura, bronchopulmonary segments)
9. Heart (blood supply, chambers)
10. Diaphragm (openings)
11. Stomach, liver, spleen, pancreas, kidney
12. Small and large intestine, appendix, anal canal
13. Testis, uterus, urinary bladder
14. Midline structures of neck, thyroid gland
15. Lateral and medial wall of nose, pharynx
16. Parotid gland, palate
17. Surfaces of the brain, brainstem

CHAPTER 7

Red Alert

OUTLINE

- Anatomy Examination Paper 1—Important Topics
- Anatomy Examination Paper 2—Important Topics
- Important Diagrams

Red Alert

This chapter includes the must study questions in anatomy before facing the final exams in order to ensure minimum pass marks.

ANATOMY EXAMINATION PAPER 1—IMPORTANT TOPICS

UPPER LIMB

1. Breast—extent, blood supply and lymphatic drainage, applied—carcinoma and metastasis, peau d'orange, etc.
2. Brachial plexus (Erb's and Klumpke's paralysis*)
3. Clavipectoral fascia
4. Axillary artery and its branches, brachial artery and branches
5. Shoulder joint (muscles producing movements*)
6. Rotator cuff
7. Intermuscular spaces (quadrangular and triangular)
8. Deltoid muscle and its applied anatomy
9. Radial and musculocutaneous nerve
10. Cubital fossa
11. Superior radioulnar joint
12. Flexor retinaculum
13. Superficial and deep palmar arches
14. Midpalmar and pulp space
15. First carpometacarpal joint
16. Axillary lymph nodes
17. Cutaneous supply of upper limb and dermatomes
18. Root value of each nerves
19. Superficial veins of upper limb
20. Intrinsic muscles of hand, nerve supply and actions
21. Axillary nerve injury
22. Carpal tunnel syndrome and Ape thumb deformity
23. Wrist drop
24. Claw hand
25. Boxers palsy
26. Tennis elbow, Golfer's elbow, and student's elbow

LOWER LIMB

1. Superficial inguinal lymph nodes
2. Femoral triangle, boundaries, contents, etc.
3. Femoral sheath
4. Great saphenous vein
5. Fascia lata, its modifications (iliotibial tract*)
6. Adductor canal/subsartorial canal/Hunter's canal
7. Popliteal fossa—boundaries, contents, popliteal aneurysm
8. Sciatic nerve
9. Structures under cover of gluteus maximus
10. Dorsalis pedis artery
11. Venous drainage of lower limb and clinical importance
12. Hip joints (relations, movements, ligaments*)
13. Knee joint (medial and lateral ligament, menisci, relations, blood supply, locking and unlocking*)
14. Muscles producing movements at the knee joint
15. Subtalar joint
16. Arches of foot (medial long arch*)
17. Inversion and eversion
18. Cutaneous supply of foot
19. Root values of all nerves

Red Alert

THORAX
1. Typical intercostal spaces—muscles, nerves and blood supply
2. Lungs—bronchopulmonary segments, blood supply and lymphatic drainage
3. Root of lung
4. Pleura and its recess
5. Sinuses of pericardium
6. Posterior mediastinum
7. Right atrium
8. Blood supply of hearts and cardiac dominance
9. Coronary sinus
10. Cardiac plexus
11. Azygos vein and hemiazygos vein
12. Openings of diaphragm
13. Arch of aorta and its development
14. Esophagus and its constrictions
15. Thoracic duct

GENERAL HISTOLOGY
1. All 3 cartilages.
2. Compact bone (LS and TS)
3. Skeletal muscle
4. Smooth muscle
5. Cardiac muscle
6. Artery (large and medium sized)
7. Vein (large and medium sized)
8. Lymph node
9. Spleen
10. Thymus
11. Palatine tonsil
12. Spinal ganglion
13. Sympathetic ganglion
14. Thick and thin skin

GENERAL EMBRYOLOGY
1. Implantation
2. Fertilization
3. Decidua
4. Yolk sac
5. Chorion
6. Amnion
7. Primitive streak
8. Intraembryonic mesoderm
9. Somites
10. Notochord
11. Neurulation
12. Neural crest
13. Placenta
14. Amniocentesis
15. Structure of spermatozoa
16. Derivatives of foregut, midgut, hindgut

GENERAL ANATOMY
1. Classification and examples of joints
2. Long bone—blood supply
3. Cartilage (hyaline cartilage*)

4. Connective tissue fibers and cells
5. Epiphysis
6. Dermatomes
7. Neuroglia

ANATOMY EXAMINATION PAPER 2— IMPORTANT TOPICS

HEAD AND NECK

1. Scalp
2. Face—nerve (motor and sensory) and blood supply (dangerous area of face*)
3. Lacrimal apparatus
4. Carotid sheath
5. Sternocleidomastoid
6. Trigeminal ganglion
7. Lymph nodes of neck
8. Deep cervical fascia
9. Posterior triangle of neck
10. Thyroid gland (blood supply*) and its development
11. Submandibular gland and its secretomotor pathway
12. Parotid gland (secretomotor pathway and parotid duct)
13. Temporomandibular joint
14. Cavernous sinus
15. Palatine tonsil
16. Lateral wall of nose (arterial and nerve supply)
17. Nasal septum—formation, arterial and nerve supply, little's area
18. Tongue (development and nerve supply*)
19. Middle ear (medial wall*)
20. Extraocular muscles
21. Pharynx—boundaries, constrictors, Killian's dehiscence
22. Relations of hyoglossus
23. Muscles of mastication (lateral pterygoid*)
24. Carotid triangle
25. Tentorium cerebelli
26. Ciliary ganglion
27. Pterygopalatine ganglion
28. Mandibular nerve
29. Palate development
30. Maxillary artery
31. Auditory tube
32. Tympanic membrane
33. Classification of dural venous sinuses
34. Hiatus semilunaris openings
35. Structures passing through superior orbital fissure, foramen ovale, carotid canal, jugular foramen

NEUROANATOMY

1. Cerebellum—subdivisions and fissures*
2. Brain—sulcus, gyrus and functional areas
3. Third ventricle
4. Interpeduncular fossa
5. Insula
6. Superior colliculus
7. Superolateral surface of brain
8. Spinal cord (blood supply*)
9. Circle of Willis

Red Alert

10. Corpus callosum
11. Internal capsule and its blood supply
12. Functional areas of brain
13. Lateral ventricle
14. Floor of fourth ventricle
15. Lateral geniculate body
16. Association fibers of cerebrum
17. Cerebellar peduncles
18. Blood supply of superolateral surface of brain
19. Crus cerebri
20. Red nucleus
21. Choroid plexus
22. Dural folds
23. Basal ganglia

ABDOMEN AND PELVIS

1. Rectus sheath
2. Inguinal canal and inguinal hernia
3. Cryptorchidism
4. Stomach—bed, lymphatic drainage and blood supply
5. Duodenum—parts (2nd*) relations and blood supply
6. Portal vein and portocaval anastomoses
7. Pancreas and its development
8. Extrahepatic biliary apparatus
9. Liver and its development (hepatic segments and relations of inferior surface*)
10. Greater omentum
11. Greater and lesser sac
12. Mesentery
13. Kidney—coverings, Morri's parallelogram, position, relations (posterior*)
14. Spleen—surfaces, relations and blood supply
15. Vermiform appendix (positions*)
16. Cecum
17. Superior mesenteric artery
18. Meckel's diverticulum
19. Urinary bladder and its development (trigone of bladder*)
20. Uterus—parts, supports (true) and development
21. Prostate and its development
22. Urethra (male urethra—parts) and development
23. Perineal body
24. Ischiorectal fossa—boundaries and contents
25. Superficial and deep perineal pouches
26. Rectum and anal canal
27. Murphy's sign, Courvoisier's sign
29. Coverings of testis

HISTOLOGY

1. Stomach (fundus and pylorus)
2. Colon
3. Appendix
4. Ileum
5. Jejunum
6. Duodenum
7. Liver
8. Pancreas
9. Gallbladder

10. Kidney
11. Urinary bladder
12. Trachea
13. Ovary
14. Uterus
15. Testis
16. Epididymis
17. Prostate gland
18. Cerebellum
19. Cerebrum
20. Spinal cord
21. Cornea
22. Retina
23. Suprarenal gland
24. Thyroid gland
25. Pituitary gland

SYSTEMIC EMBRYOLOGY

Thorax

1. Heart tube formation
2. Right atrium
3. Interatrial septum
4. Aortic arches
5. Fallot's tetralogy
6. Diaphragm

Head and Neck

1. Pharyngeal arches
2. Palate and cleft palate
3. Face
4. Upper lip
5. Tongue
6. Thyroid
7. Diencephalon derivatives

Abdomen and Pelvis

1. Derivatives of foregut, midgut and hindgut
2. Stomach
3. Meckel's diverticulum
4. Pancreas
5. Liver and gallbladder
6. Kidney
7. Urinary bladder
8. Uterus
9. Testis and descent of testis
10. Rectum and anal canal
11. Prostate
12. Development of 2nd part of duodenum

---

* is meant for giving a clue that the given part in brackets is important among the other topics coming under the main topic.

IMPORTANT DIAGRAMS

Please draw at least one diagram and try to write two applied anatomy along with each question:

UPPER LIMB

1. Axillary lymph nodes
2. Branches of axillary artery
3. Clavipectoral fascia
4. Transverse section of arm through middle
5. Sagittal section through shoulder joint
6. Brachial plexus
7. Rotator cuff
8. Superficial veins of upper limb
9. Superficial and deep palmar arches
10. Cutaneous supply of upper limb, especially hand

THORAX

11. Typical intercostal nerve
12. Mediastinal surface of right and left lungs
13. Azygous and hemiazygous veins
14. Pleural recesses
15. Root of right and left lungs
16. Bronchopulmonary segments (costal aspects and distal portion of adjacent segments)
17. Transverse section through body at the level of T4 vertebra
18. Sinuses of pericardium
19. Blood supply of heart

LOWER LIMB

20. Transverse section of upper one-third of thigh
21. Cutaneous supply of lower limb
22. Femoral triangle
23. Structures under cover of gluteus maximus
24. Hip joint
25. Transverse section of leg
26. Knee joint (tibial and fibular collateral ligaments)
27. Transverse section through knee joint showing relations
28. Popliteal fossa
29. Long and short saphenous vein
30. Extensor retinaculum
31. Arches of foot

ABDOMEN AND PELVIS

32. Boundaries of inguinal canal
33. Sagittal section through abdomen to show reflections of peritoneum
34. Stomach bed
35. Relations of 1st, 2nd, and 3rd part of duodenum
36. Inferior surface of liver and impressions
37. Tributaries of portal vein
38. Relations of pancreas
39. Anterior and posterior relations of kidney
40. Relations of cecum
41. Positions of appendix
42. Coronal section through ischiorectal fossa
43. Sagittal section through male and female pelvis

44. Anterior view of male urethra
45. Superior view of pelvic diaphragm
46. Prostate gland
47. Coronal section through anal canal

HEAD AND NECK

48. Sensory nerve supply of face
49. Layers of scalp
50. Arterial and nerve supply of scalp
51. Lacrimal apparatus
52. Carotid sheath
53. Posterior triangle of neck with contents
54. Tentorium cerebelli
55. Cavernous sinus
56. Veins of face and communications
57. Orbit with extraocular muscles
58. Carotid triangle with contents
59. Ansa cervicalis
60. Parotid gland and relations
61. Relations of hyoglossus muscle
62. Medial wall of middle ear
63. Distribution of mandibular nerve
64. Temporomandibular joint
65. Blood supply of thyroid gland
66. Styloid apparatus
67. Palatine tonsil, blood supply and relations
68. Waldeyer's ring
69. Blood supply, nerve supply of nasal septum
70. Blood supply lateral wall of nose
71. Coronal section through larynx
72. Movements of vocal cord
73. Nerve supply of tongue
74. Transverse section of medulla, pons and midbrain
75. Sulci and gyri of superolateral and medial surface of brain
76. Lateral ventricle
77. Floor of fourth ventricle
78. Blood supply of superolateral surface of brain
79. Corpus callosum
80. Functional areas of brain
81. Cerebellum—lobes and morphological subdivisions
82. Blood supply of spinal cord
83. Circle of Willis

Index

Page numbers followed by *f* refer to figure.

A

A band 23
Abdomen 163, 210, 218
    planes 210
    quadrants 210
Abundant intercellular stroma 12
Acid
    fuchsin 2
    gastric 64
    nucleic 2
Acidic properties 2
Adenohypophysis 124
Adenomyosis 107
Adrenaline 120
Adult's skeleton 178
Adventitia 59, 80, 83, 87
Air 156
Airway 155
Albuginea 147
Alimentary system 59
Amniocentesis 147
Amnion 111
Amyloid bodies 119
Anal canal 147
Anastomosis, branching 27
Angina pectoris 27
Angiogram 158
Ankle, anteroposterior view 167
Ankyloglossia 141
Anomalies 137, 139*f*, 140
Anti-Mullerian hormone 112
Antrum folliculi 103
Aorta 28
    abdominal 212
    arch of 138, 208
Aortocaval compression syndrome 32
Appendices epiploicae 71
Appendix 72, 73
Arachnoid mater 99
Arch
    arterial 138
    fourth 138
    second 138
    third 138
Arm 2
    anteroposterior view 160
Arterial system 28
Arterioles 28
Arteriosclerosis 31
Artery 28
    axillary 204
    brachial 31, 204
    central 99
    dorsalis pedis 206
    elastic 28
    facial 213
    femoral 206
    hepatic 75
    large 28, 29
    medium-sized 28, 30, 31
    popliteal 206
    radial 31, 204
    subclavian 28
    ulnar 31, 204
    umbilical 111
Atlas
    inferior view 197
    superior view 197
Atretic follicles 103
Atrial septal defect 150
Auditory canal, external 15
Auditory ossilcles 178
Auerbach's plexus 59
Autonomic nervous system 28
Autorhythmicity 27
Axillary nerve 204
Axis
    anterior view 198
    posterior view 198
Axon 44
    cylinder 45

B

B lymphocyte
    proliferation, sites of 36
    smaller mature 36
Bacteria 39
Barium
    enema 156, 157, 172
    meal 156, 157, 171, 172
    studies 156
    swallow 156, 171
Barr body 149
Barret esophagus 63
Bile canaliculi 75
Billroth cords 40
Binucleate 48
    muscle fibers 27
Blastocyst 134*f*
Blastopore 136
Blood vessels 4, 28, 47, 63, 67, 79
    tunica media of 24
Body cavities 4
Bone 19, 155, 178
    age and sex determination with 179
    compact 18, 21
    coverings of 19
    cyst, aneurysmal 20
    depressions and openings 178
    long 178
    longitudinal section 20
    markings on 178
    marrow, inflammation of 20
    matrix 19
    parts of 178
    projections and parts 178
    transverse section 19
Bowman's capsule 84
    parietal layer of 4
Bowman's glomerulus 84
Bowman's membrane 95
Brain 220
    computerized tomographic scan 174
    MRI scan 175
Bronchial glands 83
Bronchioalveolar carcinoma 83
Bronchiole 83
Brunner's gland 64, 65, 67
Brush bordered appearance 84
Buccopharyngeal membrane 138

C

Calcitonin 123
Canaliculi 19, 20
Carbohydrates 11
Cardiac muscle 26, 27
    fibers 27
Cardiac silhouette 155
Carotid artery
    common 28, 213
    external 213
Cartilage 11
    chondrocytes 12
    matrix, alternating layers of 16
Cell
    absorptive 64
    adipose 47, 51, 55, 63
    alpha 79
    beta 79
    betz 131
    blood 144
    bone consists of 19
    cartilage consists of 11
    chief 60, 123
    chondroblast 11
    chromaffin 120
    chromophil 124
    chromophobe 124
    delta 79
    dust 83
    endocrine 60

Index

enterochromaffin 64
enteroendocrine 63, 64
ependymal 127
follicular 123
fusiform 131
glial 44
interstitial 112
Leydig 112
macrophagic 75
mass, intermediate 135
oxyntic 60
oxyphil 123
parietal 60
satellite 44, 47-49
small basal 115
stellate 128, 131
stem 60, 64
trophoblast 108
types of 146
undifferentiated 60
Cement line 19
Central axon 44
Central canal 19, 20
Central nervous system 44, 47, 127
Central nucleus 47
Cerebellar folia 128
Cerebellum 128, 129
Cerebrum 130, 131
Cervical pleura 209
Cervical vertebrae
   anterior view 199
   posterolateral oblique view 199
   superior view 199
Chest
   broad 150
   lateral view 163
   posteroanterior view 163
   radiograph 155
      anteroposterior 155
      lateral 155
Cholangiopancreatogram, endoscopic retrograde 157
Cholelithiasis 76
Chondrocytes 11, 12, 15-17, 80
   cell nests of 13
Chondromas 12
Choriocarcinoma 108
Chorion 135
   epithelioma 137
   frondosum 137
Chorionic plate 108
Chorionic villi 108
   formation 137f
   primary 137
Chromosome
   banding 149
   groups of 150f
Cilia 7
   spermatozoa 7
Ciliated columnar
   cells 104
   epithelium 6
Clark's column 127
Clavicle 155
   inferior view 185
   superior view 185
Cleft palate 139
Coelomic epithelium 146

Collagen 2, 11
   bundles 17
   fibers 12, 16, 19
Colles' fracture 179
Colon 70, 71
Columnar epithelium 67
   stratified 8
Computed tomography 158
Concave mirror 2
Concentric lamellae 20
   layers of 19
Connective tissue 23, 47, 100, 112
   capsule 47, 48
      consist of 36
   cells 64, 71
   fibers 71, 80
   interstitial 112
   layer of 19, 44
   septa, interlobular 55, 79
   subendothelial 28, 32
Contractile myoepithelial cells 51, 52
Conus 142
Cornea 94, 95
Corneal endothelium 95
Corneal epithelium 95
Corneal stroma 95
Corpus
   albicans 103
   luteum 103
Cortex 36, 84, 103, 128
   outer 36
      dark 84
Costal cartilages 12
Costodiaphragmatic reflection 209
Costomediastinal reflection
   left 209
   right 209
Cranial cavity, floor of 182, 183
Crypts 39, 76
Cubital vein, median 32, 35
Cubitus valgus 150
Cuboidal epithelium 100, 103
   stratified 8
Cumulus oophorus 103
Cystogram 157
Cytoplasm 2, 91

D

Decidua 135, 135f
   basalis 108, 135, 137
   capsularis 135
   parietalis 135
   reaction 135
Deep palmar arch 206
Deep reticular layer 91
Deep stratum basalis 107
Dehydration 2
Dense connective tissue 19
   capsule 40, 51
Dense foreign bodies 154
Dermatome 136
Dermis 91
Descemet's membrane 95
Desmosomes 91
Diaphragm 143, 155
Didelphys uterus 145
DiGeorge syndrome 43

Discs, intercalated 26, 27
Distal convoluted tubule 84
Doppler studies 159
Down syndrome 151
Duct
   alveolar 83
   bile 75
   carcinomas 100
   intercalated 51, 55
   interlobular 50, 51, 53, 79
   lobar 50
   paramesonephric 145
   parotid 214
   striated 51
   system 55
   thoracic 210
Ductus epididymis 115
Duodenal ulcer 67
Duodenum 64, 65, 67
Dura mater 99

E

Ectoderm 138
Ectopia vesicae 145
Ectopic pregnancy 134
Elastic cartilage 11, 14, 15
Elastic fibers 28, 76
Elastic lamina
   external 28
   internal 28, 32
Elastic membrane, longitudinal 80
Elbow
   anteroposterior view 161
   lateral view 161
Embryogenesis 134
Embryology 133
   general 134
Embryonic development 148f
Embryonic disc 135
Embryonic germ layers 135f
Empyema 76
Enamel 154
Endochondral ossification 20
Endocrine
   part 79
   system 120
Endoderm 138
Endometrium 107
   decidua basalis of 108
Endomysium 23
Endosteum 19
Endothelium 4, 135
   consisting of 32
Enterocytes 64
Eosin 2
Epidermis 91, 92
Epididymis 114, 115
Epimysium 23
Epinephrine 120
Epiphyseal plate 12
   growth hormone 20
Epiphyses 179
Epithelia 3
Epithelial cells 3, 7, 79
   general functions of 3
   simple columnar 71
   surface specializations of 7

Index

Epithelial tissue 3
Epithelium 3, 4
    anterior 95
    lines, types of 68
    simple 3
    stratified 3, 8, 100
    surface 60
Esophageal adenocarcinoma 63
Esophagus 8, 58, 59, 143, 209
Extensor retinaculum 205
    inferior 207
    superior 207
Extracellular matrix 11, 19
Extrauterine implantation 134
Eye piece lense 2

F

Face 140
    development of 140f
Fallopian tube 7, 104, 105
Fallot's tetralogy 143
Fasciculus 23
F-cells 79
Femur 192
Fibers
    branching 26
    extracellular matrix consists of 11
Fibroblasts 100
Fibrocartilage 11, 16, 17
Fibrocytes 11
Fibromuscular stroma 119
Fibrous layer 19
    outer 11
Fibula 193
Filiform 56
    papillae 56
Film, type of 155
Finger-shaped villi 69
Flagella 7
Flattened cells, single layer of 4
Flattened dead cells, homogenous glassy layer of 91
Flexor retinaculum 205, 207
Focusing knobs 2
Foliate papillae 56
Folium 128
Follicles 123
Foot
    lateral view 168, 194
    medial view 194
    oblique view 168
Foramen
    ovale 142
    primum 142
    secondum 142
Foramina, structures passing through 182, 183
Forearm, anteroposterior view 162
Foregut derivatives 143
Fragility fracture 179
Free air 155
Frontonasal process 140
Fungiform 56
    papillae 56
Fusion, steps of 139, 140

G

Gallbladder 7, 76, 77, 144
    fundus of 211
Ganglioglioma 131
Ganglion cell
    layer 96
    parasympathetic 71
Gap junction 24
    complex 27
Gas bubble 155
Gastric glands 60, 63
Gastric leiomyosarcoma 63
Gastric pits 60, 63
Gastroesophageal reflux disease 63
Gastrointestinal tract 58
    wall of 59
Genetics 149
Germ cells, primordial 146
Germ layers 135
Germinal centers 36, 39
Germinal epithelium 103
    roots 112
Giannuzzi demilunes 55
Gland 123
    adrenal 120, 121
    lactating 100
    mammary 100, 101
    mucous 81
    nonlactating 100
    parathyroid 123
    parotid 51, 214
    prostate 118, 119
    serous 81
        salivary 50, 51
    small ducts of 4
    sublingual 52
    submandibular 55
Glandular tissue 100
    less 100
Glenoid labrum 16
Glomerulus 84
Glucocorticoids 120
Glycosaminoglycans 19
Goblet cells 6, 64, 70, 80
    depletion 71
    lie 67
Gonads, development of 146, 146f
Graafian follicle 103
Gubernaculum 147
Gut 143

H

Hair
    follicles 91
    line, low 150
Hand, dorsal view 189
Hangman's fracture 179
Hard palate 139
Hassall's corpuscle 42, 43
Haversian system 18-21
Head and neck 169, 213, 218
Heart 208
    border
        left 208
        lower 208
        right 208
        upper 208
        edges of 156
    tube 142, 142f
Heat rigor 23
Hematoxylin 2
Henle, loop 84
Hepatic lobules 75
Hepatic sinusoids 75
Hepatocytes, radiating plates of 75
Herring bodies 124
Hila 155
Hindgut derivatives 143
Hip bone
    lateral view 191
    medial view 190
Hour glass bladder 145
Humerus 155, 187
Hyaline cartilage 11-13, 80, 83
    C shaped 80
Hyaline cartilaginous plates 81
Hydroxyapatite crystals 19
Hyoid arch 138
Hypobranchial eminence 141
Hysterosalpingography 158, 173

I

I band 23
Ileum 64, 68, 69
Imaging modalities 154, 174
Imaging modalities
    with ionizing radiations 154
    with nonionizing radiations 159
Immunoglobulins, subepithelial deposit of 84
Implantation 134, 134f
Infundibulum 124
Inguinal canal 210
Inguinal ligament, midpoint of 206
Inorganic compounds, matrix consists of 19
Instrumentation 156
Integumentary system 91
Interatrial septum 142
    development of 142f
Interstitial growth 11
Interstitial implantation 134
Interstitial lamellae 19
Interterritorial matrix 12, 13
Intervertebral discs 16
Intervillous spaces 137
Intestinal atresia 67
Intestinal crypts 66
Intestinal gas 159
Intestinal glands 64
Intraembryonic mesoderm 135
Intramembranous ossification 20
Intrapulmonary bronchus 83
Intrauterine implantation, abnormal 134
Intravenous
    pyelogram 173
    pyelography 157, 158
Iodine studies 157
    types 157

J

Jaundice 76
Jejunum 64, 66, 67

Index

Jugular vein
    external 213
    internal 213

K

Karyotyping 149
Keratin 91
Keratinized sites 8
Keratocytes 94
Kidney 84, 85, 144, 212
    development of 145f
Klinefelter syndrome 150
Knee
    anteroposterior view 166
    lateral view 166
Kupffer's cells 75, 144

L

Lacunae 19, 20
Lamellae 19
    circumferential 19
    external circumferential 19
    internal circumferential 19
Lamina propria 59, 60, 63, 64, 67, 68, 71, 72, 80, 83, 88, 87, 107, 116
    projections of 64
Lamina terminalis 137
Langerhans islets 78, 79
Leg, anteroposterior view 167
Leiomyoma 107
Leiomyosarcomas 24
Lense, objective 2
Lieberkuhn crypts 64, 72
Light microscope 2
Light source 2
Limiting membrane
    internal 96
    posterior 95
Lingual glands, posterior 56
Lingual swellings 141
Liver 74, 75, 144, 211
    cirrhosis 40
    development of 144f
    border
        lower 211
        right 211
        upper 211
Lobules 112
Loose connective tissue 76
    tunica adventitia consists of 35
Lower limb 165, 206, 216
Lumbar vertebrae
    anteroposterior view 164
    lateral view 201
    posterior view 201
    superior view 201
Lumen 35, 100
    congenital absence of 67
    narrowing of 67
Lung 82, 83, 141, 154, 208
    anterior border 208
    apex 208
    disease, interstitial 83
    fields of 155
    inferior border 209
    posterior border 209
Lymph node 36, 37
Lymphatic cells 64
    aggregations of 71
    lamina propria consists of 67
Lymphatic nodule 37, 71, 72
    occasional 63
Lymphatic tissue 80
Lymphocyte 100
Lymphocytic lymphoma, chronic 36
Lymphoid
    infiltrates 51
    nodule, subepithelial 38
Lymphoreticular system 36

M

Macrophages 64, 67, 83
Macrostomia 140
Magnetic resonance imaging 159
Malpighian corpuscles 40
Mandible
    anterior view 184
    lateral view 184
    posterior view 184
Mandibular arch 138
March fracture 179
Martinotti cells 131
Mastication, muscles of 138
Matrix 12, 15
McBurney's point 212
M-cells 64
Meckel's cartilage 138
Meckel's diverticulum 144, 144f
Median nerve 204
    arm 204
    forearm 204
Medulla 36, 43, 120
    inner lighter 84
    lighter staining inner 43
Medullary cords 37, 146
Medullary sinus 36
Meissner's nerve plexus 59, 60
Membrana granulosa 103
Merkel cells 91
Mesoderm 23, 138
    intermediate 146
Mesothelium 4, 59
Metaplastic columnar epithelium 63
Methylene blue 2
Microscope 2
    parts of 2
Microvillus 7
Midgut derivatives 143
Mineralocorticoids 120
Mitochondria 2
Molecular layer, external 128
Molecules
    diffusion of 4
    filtration of 4
Mood swings 48
Mossy fibers 128
Motile structures 7
Mucocele 76
Mucosa 59, 64, 104, 107, 116
    consist of 76
    folds 76
Mucous acini 52, 53, 55
Mucous filled goblet cells, number of 71
Mucous neck cells 60
Mucous salivary gland 52, 53
Müllerian ducts 145
Multipolar cells, small 131
Muscle 23
    cells, multinucleated 23
    coat 87, 88, 104, 107
    fibers, cylindrical 22
    involuntary 24, 27
    striated 138
    trachealis 80
    voluntary 23
Muscular arteries 31
Muscular patches 32
Muscularis 76
    externa 59, 60, 63, 64, 67, 68, 71, 72
    interna 76
    mucosa 59, 60, 64, 68, 71, 72, 76
Musculocutaneous nerve 205
Myelin sheath 44
Myenteric nerve plexus 59, 60
Myenteric plexus 67
    parasympathetic ganglia of 72
Myoblasts 23
Myocardial infarction 27
Myometrium 107
Myosin 23
Myotome 136

N

Nasal pits 140
Nasal placodes 140
Nasal process
    lateral 140
    medial 140
Nasal septum 12
Nasolacrimal groove 140
Natural light 2
Neck
    lateral view 170
    webbing of 150
Necrosis, areas of 76
Nerve 47
    facial 214
    fiber 35, 44-46, 99
        bundles 98
        numerous fascicles of 47
    sciatic 207
Nervous tissue 44
Neural crest 137
Neural folds 136
Neural groove 136
Neural plate 136
Neural tube 136
    formation 136f
Neuroglia 131
Neurohypophysis 124
Neuronal bodies 47
Neuropore
    anterior 136
    posterior 136
Neurulation 136
Noradrenaline 120
Norepinephrine 120
Notochord 136, 136f
Nucleus
    dorsal 127
    eccentric 48
    pulposes 136
Numerous elastic fibers 15

Index

O

Olfactory pits 140
Olfactory placodes 140
Oligodendrocytes 44
Oocytes 103
Optic nerve 98, 99
    fiber layer 96
Oral cavity 8, 51
Oral lichen planus 56
Osmotic barrier 88
Osteoblasts 19
Osteoclasts 19
Osteocytes 18-20
Osteogenic layer 19
Osteology 177
    clinical aspects of 179
Osteons 19
Ovarian follicles 103
    primary 103
Ovary 102, 103, 146, 147
    mucinous tumor of 103

P

Pacinian corpuscle 91
Palatal process 139
Palate 138
    anomalies of 139*f*
    development of 138*f*
Palatine tonsil 38, 39
Palmar arch, superficial 206
Pancreas 75, 78, 79, 144
    annular 144
    development of 144*f*
Pancreatic acini 78
Pancreatic islets 79
Paneth cell 64
    metaplasia 71
Papillae, circumvallate 56
Papillary layer, superficial 91
Parathyroid hormone, action of 20
Paraxial mesoderm 135
Parenchyma 83, 100, 119, 123
Pars cystica 144
Pars hepatica 144
Pars nervosa 124
Patella 191
Peg cells, nonciliated 104
Pelvis 210, 218
    anterior view 189
    anteroposterior view 165
    posterior view 190
Peptic ulcer 63
Periarterial lymphatic sheaths 40
Perichondrium 11, 12, 15-17
Perimysium 23
Periosteum 19
Peripheral nervous system 44
Perisinusoidal space 75
Peyer's patches 64, 68
Pharyngeal arches 138, 138*f*
Pheochromocytoma 120
Philtrum 140
Pia mater 99, 128
    superficial 131
Pituitary
    adenomas 124
    gland 124, 125
Placenta 108, 109, 137
    previa 134
    site trophoblastic tumor 108
Plane radiographs 154, 160
Plasma cells 64, 100
Plate mesoderm, lateral 135
Pleural reflection 209
Plica circularis 64
Podocytes 84
Poliomyelitis 127
Polycystic ovary 103
Portal canal 75
Positron emission tomography scan 159
Postganglionic axons 48
Postganglionic parasympathetic neurons 59
Preganglionic axons 48
Primitive streak 135
Prochordal plate 135
Proliferated tubules 100
Prosencephalon 137
Prostate 119, 147
Prostatic concretion 119
Proteoglycans 19
Pseudostratified columnar epithelium 8, 9, 115, 116
Pseudounipolar neurons 47
Pubic symphysis 179
Pulp, red 40, 41
Purkinje cell 128
    layer 128
Pyelography, retrograde 157
Pyloric sphincter 63
Pyramidal cells
    large 131
    small 131
Pyramidal shaped protein, acinus consists of 79

R

Radial nerve 205
    arm 205
    forearm 205
Radiology 153
Radio-opacity, concept of 154
Radius and ulna 188
Ranula 52
Ranvier nodes 44, 45
Rectum 147
Renal corpuscle 4, 84
Renal pelvis 158
Renal pyramids, medulla consists of 84
Renal system 84
Reproductive system 8
    female 100
    male 112
Respiratory
    bronchiole 83
    system 80
    tract 24
Reticular connective tissue 19
Reticular fibers, layer of 79
Retina 96, 97
Retinoblastoma 96
Rib 155
    lateral view 196
    medial view 196
    superior view 196
Right atrium 142
Root of mesentery 212

S

Sacrum
    anterior view 202
    posterior view 202
Saliva 52
Salivary gland, mixed 54, 55
Saltatory conduction 44
Saphenous
    opening 206
    vein, great 206
Sarcolemma 23
Sarcoplasm 23
Sarcoplasmic reticulum 23
Scaphoid nonunion 179
Scapula 155
    anterior view 185
    lateral view 186
    posterior view 186
Sclerotome 136
Secretion 3
Secretory acinar tissue 101
Secretory serous acini 79
Seminiferous tubules 112
Sensory
    perception 3
    receptor 91
Septa 51
Serosa 59, 60, 63, 76, 104, 107
Serous acini 50, 51, 55
Sertoli cells 146
Sex chromatin 149
Sex cords 146
Sex corticoids 120
Sharpey's fibers 19
Short stature 150
Shoulder 160
    anteroposterior view 160
Sialadenosis 52
Sialosis 52
Simple columnar epithelium 4, 5, 6, 7, 63, 64, 76
Single central nucleus 27
Sinus, marginal 36
Sinusoids 75
    radiating plates of 75
Skeletal element 138
Skeletal muscle 22, 23
    development of 23
    fibers 23, 56, 57
        intercalated 56
Skeleton
    appendicular 178
    axial 178
    costal 12
Skin 91
    thick 90, 91
Skull 180
    anterior view 180
    anteroposterior view 169
    inferior view 181
    lateral view 170, 181
    occipitomental view 169
    posterior view 180
Small bowel enema 156

Small intestine 64
Smiths fracture 179
Smooth muscle 24, 25, 83
    bundles, muscularis layer consists of 76
    cells 64, 67
    fibers, consisting of 87
    lack striations 23
    layers, outer longitudinal 59
    malignant tumors of 24
    small layer of 83
Soft palate 139
Soft tissues 154
    external 155
Space of Disse 75
Spermatogenic cells 112, 146
Spherical lymphoid nodules 36
Spinal artery, anterior 127
Spinal cord 126, 127
Spinal ganglion 46, 47
Spindle cells, tumor consists of 24
Spine 155
Spleen 40, 41, 212
Splenic cords 40
Splenic nodules 40
Splenic parenchyma 40
Spotters 216
Squamous cell
    carcinoma cells 92
    nonkeratinized 57
Squamous epithelium 82
    keratinized stratified 10, 91
    nonkeratinized stratified 10
    simple 4, 5
    stratified 8
        nonkeratinized 39, 59
Stenosis 67
Stereocilia 7
Sternum
    anterior view 195
    lateral view 195
Stomach 143, 211
    cardiac orifice 211
    development of 143f
    fundus 60, 61, 211
    greater curvature 211
    pylorus 62, 63, 211
Stratum basale 91
Stratum corneum 91, 92
Stratum functionalis, superficial 107
Stratum granulosum 91
Stratum lucidum 91
Stratum spinosum 91, 92
Stroma 100, 103, 123
Subcapsular sinus 36
Submucosa 59, 60, 64, 71, 72, 83
    absence of 77
Substantia propria 95
Sulci 128
Surgical trauma 51
Sweat glands 91
Sympathetic ganglion 48, 49
Symphysis pubis 16
Syncytiotrophoblast 108
Synovial joints, chronic disorder of 20
Systemic circulation 43
Systemic embryology 138

T

T lymphocyte
    consists of 36
    maturation 43
Taeniae coli 71
Tall columnar cells 115
Terminal bronchiole 83
Territorial matrix 12, 13
Testis 112, 113, 146
    descend of 147
Theca folliculi 103
Thigh, anteroposterior view 165
Thin skin 92, 93
Thin tunica intima 34
Thoracic vertebrae
    anteroposterior view 164
    lateral view 200
    posterior view 200
    superior view 200
Thorax 163, 195, 208, 217
Thromboangiitis obliterans 31
Thymic corpuscle 43
Thymic follicular hyperplasia 43
Thymus 42, 43
Thyroid
    diverticulum 141
    follicles 4
    gland 122, 123, 141, 141f
Tibia 193
    artery, posterior 206
Tissues, adipose 52
Toluidine blue 2
Tongue 56, 57, 141, 141f
    geographical 56
    shape 67
    shaped villi 66
    tie 141
Trabeculae 36, 40, 43
Trabecular arteries 40
Trachea 80, 81, 154
Tracheal rings 12
Tracheostomy 80
Transitional cell carcinoma 87
Transitional epithelium 8, 9, 86-88, 119
Truncus arteriosus 142
Tubular organ 32
Tubules, collecting 84
Tubuloacinar seromucous tracheal gland 80
Tunica
    adventitia 28, 32, 35
    albuginea 103, 112
    intima 28, 32
    media 24, 28, 32, 35
    vasculosa 112
Turner's syndrome 150

U

Ulnar nerve 205
    arm 205
    forearm 205
Ultrasonograph 159
    antenatal scanning 174
Umbilical cord 110, 111
Undertaker's fracture 179
Unicornuate uterus 145
Upper limb 160, 185, 204, 216
Upper lip 140

Ureter 86, 87, 212
Ureteric bud 145
Ureteropelvic junction 158
Ureterovesical junction 158
Urinary bladder 88, 89, 145
    layer of 88
Urinary tract 24
    cancers 87
Uterine tube 145
    development of 146f
Uterus 7, 106, 107, 145
    development of 146f
    one-half of 145

V

Vas deferens 116, 117
Vasovasorum 28, 32, 35
Vein 32
    central 75, 99
    cephalic 32, 35
    facial 213
    large 32, 33
    medium-sized 32, 34, 35
    portal 75
    saphenous 32, 35
    umbilical 111
Vena cava
    inferior 32
    superior 32
Venous sinuses 40
Venous system 32, 35
Venules 32, 55
Verhoeff's method 15
Vertebra 197
    column 178
Vesicourethral canal 145
Vice versa 2
Visceral peritoneum 63
Vitamin
    D, deficiency of 20
    deficiencies 56
Vocal folds 8
Volkmann's canal 20, 21

W

Water-soluble contrast study 158
Wavy bundles 16
Wharton's jelly 111
White fibrocartilage 16
White pulp 40, 41
Wrist and hand, anteroposterior view 162

X

X-chromosome 149

Y

Y-chromosome 149
Yellow fibrocartilage 15

Z

Zona
    fasciculata 120
    glomerulosa 120
    pellucida 103
    reticularis 120
Zymogenic cells 60, 79
Zymogens 64, 79